Discovering
LIFETIME FITNESS

Discovering
LIFETIME FITNESS

CONCEPTS OF EXERCISE
AND WEIGHT CONTROL

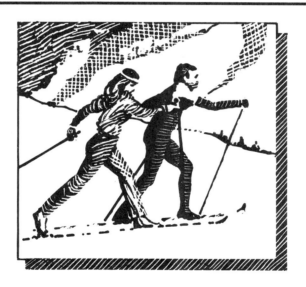

George B. Dintiman
Robert G. Davis
Jude C. Pennington
Virginia Commonwealth University

Stephen F. Stone

WEST PUBLISHING COMPANY
St. Paul   New York   Los Angeles   San Francisco

Composition: Parkwood Composition
Copyediting: Susie Blackmun
Cover Illustration and Design: Judi Rettich
Text Design: Judi Rettich

LIBRARY OF CONGRESS
Library of Congress Cataloging-in-Publication Data

Discovering lifetime fitness: concepts of exercise and weight control
    George B. Dintiman . . . [et al.].—2nd ed.
        p. cm.
    Bibliography: p.
    Includes index.
    ISBN 0-314-48120-6
    1. Exercise.   2. Reducing diets.   3. Physical fitness.
I. Dintiman, George B.
RA781.D547 1989
613.7—dc 19   88-25150
                                                                              CIP

THE AUTHORS

George B. Dintiman is a professor in the Division of Health and Physical Education at Virginia Commonwealth University, where he previously served as Division Chair for eighteen years. His educational background includes a B.S. from Lock Haven University, M.S. from New York University, and Ed.D. from Columbia University.

Dr. Dintiman is an NFL speed consultant, a founder and president of the NASE (National Association of Speed and Explosion) and a national network of speed clinics and camps, and is internationally known for his work in speed improvement with team sport athletes. He is author of twenty-one books on fitness, health, sports, nutrition, and weight control, and has lectured nationally on various subjects. A former member of the Governor's Council on Physical Fitness, Dr. Dintiman is a dedicated physical fitness enthusiast, playing competitive rugby until the age of 38, running 3–4 times weekly for the past 28 years, and playing competitive age group tennis.

Robert G. Davis received his undergraduate education at West Chester State College in Pennsylvania, a Master's degree from Pennsylvania State University, and his Ph.D. from the University of Maryland. Prior to joining Virginia Commonwealth University in 1973, he taught public school for six years, five at the elementary level.

An associate professor of Physical Education at Virginia Commonwealth University, Dr. Davis is in charge of the physical education graduate program, and specializes in the elementary area.

He has authored two books dealing with elementary physical education. He has also written a book on conditioning for tennis, which he has played for over 25 years and is a past club professional.

Jude Cole Pennington received his B.S. degree from Lock Haven State University, M.A. from Temple University, and Ph.D. from Florida State University. As a faculty member in the Health and Physical Education Division at Virginia Commonwealth University, he is regularly involved in teaching fitness and exercise classes. He has lectured extensively on health and physical fitness topics throughout Virginia, and is a frequent clinician and presenter at the annual Virginia Fitness Institute and Virginia State Blue Ridge Health Education conferences.

Stephen E. Stone is currently a wellness consultant residing in Richmond, Virginia. His educational background includes a B.S. from Lock Haven University, M.Ed. from East Stroudsburg University, and Ph.D. from Texas A & M University. Dr. Stone has been an associate professor of Health Education at the University of Maryland, College Park, and Virginia Commonwealth University in Richmond, Virginia. He is well known for his work in childhood obesity, nutrition, and aerobic fitness. His innovative techniques in fitness for adults and senior citizens have attracted considerable attention throughout the East Coast. He has lectured nationally on various subjects.

CONTENTS

The second edition of *Discovering Lifetime Fitness: Concepts of Exercise and Weight Control* is a basic health–related physical fitness text designed to help college students make conscious decisions about a variety of behaviors that can make a difference in their health status. The book is designed for students in courses such as Wellness, Fitness and Weight Control, Conditioning, Foundations of Physical Activity, and similar courses. It is written in a nontechnical, easy–to–read style, and is a complete resource text. This completeness enables students to select and apply concepts and programs to their exercise and weight control needs and interests in a sound, safe manner.

Special features of the second edition include:

1 A handy chart covering all types of exercise-related injuries and their prevention and emergency treatment

2 Self-testing instruments to allow students to compare their aerobic fitness, muscular strength and endurance, flexibility, and body fat to national standards

3 Two Laboratories in each chapter to allow students to discover additional information about themselves

4 Motivational and behavioral modification techniques to help students begin a total fitness program

5 Myths and Fallacies section in each chapter

6 Fitness starter programs in aerobic activities that allow students to begin at their individual fitness level

7 Lead-in content areas and Key Terms at the beginning of each chapter

8 A question-and-answer section at the end of each chapter to respond to common concerns that were not previously covered

9 An extensive Appendix section to provide an easy reference to important information for the college student such as girth control to flatten the stomach, lower back exercises, and numerous nutritional tables.

The Introduction and Chapters 1 and 2 are designed to motivate students to exercise through a discussion of health and wellness, an examination of the benefits of exercise including the prevention of cardiovascular disease, and a discussion of exercise and weight control values, and motivational techniques. Chapter 3 contains a comprehensive discussion of the basic concepts of conditioning to help students begin an exercise program at their level of fitness and progress steadily and safely to higher levels. Various forms of aerobic exercise, the foundation of a sound program, are presented. Chapters 4 and 5 cover the key areas of muscular strength and endurance, and flexibility training. Self-testing activities allow students to evaluate their current status before beginning a sound program that meets their exercise objective. Chapters 6 and 7 provide extensive coverage in the areas of nutrition and weight control, and are concerned with sound eating practices that contribute to improved health, improved performance, improved fitness, and the safe management of body weight and fat throughout life. Chapter 8 provides a model for the prevention of exercise-related injuries and illnesses and the safe use of exercise in a student's daily routine. Chapter 9 applies the information presented in previous chapters to individualize fitness programs in aerobic activities and sports, and help the student begin his or her program by tailoring exercise to current fitness levels. Chapter 10 discusses the merits of the sports approach to fitness, and evaluates a number of sound sports choices that have the potential to improve health and wellness. The final chapter, Beyond Fitness, is designed for students interested in competitive fitness activities and sports, and deals with advanced training programs in strength, flexibility, aerobics, anaerobics (or speed endurance), and sprinting speed improvement. The book's appendices provide an excellent resource for students by supplementing text material in the areas of fitness testing, nutrition, calorie counting, caloric expenditure, injury prevention and treatment, posture, lower back problems, and girth control. A "Fitness Profile Card" is provided to allow students to record test results in all areas, and to plot their progress.

The authors are indebted to several individuals who have assisted in the preparation of the manuscript. We are grateful for the thoughtful criticism and helpful suggestions of the following individuals: George Borden, M.S., Athletic Trainer, Director of Sportsmedicine, Virginia Commonwealth University; Brenda Dintiman-Shanahan, M.D., Department of Dermatology, University of New Mexico; Barney Groves, Ph.D., strength coach, Virginia Commonwealth University; Virgil May, M.D., Orthopedic Surgeon and Virginia Commonwealth University Team Physician.

We would also like to thank Fran Myers for her contribution in the discussion on flexibility, and Cheryl Valenti, Manager of the Raintree Swim and Fitness Club, where many of the text photos were taken.

Finally, we express our gratitude to the following reviewers:

Richard Borstad
Augsburg College

William Considine
Springfield College

Tom Crum
Triton College

Jean Dudney
San Antonio College

Harry DuVal
University of Georgia

Joe Ross
Normandale Community College

Patricia Taylor
University of Akron

Ray Webster
William Jewell College

A complete instructor's manual is available.

George B. Dintiman
Robert G. Davis
Jude C. Pennington
Stephen F. Stone

Discovering
LIFETIME FITNESS

The
The Wellness
Concept

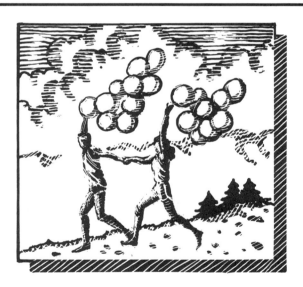

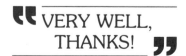
**"VERY WELL,
THANKS!"**

? HAVE YOU EVER WONDERED ABOUT:

The meaning of health and wellness?
How specific behavioral choices affect your health?
The relationship of lifestyle to wellness?
The factors associated with a long, healthy life?
How healthy a life you are living?

KEY TERMS

Emotional health
Good health habits
High-level wellness
Lifestyle changes
Mental health

Morbidity
Mortality
Social health
Spiritual health
Wellness

In the past decade, we have seen considerable change in the health behaviors of many Americans. More and more people are engaging in regular, aerobic exercise such as walking, backpacking, jogging, swimming, cycling, aerobics, and vigorous recreational sports (tennis, racquetball, handball, squash, full-court basketball, cross-country skiing, soccer). Many combine some form of aerobic exercise with strength and flexibility training. An informed public is learning to control body weight and fat; to purchase food wisely; eat nutritiously; and prevent cardiovascular disease, some forms of cancer, and other disorders. Quick fixes such as fad diets, drugs, exercise gadgets, and programs that promise slimness and fitness overnight are having less impact on an informed public who realize there are no shortcuts to health and wellness.

This introduction is designed to stimulate your thinking about health (which is nothing more than a matter of personal choice), define and differentiate between health and wellness, evaluate the health and wellness of the American people, show the association of lifestyle to health and wellness, and provide a means for you to evaluate your lifestyle and predict your future health and wellness.

HEALTH AND WELLNESS

Definitions of health vary from individual to individual. Some measure health by the quality of life; others, by the quantity (length). Definitions of health range from the simple absence of disease, illness, and injury to the more difficult level of peak physical fitness. All definitions center around deriving satisfaction from life.

The majority of college students want this satisfaction, but need information to accurately weigh the benefits and costs of health decisions. The simple fact is that your definition of health affects your behavior: if you want to achieve health, your habits must be a reflection of this pursuit. The chapters that follow serve as valuable information to evaluate your present condition, and to guide future health decisions.

The chapters that follow also address a larger concern. It is important to realize that the total health picture is more than exercise decisions. Our views of health tend to center around *physical health,* but total health (wellness) involves four other components:

Social health. The ability to interact and develop satisfying interpersonal relationships.

Mental health. The ability to learn and develop intellectual capabilities.

Emotional health. The ability to control emotions, expressing them when appropriate, and avoiding the showing of emotions when inappropriate.

Spiritual health. The belief in a unifying force; a god-like force for some, nature or scientific laws for others.

Wellness is the integration of these five components at any level of health or illness (see Figure I.1). In other words, you can be well regardless of whether you are physically ill or healthy. A paralyzed accident victim, for example, can achieve wellness by maximizing and integrating the five health components within the physical limitations of paralysis (and thus achieve **high-level wellness**).

Everyone has some degree of wellness. You may be ill and still possess high-level wellness, or

FIGURE I.1   Wellness is the integration of these five health components.

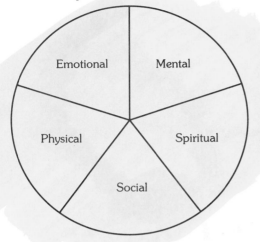

be healthy but have low-level wellness. The integration of the five components is important. Your values affect the way you perceive and approach health and wellness.

The way you judge specific behavior as healthy or unhealthy depends both upon your values, and upon the factors surrounding each situation. Values also influence your attempt to change behavior such as starting a desirable health habit, or eliminating an unhealthy habit. Techniques to help you make healthy choices are presented in Chapter 2.

WELLNESS AND THE AMERICAN PEOPLE

Although there are considerable references to an unhealthy America, the truth is that American people in the 1980's are healthier than ever before. They are better informed about proper exercise, nutrition, weight control, drug use and abuse, and other lifestyle behaviors that affect health and wellness.

The two most common ways to measure our nations health—**mortality** (life expectancy and death rates) and **morbidity** (incidence or prevalence of disease and illness) are indicators of the health and wellness levels of today's Americans. Researchers have found that death rates are down,

that significant gains have been made in life expectancy, and that infant mortality rates are improving. Since the turn of the century death rates have declined 67 percent: from 18 deaths per 1,000 in 1900, to 8 deaths per 1,000 in the period 1900–1950; and, from 8 deaths per 1,000 in 1950, to 6 deaths per 1,000 in 1977. Life expectancy, or the number of years newborn can expect to live, has risen from 47 years in 1900, to 74.6 years in 1982. Gains in the first half of this century were due largely to the control of infectious and parasitic diseases. The eight percent increase over the past 30 years is a result of a decline in death from cardiovascular disease (Whelan 1987).

Although life expectancy is increasing, the maximum lifespan of Americans is not. Some experts feel that the biological limit under ideal conditions is approximately 85 years of age. When accidental death (responsible for three lost years of life) is eliminated, we are currently only eight years or so off this limit.

The control of infectious diseases (polio, smallpox, typhus, tuberculosis, bubonic plague, measles, rubella, whooping cough, mumps, influenza, and pneumonia) has also significantly reduced deaths per 1,000 population in the United States. This decrease in morbidity, however, may be reversed by the current AIDS epidemic unless a vaccine or cure is found.

Table I.1 compares the ten leading causes of death in the year 1900, and today. Unlike the early part of the century when infectious diseases were the leading killers, today's health problems are strongly related to lifestyle. Cardiovascular disease (heart disease, stroke, and arteriosclerosis), chronic lung disease, diabetes mellitus, cirrhosis of the liver, suicide, and several forms of cancer are all related to lifestyle and health behaviors. Although there are no guarantees, it is known that you can significantly reduce your chances of premature death by having a healthy lifestyle. Death from heart disease, for example, has declined 30 percent in the past 15 years. This decline is mainly a result of **lifestyle changes** such as the elimination of smoking in males, decreased intake of dietary fat, increased exercise, and control of body weight (Whelan 1987). Early findings also suggest that diet may help prevent some forms of cancer (see Chapter 6). Research findings continue to suggest

TABLE I.1 LEADING CAUSES OF DEATH IN THE UNITED STATES: 1900 AND TODAY	
1900	**Today**
1. Tuberculosis	1. Heart Disease
2. Pneumonia and influenza	2. Cancer
3. Enteritis, gastritis, colitis	3. Stroke
4. Diseases of the heart	4. Accidents
6. Kidney diseases	6. Pneumonia and influenza
7. Accidents	7. Diabetes Mellitus
8. Cancer	8. Cirrhosis of the liver
9. Diseases of early infancy	9. Arteriosclerosis
10. Diphtheria	10. Suicide

SOURCE: National Center for Health Statistics, *Monthly Vital Statistics Report* 30, no. 13 (December 20, 1982): 22–23.

a significant relationship between the incidence of illness and premature death, and lifestyle.

HIGH-LEVEL WELLNESS AND YOUR LIFESTYLE

Lifestyle during the college years often carries over into old age. Inactive college students who overeat, eat the wrong kinds of foods, fail to control their body weight and body fat, and overuse alcohol, tobacco, and other drugs form habits that are difficult to break in later years. Even more unfortunate is the fact that during the third and fourth decades of life (age 20 to 40) the silent killers such as hypertension and atherosclerosis are progressing with few recognizable signals. Youth, and a substantial reserve built into the body systems lures young adults into a false sense of security. When a commitment is made to wellness, this problem is eliminated. As discussed previously, wellness is not just exercise, but a holistic

approach to health-related fitness that leads to feeling and looking good. It involves a commitment to making correct health choices in all the areas discussed in this book. Following an aerobic exercise program seven days per week for several hours daily, while neglecting other health behaviors, for example, is not the way to obtain wellness. Wellness involves regular exercise; proper nutrition; control of body weight and body fat; limited use of food drugs; and good emotional and mental behavior.

Studies have shown that a number of **good health habits** are associated with wellness, and actually predict longevity (Breslow 1980):

Sleeping 7–8 hours daily

Eating breakfast regularly

Eliminating or limiting snacking between meals

Maintaining normal ideal weight for height

Not smoking tobacco

Moderate use or elimination of alcohol

Regular physical activity

In support of such studies, the Center for Disease Control of the U.S. Public Health Service estimates that unfavorable lifestyle factors are the major cause of premature death before age 65 (Montoye, Christian, Nagle and Levin 1988).

As we can see, high-level wellness is obviously a function of lifestyle. A healthy lifestyle during the college years and throughout life can easily be obtained by:

Engaging in an aerobic exercise program at least four times weekly (see Chapter 3)

Eating a balanced, nutritionally sound diet, and drinking alcohol only in moderation (see Chapter 6)

Controlling body weight, and maintaining minimal body fat (see Chapter 7)

Controlling high blood pressure and atherosclerosis (see Chapter 1)

Avoiding smoking cigarettes, or using tobacco in any form (see Chapter 8)

Adopting a healthy lifestyle conducive to the

prevention of chronic and degenerative diseases (see Chapter 3, 4, 5, and 8)

Learning to live with yourself, and accepting your limitations (mental, physical, and economic)

EVALUATING YOUR LIFESTYLE

Take a moment to examine your current behaviors by completing the health questionnaire in Table I.2. There are no right or wrong answers. The behaviors mentioned are recommended for most Americans. The questionnaire merely tells you how likely it is that your current behaviors will keep you healthy. The questionnaire has six sections: smoking, alcohol and drugs, eating habits, exercise and fitness, stress control, and safety. Complete one

section at a time by circling the number corresponding to the answer that best describes your behavior:

Scale
2 = Almost always
1 = Sometimes
0 = Almost never

Add the numbers you have circled to determine your score for that section. Write the score on the line provided at the end of each section. (Note: The following section "Your Health Style Scores," and the Lifestyle Evaluation Table are taken from U.S. Department of Health and Human Services 1981.)

YOUR HEALTH STYLE SCORES

After you have figured your score for each of the six sections, evaluate the score comments listed

---

TABLE I.2   LIFESTLE EVALUATION

Cigarette Smoking

NOTE: If you never smoke, enter a score of 10 for this section and go to the next section, "Alcohol and Drugs."

1. I avoid smoking cigarettes.	2	1	0
2. I smoke only low-tar and -nicotine cigarettes, *or* I smoke a pipe or cigars.	2	1	0

"Cigarette Smoking" Score: __10__

Alcohol and Drugs

1. I avoid drinking alcoholic beverages, *or* I drink no more than one or two drinks a day.	(4)	1	0
2. I avoid using alcohol or other drugs (especially illegal drugs) as a way of handling stressful situations or the problems in my life.	(2)	1	0
3. I am careful not to drink alcohol when taking certain medicines (for example, medicine for sleeping, pain, colds, and allergies).	(2)	1	0
4. I read and follow the label directions when using prescribed and over-the-counter drugs.	(2)	1	0

"Alcohol and Drugs" Score: __10__

Eating Habits

1. I eat a variety of foods each day, such as fruits and vegetables, whole grain breads and cereals, lean meats, dairy products, dry peas and beans, and nuts and seeds.	(4)	1	0
2. I limit the amount of fat, saturated fat, and cholesterol I eat (including fat on meats, eggs, butter, cream, shortenings, and organ meats such as liver).	(2)	1	0
3. I limit the amount of salt I eat by cooking with only small amounts, not adding salt at the table, and avoiding salty snacks.	2	(1)	0
4. I avoid eating too much sugar (especially snacks of sticky candy or soft drinks).	(2)	1	0

"Eating Habits" Score: __9__

TABLE I.2   LIFESTLE EVALUATION—Continued

Exercise and Fitness

1. I maintain a desired weight, avoiding overweight and underweight.   (3)   1   0

2. I do vigorous exercises for fifteen to thirty minutes at least three times a week (examples include running, swimming, brisk walking).   (3)   1   0

3. I do exercises that enhance my muscle tone for fifteen to thirty minutes at least three times a week (examples include yoga and calisthenics).   (2)   1   0

4. I use part of my leisure time participating in individual, family, or team activities that increase my level of fitness (such as gardening, bowling, golf, and baseball).   (2)   1   0

"Exercise and Fitness" Score: __10__

Stress Control

1. I have a job or do other work that I enjoy.   (2)   1   0

2. I find it easy to relax and express my feelings freely.   (2)   1   0

3. I recognize early, and prepare for, events or situations likely to be stressful for me.   2   (1)   0

4. I have close friends, relatives, or others whom I can talk to about personal matters and call on for help when needed.   (2)   1   0

4. I participate in group activities (such as church and community organizations) or hobbies that I enjoy.   (2)   1   0

"Stress Control" Score: __9__

Safety

1. I wear a seat belt while riding in a car.   (2)   1   0

2. I avoid driving while under the influence of alcohol and other drugs.   (2)   1   0

3. I obey traffic rules and the speed limit when driving.   (2)   1   0

4. I am careful when using potentially harmful products or substances (such as household cleaners, poisons, and electrical devices).   (2)   1   0

5. I avoid smoking in bed.   (2)   1   0

"Safety" Score: __10__

LIFESTYLE EVALUATION SOURCE: Department of Health and Human Services. *Health Style: A Self Test.* 1981.

below. Remember, there is no total score for this test. Consider each section separately. You are trying to identify aspects of your lifestyle that you can improve in order to be healthier and to reduce the risk of illness.

Scores of 9 and 10. Excellent! Your answers show that you are aware of the importance of this area to your health. More important, you are putting your knowledge to work for you by practicing good health habits. As long as you continue to do so, this area should not pose a serious health risk. It's likely that you are setting an example for your family and friends to follow. Although you received a very high score on this part of the test,

you may want to consider other areas where your scores could be improved.

Scores of 6 to 8. Your health practices in this area are good, but there is room for improvement. Look again at the items you answered with a "Sometimes" or an "Almost Never." What changes can you make to improve your score? Even a small change can often help you achieve better health.

Scores of 3 to 5. Your health risks are showing! Would you like more information about the risks you are facing and about why it is important for you to change these behaviors? Perhaps you need help in deciding how to make the changes you desire. In either case, help is available.

Scores of 0 to 2. You may be taking serious and unnecessary risks with your health. Perhaps you are not aware of the risks and what to do about them. You need to acquire information to help you improve your scores and, thereby, your health.

SUMMARY

It is important to remember that heart disease, cancer, and other chronic and degenerative diseases are multi-causal. No single behavior can account for either the cause, or the prevention of the disease. Genetics are also important to morbidity and mortality. Heredity deals the cards, and environment plays the hand, which allows individuals with a poor genetic makeup to overcome some heredity deficiencies. Those who inherit the tendency for a long life can also negate genetic factors with an unhealthy existence of smoking, drug and alcohol abuse, sedentary living, overeating, obesity, and excessive emotional stress. To increase your chances of living a long, healthy life, experts agree that you should choose a healthy lifestyle.

BIBLIOGRAPHY

Whelan, Elizabeth M. "The Truth About Americans' Health." *USA Today Magazine* Society for the Advancement of Education, May, 1987; 55–58.

Breslow, L., and L. E. Enstrom. "Persistence of Health Habits and Their Relationship to Mortality." *Preventive Medicine,* 1980, 9:469–483.

Dintiman, George B., and Jerrold Greenberg. *Health Through Discovery.* 4th ed. New York: Random House, 1989.

Dintiman, George B., and Robert Ward, *Train America! Achieving Peak Performance and Fitness for Sports Competition* Dubuque, Iowa: Kendal Hunt, 1988.

Knowles, John H., ed. *Doing Better and Feeling Worse: Health in the United States.* New York: W. W. Norton, 1977.

Montoye, Henry J., Janet L. Christian, Francis J. Nagle, and Saul M. Levin. *Living Fit.* Reading, Mass.: Benjamin Cummings, 1988.

U.S. Department of Health and Human Services. *Health Style: A Self Test.* Washington, D.C.: Public Health Service, 1981.

CHAPTER ONE

Benefits of EXERCISE

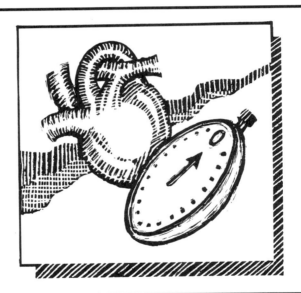

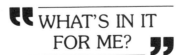 WHAT'S IN IT FOR ME?

? HAVE YOU EVER WONDERED ABOUT:

The meaning of fitness?
The components of fitness?
The term aerobics?
Exercise and your looks?
The physical benefits of exercise?
The importance of blood pressure?
The effects of exercise on blood pressure?
Whether exercise will help you live longer?
Heart disease and exercise?
The physiological benefits of exercise?

KEY TERMS

Aerobics
Aging
Anaerobic activities
Blood pressure
Body composition
Calorie
Cardiovascular efficiency
Flexibility
Health-related fitness
Heart rate

High density lipoproteins
(HDL)
Low density lipoproteins
(LDL)
Motor fitness
Muscular endurance
Muscular strength
Risk factor
Stroke
Stroke volume
Total serum cholesterol

A 1978 nationwide survey by Louis Harris indicated that many American adults practice some habits that are hazardous to their health and live unhealthy lives. In spite of these widespread destructive behaviors, Americans also believe that certain lifestyle changes will improve their health. Ninety-two percent of those surveyed believed that if they ate more nutritious food, smoked less, maintained proper weight, and exercised regularly it would do more to improve their health than regular physician care.

Public confusion over the role of behavior and lifestyle in maintaining health is echoed by medical authorities. Opponents of the "lifestyle" approach to health believe that most chronic diseases like cancer and heart disease have many causes. The biological disease mechanisms responsible for chronic illness have received the most attention in research and clinical settings. Behavioral influences on health and disease have had less medical emphasis until recently.

Before age 30, the human body seems to be able to absorb large amounts of abuse and neglect without any overt signs of harm. Later in life, the results of abuse begin to appear in the form of premature illness, increased injuries, and even death. Some experts argue that it

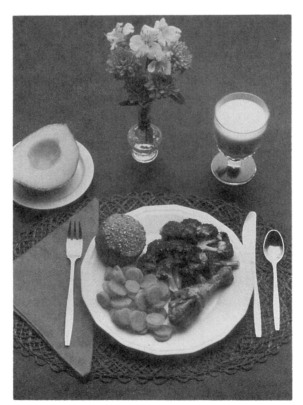

Figure 1.1   A healthy lifestyle includes good nutritional habits.

is the time lag of 20 or 30 years between body abuse and the appearance of disease from such abuse that encourages us to neglect our health. We demand instant gratification, live day by day, and neglect the consequences because they are so far in the future. Both disease lag and medical emphasis lead to a certain fatalism. Since disease can be prevented and death delayed through the use of scientific and technological advances, some people think, "Why worry about cancer? A cure will soon be found." For others, genetic fatalism takes hold: "The genes will decide your fate no matter what you do."

Those who favor the role of leading a healthy lifestyle in preventing disease and promoting health argue against fatalistic conclusions. A number of chronic and degenerative diseases (7 out of the 10 leading causes of death) have been strongly linked to behaviors such as drinking in excess, lack of exercise, smoking habits, drug abuse, stress, eating habits, and obesity. Lifestyle changes in some of these areas have also been shown to improve health and prevent some diseases such as early heart disease and stroke.

WHY PEOPLE EXERCISE

Based upon what is known about exercise and health, one might believe people exercise for the health of it, but researchers have found that most people exercise merely to look better. In a survey to determine why college students took fitness and weight control classes, aesthetics topped the list, followed closely by health benefits and social and emotional well-being (Kaslow 1988). No matter what your reasons for exercising, a total wellness program will provide numerous health benefits on your road to fitness. This chapter contains the short-term and long-term benefits of regular exercise for college students of all ages.

EXERCISE AND HEALTH

Exercise has many health benefits associated with it, such as maintaining a healthy heart and circulatory system, delaying the onset of early heart disease, and lessening the severity of a heart attack should one occur. In addition, exercise aids weight control, helps the body handle blood fat, and improves most bodily functions. Although exercise is no guarantee of a disease-free or illness-free life,

it will provide an improved quality of life while living.

EXERCISE AS A LIFESTYLE HABIT

Since exercise benefits cannot be stored, exercise must be a part of daily lifestyle. Scientists working with astronauts found that physical inactivity and weightlessness leads to fitness deterioration; skeletal mass gets weaker, and after only 18 hours of total bed rest some cardiovascular deconditioning occurs. The experience of the astronaut is similar to **aging,** which is the process of deterioration. Inactivity significantly contributes to aging; it appears that aging does not accelerate from overuse but from underuse. Those who adopt regular exercise as a lifestyle can maintain a fairly high fitness level throughout life.

WHAT IS FITNESS?

There is really no one answer to the question, what is fitness? Fitness is a personal matter. What is it you want to do? What quality of life do you want? How concerned are you about your looks? Do you like to participate in recreational activities?

How about dancing? Do you want an active sex life? Fitness affects every aspect of life including what employment you can accept, how prepared you will be for emergencies, your recreational activities, and even some of the friends you will have. Your fitness activities, or lack thereof, may also affect how long you will live as well as how happy you will be while living.

THE COMPONENTS OF FITNESS

There are two basic classifications of fitness: health-related and motor. The most important of these, **health-related fitness,** includes five key components: cardiovascular efficiency, muscular strength, muscular endurance, flexibility, and body composition. **Motor fitness** components such as speed, coordination, reaction time, and agility are less important and have little affect on your physical health (i.e., speed is not necessary to a healthy life). This chapter contains a discussion of each health-related fitness component.

Exercise benefits you physically, psychologically, and even intellectually. Listed below are several outcomes of a total fitness program. What you will receive from your exercise program, however, will be dependent upon what you put into it.

PHYSICAL BENEFITS OF EXERCISE

GOOD LOOKS

A major motivation for exercising, as well as an exercise benefit, is improved looks. Aerobic exercise can help maintain body weight or aid a weight reducing program. It has been reported that 27 percent of college females are terrified of becoming fat (Bartley, 1987). Some researchers report that more than one in four college students already have a weight problem. By exercising, these students could help eliminate their problem. Over a year's time, three 30-minute sessions of aerobic activity each week can remove or keep off 25 pounds of unwanted fat without any dietary changes.

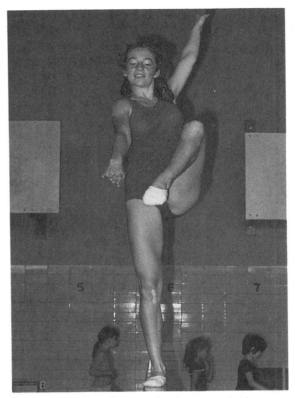

Figure 1.2   Regular exercise improves both physical appearance and emotional health.

IMPROVED POSTURE AND BODY MECHANICS

Exercise can improve posture and body mechanics. Can good posture make you more attractive? Figuratively speaking, yes. At any age the main obstacle is gravity. Gravity pulls down anything you do not hold up. To combat it, you must strengthen the postural muscles—those muscles that, when fatigued or weakened, allow your body to sag and slump. Without exercise you may begin to look and move like an older person.

BODY CONTOURING

Exercise can also help you to develop aesthetically pleasing lines. Although it is not possible to spot reduce, a total fitness program will help to firm the body. For both sexes there is a trend toward a thinner, firmer body.

BODY COMPOSITION

Your **body composition** is important to your health. The body is made up of many substances, including fat. The percent of fat in relation to lean muscle mass and bone is an indicator of one's health; certain health problems, such as high blood pressure and heart disease, are associated with high fat levels. The best way to estimate body fat is to be weighed underwater. Since such a test is impractical for most people, fat percentage is estimated using other methods, the most common of which is measuring skin thickness.

Exercise is an excellent way to maintain or lose body fat. The basic measure of heat (energy) is the **calorie,** and all foods contain calories. If you take in more food (calories) than your body needs, you gain fat. Conversely, if you consume fewer calories than your body needs, you lose fat. When exercising, your body burns more calories than when you are sedentary. If you make no dietary changes, you can lose fat by just increasing your exercise level.

It takes considerable exercise to lose one pound or fat, but combining exercise with good nutrition is the best way to control weight. Yearly goals should be set. To accomplish a long-term fat-loss goal, you should strive to lose no more than 1½ to 2 pounds a week. (See Chapter 7 for more information on weight control.)

CARDIOVASCULAR EFFICIENCY

The foundation for fitness is an efficient cardiovascular system—heart, lungs, and blood vessels—which supplies fuel to the working muscles while removing waste products. A test commonly used to estimate cardiovascular efficiency is the 1.5-mile run (see Chapter 3).

A word closely associated with health-related fitness is **aerobics.** Aerobics means "with air" and is used to describe those fitness activities such as jogging, cycling, and lap swimming that last 20 or more minutes and are done at a low enough intensity to allow the circulatory system to provide working muscles with oxygen. High-intensity activities, such as sprinting, which prohibit the exchange of oxygen with the working muscle, are called **anaerobic activities.**

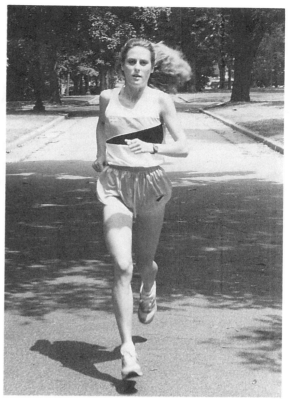

Figure 1.3   The key to fitness is an efficient cardiovascular system.

Aerobic exercise will improve **cardiovascular efficiency.** With exercise, the heart muscle grows in size and strength and improves its **stroke volume**—with each beat, the heart pumps more blood, resulting in a lower resting **heart rate.** It is not unusual for the normal heart rate of 72–80 beats per minute (BPM) to be lowered 10 to 20 BPM after only six to eight months of aerobic activity. This reduction in heart rate begins soon after an aerobic program is initiated, and is an early sign that your exercise program is working. Although the overall cardiovascular system takes nearly three months to condition, a lower resting heart rate can occur in as little as two weeks.

HEALTHY BLOOD

People usually worry about fat they can see, but a greater health risk is fat in the blood. HDL, or **high density lipoprotein,** takes fat entering the system though the diet and transports it to the liver where it is metabolized for use as fuel. LDL, or **low density lipoprotein,** is like a glue that takes dietary fat and deposits it on arterial walls, clogging the vessels which can lead to cardiovascular problems. Aerobic exercise increases the beneficial blood fat (HDL). In order to most effectively maintain high HDL, aerobic exercise should be performed at least once very 48 hours. It also helps to reduce saturated fats and cholesterol in the diet (see page 17 for a more detailed discussion of cardiovascular health).

RECOVERY TIME

As the cardiovascular system becomes more efficient, the body's recovery rate from strenuous exercise improves. Following exercise, a conditioned individual's heart and breathing rates return to resting levels sooner than those of the unfit person.

DECREASED BREATHING RATE

Although the reduction is not as dramatic as resting heart-rate, both resting and exercise breathing rates decline as fitness improves. The conditioned individual will also experience less labored breathing during exercise than will the unfit individual. Breathing rate reduction reflects a more efficient cardiovascular system. When blood leaves the lungs of both the fit and unfit person, the oxygen level for both is nearly identical, but the fit individual's body is better able to transfer the oxygen to the working muscles.

BLOOD PRESSURE

The term **blood pressure** is familiar to everyone, but some people do not understand the numbers associated with it. Ideal blood pressure is 120/80; the two numbers signify systolic pressure and diastolic pressure. *Systolic pressure* is the force on the blood vessel walls during the heart's contraction phase. When the heart is at rest, there is also pressure on vessel walls, and this is known as *diastolic pressure.* It is this resting pressure that can be the greater risk factor.

Although improved fitness does not affect blood pressure as dramatically as heart or breathing rates, it does help to maintain proper levels. Excess weight, a leading cause of high blood pressure, can be significantly reduced through exercise. Anyone diagnosed with high blood pressure must exercise cautiously, but the combination of exercise and medication will usually result in lower blood pressure.

MUSCULAR STRENGTH

Strength is a muscle's ability to exert maximum force and this can be measured several ways. It is possible to evaluate strength using a weight training machine, or with special strength testing devices such as the hand dynomometer or cable tensionmeter. On most fitness tests, strength items such as pull-ups or sit-ups are actually muscular endurance tests. (See chapter 4 for strength tests.)

Skeletal muscle responds rapidly to exercise, and most exercisers find this highly motivating. The best results are achieved through weight training. Identical weight training programs, however, have varying effects on individuals. While some improve more than others, everyone will experience gains. Beginners generally gain strength after only a few workouts, with rapid improvement over the first four to six weeks. Additional gains occur much less dramatically.

Strength is a key component to other fitness benefits. For example, improved strength in the musculature as well as in the tendons and ligaments surrounding the joints helps prevent certain injuries. Strength also shortens recovery time following certain injuries. And added strength usually enhances the performance of any sport. (For more on strength development, see Chapter 4.)

MUSCULAR ENDURANCE

Muscular endurance is the ability to repeat a high number of muscular contractions, and is evaluated using tests such as the number of pull-ups or sit-ups that can be performed. The most frequently used endurance test is the number of sit-ups that can be completed in one minute. As with muscular strength, immediate endurance gains will be realized through a weight training or calisthenic program.

FLEXIBILITY

Flexibility is the range of motion of a joint, and is important for efficient movement and injury prevention. The *sit and reach* is the most commonly used flexibility test (see Laboratory 5.1). Flexibility exercises will help maintain or improve joint motion as you age. With aging, activity normally decreases, resulting in loss of flexibility. By including flexibility exercises, an active lifestyle can be maintained. Improved flexibility will allow you to move more freely and efficiently with minimal resistance. Stretching exercises can prevent the joint stiffening and muscular shortening that occur with injury, disease, inactivity, aging, and fatigue. Remaining flexible throughout life adds to graceful movement and a youthful appearance. Increased flexibility also aids performance in sports, and relieves some forms of muscle soreness. Stretching exercise helps condition the muscles, tendons, and ligaments.

EXERCISE AND AGING

There has been a perpetual search for the fountain of youth, but no one has been able to stop or reverse the aging process. Exercise, however, makes it possible to slow down the process and thus improve the quality of life (see Figure 1.4). Whether we like it or not, we go into the declining years sometime between 25 and 30 years of age. During this time span, the number of cells being destroyed begin exceeding the number produced.

The rate of physical deterioration varies among individuals. A person who participates in a comprehensive fitness program throughout life will age more slowly than an inactive individual. Regardless of even herculean efforts, however, fitness will decline. Muscular efficiency diminishes about 1 percent annually beginning in the late 20's. By age 50 most sedentary individuals will be approximately 75 percent as muscularly effective as they were at 25.

BONE GROWTH

Exercise is essential for proper bone growth among the young. For those over 30, exercising at least

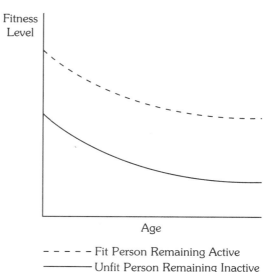

Figure 1.4   **Age-related decline in fitness level can be influenced with exercise.**

½ hour three time a week is recommended to keep bones strong. Bone mass drops about 1 percent a year after age 30, with women experiencing an increased rate for several years after menopause. Among senior citizens, osteoporosis or "brittle bones" is the leading cause of fractures, particularly in the hip.

HANDLING EMERGENCIES

Fitness is often defined as having acceptable levels of conditioning in the health-related areas with sufficient resources left over for emergencies. These emergencies could be either mental or physical stress. How well could you handle eight flights of stairs when the dorm elevator breaks? Could you push your car out of the snow to make that trip to Florida? How will your body react when the officer pulls you over? What will happen when you find out you have three final exams on the same day? Fit people handle stress and sudden physical bursts better than the unfit.

HANDLING ROUTINE TASKS

A fit person can handle routine tasks such as stair climbing and garden work with little muscle soreness and a quick recovery period. Tasks that are done seasonally or only occasionally, such as shoveling or raking, will normally result in muscle soreness even for fit individuals, but they are less likely to cause a major injury. It is not uncommon, however, for unfit individuals to suffer severe back injuries or have a heart attack while shoveling snow.

IMPROVED SEX LIFE

If you agree with Maslow's hierachy of needs, an improved sex life is an important exercise benefit; it could also be included under the psychological benefits of exercise. To participate fully in sexual activity, you need to be in good physical condition. To continue sexually into old age you should maintain that conditioning. Fitness is important to the duration, frequency, and variety of sexual activity.

PSYCHOLOGICAL BENEFITS OF EXERCISE

STRESS REDUCTION AND FEELING OF WELL-BEING

Physically fit people tend to be more emotionally stable, more extroverted, and have a better self-concept than their inactive counterparts. Feelings or attitudes about one's physical condition are positively related to feelings of self-acceptance. There is ample evidence to support the use of physical activity to improve self-concept. Individuals who have made the commitment to a lifetime of regular physical activity have been shown to possess greater self-confidence, emotional stability, and feelings of worth.

Researchers found that a physical activity program of jogging, calisthenics, and swimming not only increased the physical fitness of obese teenagers but also significantly improved their attitudes toward their bodies and themselves. A study of college students learning to swim had similar results. Participation in Outward Bound programs has been shown to create a significant attitude change in young people. After attending a course they saw others as individuals in their own right and themselves as having more mature goal orientation. They had a more positive attitude toward participation and believed they had a greater potential to reach positive goals.

Regular physical activity has also been shown to reduce depression and elevate mood. A study of 100 college professors revealed a reduction in the occurrence of depression through participation in programs such as jogging, swimming, cycling, and weight lifting. Female college students who improved their cardiovascular endurance through a jogging program became less depressed, more confident, more efficient at work, and experienced more restful sleep. It also has been demonstrated that physical activity can be effective in repelling the depressed and pessimistic moods that healthy people occasionally experience.

A number of factors related to regular exercise may account for its value in reducing stress. Exercise is a strong motivator toward developing a routine; it also is frequently done in sessions with others, thereby providing opportunities to develop friendships. Such sessions often lead to a sharing of common interests and problems as well. The relaxed atmosphere created by aerobic exercise fosters open communication and is unlike the tension experienced in most competitive sports.

Another stress reduction factor may be the feeling of doing something good for yourself. Such positive indulgence can lead to enjoyment, a feeling of controlling one's health, self-discipline, and a feeling of accomplishment. It can lead to released tension and a general improvement in self-concept.

The psychological benefits that nearly every regular exerciser feels may be related to chemical changes brought on by physical activity. The so-called exercise high may be due to natural tranquilizers—endorphins, and enkephalins—in the brain. Although not fully understood, the phenomenon appears most frequently in those who exercise beyond normal fitness limits (45 minutes or more). Those who stay in the general recognized fitness range of 20 to 30 minutes of aerobic activity do not experience a high.

INTELLECTUAL BENEFITS OF EXERCISE

Nearly every great philosopher has expounded on the "sound mind in a sound body" concept. The relationship between fitness and intelligence is positive, and although this relationship is too low to be of scientifically predictive value, it can certainly be said that a keen mind can only function at its full potential in a fit body. Even though exercise will not make you more intelligent, it is recognized as an essential element if you want to make full use of your intellectual capacity.

EXERCISE, DIET, AND CARDIOVASCULAR HEALTH

Few health-related areas are more controversial than the role of exercise in the prevention of early heart disease, a disease many experts feel is brought on by poor lifestyles such as smoking, sedentary living, overeating of the wrong kinds of foods, and stress. The controversy centers around several areas: the role of cholesterol in heart disease, the effects of exercise in managing blood serum cholesterol, and other physiological changes brought on by aerobic exercise that may provide protection from heart disease.

CHOLESTEROL AND HEART DISEASE

Research findings strongly link cholesterol levels and early heart disease. Far more important than **total serum cholesterol** (total blood cholesterol measurement including both HDL and LDL levels) is the amount of HDL (high denisty lipoproteins) or "good" cholesterol in the blood. The HDLs appear to serve two important functions: the coating of the inside of the artery walls to provide a protective layer of grease to prevent fatty deposits from building up, and the role of a scavenger that helps transport fatty deposits to the liver for dissolution. LDLs (low density lipoproteins) or "bad" cholesterol are responsive to dietary habits, form deposits on the walls of blood vessels, and are the culprits in clogged arteries and atherosclerosis.

High HDLs reduce the risk of heart disease. The key factor recently identified is the ratio of HDLs to total serum cholesterol. The ratio of total cholesterol to HDL cholesterol should be less than 5 and preferably less than 4.5. In other words, a minimum of 20 percent for men and 25 percent

for women of cholesterol should be HDLs. With a total serum cholesterol of 200 milligrams per 100 milliliters, a man's HDLs should be at least 40 mg per 100 ml and a woman's at least 50.

Cholesterol has emerged as a major villain in heart disease. Total serum cholesterol may be insignificant, however, and high levels may be tolerated providing the ratio of HDLs to total cholesterol is low. A simple blood test will provide you with LDL, HDL, total blood cholesterol, and cholesterol/HDL ratios. The following chart shows your estimated risk for heart disease based on these data.

Cholesterol/ HDL Ratio	Equivalent HDL, %	Estimated Risk
6:1	16	Very high risk
5:1	20	Some protection from early heart disease
4:1	25	Good protection from early heart disease
3.5:1	28	Excellent protection
3:1	33	Excellent; ratio present in very few individuals

THE INFLUENCE OF DIETARY CHANGES ON CHOLESTEROL

There are individuals from the medical profession who argue that little can be done to alter the course of heart disease in humans. Part of their argument comes from early studies that indicated very little reduction in total serum cholesterol following dietary changes. Since that time, however, it has been demonstrated that LDL cholesterol can be significantly influenced by dietary changes. If you lower your LDLs through dietary changes, you will lower your total cholesterol and improve the ratio of HDL to total cholesterol.

To lower your LDLs, you need to decrease saturated fat intake (animal fats) or increase your consumption of polyunsaturated fats (plant origin fats such as safflower, corn, sunflower, soybean, and cottonseed oils). In addition, there is some evidence that the fibers of legumes may be especially effective in binding bile salts and carrying them out of the body, thus reducing cholesterol. In one study, subjects on a diet with chick peas as a major item reduced cholesterol levels from 206 to 160 mg per 100 ml in 20 weeks. Daily intake of oat bran has also been shown to significantly lower cholesterol levels. In addition, a number of cholesterol-lowering drugs are now available by prescription. Diet and regular exercise are recommended in most cases, except for high risk individuals—those with exceptionally high cholesterol levels.

Cholesterol is a major factor in the prevention of early heart disease, and it is advisable to be concerned about the high intake of saturated fats and cholesterol, and the limited use of polyunsaturates in the American diet.

THE INFLUENCE OF EXERCISE ON HDL CHOLESTEROL

Exercise has been shown to affect HDLs. Active individuals with low body fat have the best ratios (1:4 or higher) and the highest HDLs. HDL readings of inactive individuals average approximately 45/200; of 10 to 12 mile-per-week runners, 55/200; and of marathon runners, 65/200. The higher the fitness level, the more likelihood of a high ratio of HDL to total serum cholesterol and high protection from heart disease. Jogging, running, and tennis have been shown to significantly increase HDLs. The greater the exercise volume weekly, the higher the HDL count. Although women have a higher HDL count than men, exercise produces still further increases. After menopause, HDL levels of women drop to the average amount of men. Running 11 miles per week was shown to increase HDLs by 35 percent and it is safe to assume that other kinds of aerobic exercise such as aerobic dance, cycling, swimming, rope jumping, and so on will produce the same effect.

It is also helpful to avoid practices that are known to lower HDL cholesterol such as cigarette smoking, certain medications used to manage high blood pressure (such as betablockers—drugs that lower cardiac output), and the use of the birth control pill.

ACTIVITY PATTERNS AND THE INCIDENCE OF HEART DISEASE

A few years ago, some experts were of the opinion that marathon runners were immune to heart disease. This feeling was based on data obtained on marathon runners in the early 1970s, before the running boom. As the number of marathon runners increased, a few instances of death from heart disease appeared. Although it is now safe to say that marathoners are not immune to heart disease, the incidence is much lower than among the nonfit population. Numerous researchers have found a relationship between inactivity and heart disease. Research has focused on occupational activity, recreational pursuits, and sports participation. In all cases, there has been a relationship between sedentary living or inactivity and cardiovascular disease. There is also considerable empirical evidence to support the value of aerobic exercise in preventing heart disease: heart disease is virtually unknown to the Tarahumara Indians of Mexico who begin distance running in childhood and continue throughout life; and for the Masai in Africa who trot up to 50 miles daily in search of food. Additional examples support the association of the active individual with the absence of heart disease.

There is also evidence linking aerobic exercise to

1. Reduced plaque buildup in the coronary arteries and their branches
2. Larger arteries to supply the heart muscle
3. Improved blood pressure
4. Improved stroke volume (amount of blood ejected per beat)
5. Improved circulation throughout the body
6. Improvement in the way the body handles fats

Proponents of exercise argue that these factors are additional proof of the preventive value of regular exercise.

Opponents of exercise as a preventive heart disease technique point out that cause-effect studies are nonexistent. They argue that statistical evidence comparing different populations and correlating different behaviors with heart disease is the only available evidence and is far from conclusive.

HEART ATTACKS

When a typical heart attack occurs, the heart muscle is rarely at fault; rather, inadequate supply of blood to the heart, usually due to clogged coronary arteries and their branches, causes tissue death to certain areas of the heart that are left temporarily or permanently without blood and oxygen.

The heart receives nourishment from two main arteries. These coronary arteries branch off from the aorta and carry oxygenated blood from the heart to the rest of the body. The right coronary artery covers the back side of the heart by branching into smaller and smaller arteries, which penetrate the heart muscle. The left coronary artery is divided into two parts, which nourish the front and left side of the heart. These coronary arteries are quite susceptible to fatty deposit buildup, atherosclerosis, and clogging.

The following list describes some major threats to a healthy heart.

Coronary thrombosis may occur due to a clot in a coronary artery with artery closure caused by an accumulation of atheromas (plaquelike lesions in the inner lining of an artery). In most cases, only a branch of an artery supplying a portion of the heart muscle is affected. Keep in mind that the heart muscle must be properly nourished second by second to function.

Angina pectoris refers to a symptom of heart disease caused by diminished blood supply to a portion of the heart muscle. When any muscle fails to receive adequate blood supply (oxygen and nutrient material), pain results. This condition is referred to as ischemia. When the heart is involved, the victim experiences a tightness or pressure in the chest and pain that may radiate to the shoulders or arms (see Appendix G for heart attack symptoms).

Arteriosclerosis (hardening of the arteries) and *atherosclerosis* (plaque buildup inside arterial blood vessels) identify a disease process occurring in the arteries of systemic circulation; rarely does the disease involve the veins or blood vessels to the lungs. If arteries supplying the brain are involved, a stroke

occurs; if the arteries supplying the legs are involved, leg pain (claudication) occurs; and if the coronary arteries are involved, chest pain (angina pectoris) and heart attack result.

Congenital heart disease involves one of four major groups of problems: (1) narrowing or constriction of a blood vessel or heart valve; (2) abnormal holes between the two blood vessels, in the muscle, or in the septum that separates the two chambers of the heart; (3) a combination of items 1 and 2; and (4) abnormal connections of the blood vessels leading to or from the heart.

Heart rhythm disturbances may involve irregular blood flow (heart murmur) caused by an impaired valve orifice that is narrowed enough to slow the flow of blood. Valve defects place a greater load on the heart, heart walls may increase in size, and tension increases inside the walls. In effect, the heart is less efficient and, in a sense, has to regurgitate blood twice. Functional murmurs involve no structural defect and are not indicative of physiological impairment or disease.

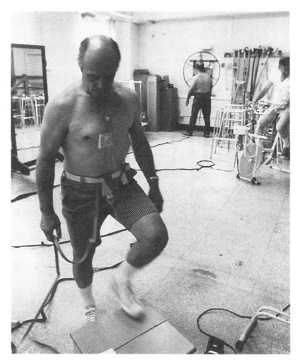

Figure 1.5   Regular exercise has been shown to benefit those who have already suffered a heart attack.

Rheumatic fever is a leading cause of valvular or rheumatic heart disease. Generally regarded as a disease of children and young people, it accounts for about 95 percent of all heart disease in patients under 20 years of age. Rheumatic heart disease is largely preventable. When sore throat persists for more than a few days, the individual should have a throat culture to determine whether there is a strep infection. If an infection exists, antibiotic therapy can prevent rheumatic fever and secondary valve damage.

Heart disease in adults is largely due to plaque buildup in the coronary arteries and their branches. When a partial or complete block occurs, the heart muscle is deprived of oxygen and the classic heart attack occurs.

CAUSES OF HEART ATTACKS

Although capsule form has the effect of greatly oversimplifying a complicated problem, it is helpful to summarize four common theories.

1. *The Lipid Theory.* A high number of fatty particles (lipoproteins) in the bloodstream cause atherosclerosis, or the accumulation of these particles on arterial walls. Particles increasing the tendency for atherosclerosis are called lipoproteins, which consist of fat (triglyceride), a blood protein (to make the fat soluble), and cholesterol (actually a steroid that has many traits of fat). Atherosclerosis is considered the major cause of heart attacks.

2. *The Personality Behavior Theory.* Individuals are classified by either Type A behavior: in a hurry, pressed for time, clock watcher, competitive, aggressive, hate to lose, lack of patience, and an underlying hostility; or Type B behavior: unaggressive, not concerned with job advancement or time pressures, a contented "cow" enjoying life as it is. Individuals exhibiting Type A behavior patterns are supposedly more likely to suffer an early heart attack.

3. *The Fibrin Deposit Theory.* Sticky fibrin deposits on the insides of artery walls are the cause of atherosclerosis. Eventually, reduced blood flow or a complete block due

to clotting or narrowing of coronary artery branches results in a heart attack.

4. *The Risk Factor Theory.* A number of **risk factors** in combination make one more susceptible to heart disease.

HEART DISEASE RISK FACTORS

A number of factors have been linked with a high risk of heart disease. Among the factors that cannot be controlled are sex, race, age, and heredity. Controllable factors include hypertension, obesity, inactivity, hyperlipidemia, smoking, contraceptive pills, and diabetes. With normal blood pressure and blood fat levels and in the absence of smoking and diabetes, the chances of a male having a heart attack prior to age 65 are fewer than one in 20. With one of these risk factors, the risk doubles; with two, the chances become one in two, or 50 percent.

Risk Factors	Comment
Hereditary Traits	The genetic tendency to develop atherosclerosis early in life greatly increases the risk of heart disease.
Hypertension	High blood pressure accelerates arteriosclerosis and atherosclerosis. It forces the heart to work harder and can lead to kidney damage. Heart disease and high blood pressure are directly related. A nine-member group sponsored by the National High Blood Pressure Coordinating Committee has redefined normal and abnormal readings based on recent research: *Systolic Pressure* at 140 or less is normal; at 140–154 produces borderline isolated systolic hypertension; at 160 and above produces isolated systolic hypertension; *Diastolic Pressure* at 85 or less is normal; at 85–89 is high normal; at 90–104

	produces mild hypertension; at 105–114 produces moderate hypertension; at 115 and above produces serious hypertension.
Obesity	Obesity is often accompanied by high fat levels in the blood, a higher incidence of arteriosclerotic disease, and high blood pressure.
Inactivity	Inactivity appears to contribute to early heart disease in a number of ways; obesity, high blood fat levels, and plaque accumulation.
High Cholesterol	High cholesterol levels increase one's risk of heart disease.
Cigarette Smoking	Smoking, in combination with some of the other risk factors, is a strong contributor to heart disease. Statistically, the incidence of heart disease is 70 to 200 percent higher among smoking males. The risk is also higher for smoking females. The risk of heart disease increases with number of cigarettes smoked and the degree of inhalation. Cigarette smoking appears to produce several changes, each with implications for heart disease: the amount of cholesterol deposits in the arteries are increased, chest pain in heart patients is increased, the clumping of platelets which may be associated with clotting is increased, and heart rate and blood pressure are increased.
The Pill	Use of the contraceptive pill in combination with cigarette smoking has been associated with a higher incidence of early heart disease.
Diabetes	Individuals who suffer from diabetes are more apt to suffer an early heart attack or stroke.

STROKE

The causes of a **stroke** are similar to those discussed previously for a heart attack. Like the heart, the brain must be continuously nourished. When blood supply to any portion of the brain is greatly reduced or cut off completely, nerve tissue in the brain is unable to function, and body tissue controlled by this nerve tissue also ceases to operate. This occurrence is known as a cerebrovascular accident (CVA) or stroke. A stroke may be caused by a hemorrhage (bleeding from a vessel that supplys the brain), thrombosis (a clot that clogs a vessel), embolus (a clot that shifts and eventually lodges in one of the small vessels), or compression (when blood is prevented from passing through a vessel supplying the brain).

HEART ATTACK AND STROKE PREVENTION

Reducing the risk of a heart attack or stroke involves aggressively dealing with all the risk factors. In general, measures include:

1. Elimination of tobacco smoking

2. Elimination of alcohol consumption or reduction to one or two drinks per day

3. Elimination of obesity by controlling caloric intake (see Chapter 6), total fat, saturated fat, and cholesterol consumption (see Chapter 7)

4. Initiation of a sensible exercise program to control weight, improve cardiovascular condition, and change the way your body handles fats

5. Scheduling regular medical checkups for contributing factors such as anemia, diabetes, high blood pressure, and compression on arteries in the neck

FREQUENTLY ASKED QUESTIONS

What is a normal heart rate?

Although heart rates between 50 and 100 beats per minute are not uncommon, the normal heart rate is between 72 and 80 BPM. With the increase in aerobic activity over the past 10 to 15 years, heart rates as low as 30 beats have been found in many distance runners and cross–country skiers.

The resting heart rate should be taken after you have been lying down for at least 15 minutes. Many factors such as age, body position, emotions, smoking, and food affect resting heart rate.

There is an inverse relationship between age and heart rate, i.e., as one grows older, the rate goes down. To estimate your maximum heart rate, subtract your age from 220.

Does a low heart rate mean a person is in good physical condition?

A low resting heart rate does not necessarily mean a high fitness level, in fact one form of heart disease causes a dangerously low heart rate. A decrease in heart rate while participating in an aerobic program, however, is an early sign that your conditioning level is improving. Use a change in resting heart rate as an indication of "getting in shape."

Can a person with a heart murmur exercise safely?

A person with a heart murmur should consult a sports medicine physician before beginning an exercise program. A heart murmur is caused by a heart valve's failure to close completely, allowing blood to flow back through it. Most murmurs are slight and should not affect a fitness program, but caution should be taken. Remember, exercise cannot hurt a normal heart but can damage an unhealthy one.

Are some people allergic to exercise?

Although it is rare, some people do experience an allergic reaction to exercise. The cause is not fully understood, but it is theorized that such a person's immune system does not fully destroy the histamines produced when exercising. Most allergic reactions to exercise can be treated. Those who have a "mental allergy" may find it more difficult to find a cure.

Can asthmatics exercise safely?

Yes. Exercise Induced Asthma (EIA) may occur in some individuals requiring premedication before exercising. The symptoms of generalized wheezing; coughing; chest tightness; rapid, shallow breathing; labored indrawing of air; and prolonged expiration last only a short time and will terminate even without medication in most cases. Athletes who experience some of these symptoms should work with their physicians to prevent such occurrences through self-administered medication. Don't stop exercising.

How does age affect fitness?

Physical performance declines as people get older. The rates of deterioration differ among individuals. The person who has been involved in a continual, vigorous exercise program throughout life will decrease in performance at a much slower rate than the inactive individual.

More specific charges are:

1. Oxygen consumption during strenuous exercise declines slowly with age, with a 29 percent decline by age 40.
2. The maximum heart rate declines with age. A maximum rate of about 190 to 210 beats per minute between the ages of 18 and 25 declines to approximately 160 to 210 beats per minute at age 50.
3. The capacity for endurance exercise suffers a much slower rate of decline after age 30 if aerobic training is continued on a regular basis.
4. Maximum anaerobic power (capability of sprinting full speed for extended distances), reaches a peak at about age 20, declining slowly thereafter.
5. Muscular strength decreases very slowly with age; weight training can improve strength at practically any age. Even at age 60, only a 15 to 20 percent decrease is evident.
6. Coordination is not greatly affected by age.
7. Stroke volume (amount of blood ejected per heartbeat) decreases at about 1 percent per year after maturity.
8. The amount of fat-free weight decreases with age. To maintain a constant fat/muscle ratio throughout life, body weight must be reduced. The change is due to inactive living which leads to muscle tissue atrophy.

It is nearly impossible to determine how much physical deterioration is due to aging and how much is due to inactive living. It is known, however, that the best protection against rapid or even normal physical decline is daily exercise, sensible eating, normal weight, and adequate sleeping habits. The fact that some loss of physical potential is inevitable with aging is not grounds for giving up on vigorous exercise as you get older. It is obvious that long-term exercise and proper eating habits will help prevent weight gain, aid in the maintenance of a healthy appearance, improve ability to exert a physical effort, slow the aging process, and provide a healthier life.

MYTHS AND FALLACIES

Exercise will cause athlete's heart.

"Athlete's Heart" or "sporterz" is a term used by a Swedish researcher who detected enlarged heart muscles among skiers in 1899. As the years passed, the term has gained momentum and is now used incorrectly to refer to an abnormally enlarged heart muscle brought about by exercise or athletic participation. Because of this myth, some people have the fear that heavy exercise will cause heart damage resulting in disability or premature death.

A sound heart cannot be damaged by exercise. The few cases of death or heart damage associated with strenuous exercise have usually occurred where there was an undiagnosed heart or vascular condition.

Physical training that is vigorous improves the efficiency of the heart muscle. Exercise does develop the heart muscle more fully and cause it to become heavier, larger, and slower (fewer beats per minute). It pumps much more blood per beat than the untrained heart. These changes are natural and healthy. It is also important to note that the heart size in champion athletes gets smaller after training is discontinued. The changes that occur from athletics and exercises are normal and desirable.

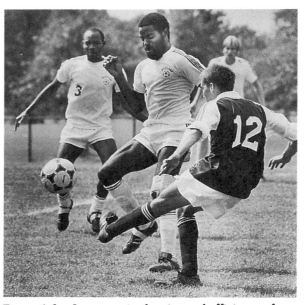

Figure 1.6 Increases in the size and efficiency of the heart, produced by regular exercise, are both natural and healthy.

Vigorous physical activity is harmful for children under 10 years of age.

Under competent leadership, almost any noncontact sport or activity is safe for children. Children between the ages of 6 and 10 should be encouraged to work on basic motor skills such as running, throwing, jumping, and catching that have carry-over value to many sports. Elementary school children, ages 6 to 12, are extremely weak in the upper body. A calisthenic program will allow more rapid development in physical skills requiring above-average strength. For the child under 10, certain pitfalls of training should be recognized. Heavy weights can overstress weight-bearing joints. The shoulder and elbow joints are growing quickly during these ages and should not be subjected to heavy weights. Injuries due to faulty lifting form or careless use of equipment may occur. Training precautions for the young follow.

1. Distance running (beyond 20 minutes) for children of this age group is a questionable activity, for it produces con-

siderable joint stress during training and requires excessive energy at a time when surplus calories are needed for growth and development.

2. Boxing is inappropriate for this age group, primarily for physical reasons.
3. Children should have a thorough physical examination prior to any participation and should undergo a good conditioning program before competition begins.
4. Contact sports and weight training are not recommended prior to age 10 because of the increased risk of injury.

Elementary school age is a time for the development of general coordination, basic motor skills, flexibility, and strength building activities. Active sports and physical pursuits are life-long possibilities, and the young or old should not be excluded from these joys simply because of age.

Exercise makes women less feminine.

This myth continues to flourish in the minds of both men and women. People worry that exercise will increase growth rate, muscle bulk, and body weight. There is no evidence to support any of these beliefs. Tradition, custom, prejudice, and ignorance retard the positive influence of physical activity for women.

Title IX is that section of the Educational Amendments Act of 1972 that forbids discrimination on the basis of sex in educational programs in schools receiving federal funds. This law requires that members of each sex have equal opportunity to participate in intramural and interscholastic programs. Title IX recognizes that the values inherent in developing physical prowess apply to women as well as to men, and that the educational benefits override irrational fears that participation makes women less feminine.

Weight training is harmful for women.

Lack of strength is the main limiting factor for women in many physical activities. Women possess a heavier layer of fatty tissue than men and also have 15–20 percent less muscle mass. To overcome these disadvantages, some form of strength training is needed.

Weight training is not dangerous for women. It will not produce an Amazon or detract from feminine appearance. It will, however

1. Improve strength
2. Develop endurance and muscle tone
3. Firm sagging areas
4. Improve appearance
5. Improve posture
6. Improve physical efficiency.

In sports where strength and explosive power are important (basketball, field hockey, badminton, track and field, swimming, and volleyball), weight training is absolutely necessary for high-level performance. A woman's best protection from injury is adequate strength. Such programs should improve the strength of supporting muscles in critical areas—ankle, knee, shoulder, and neck.

Women should not exercise during their menstrual period.

Engaging in exercise during the menstrual flow is not harmful. Depending upon the individual, performance may be completely unaffected. Do not stop exercise or training completely during menstruation, because loss of five or more days will lower your conditioning level. An iron supplement may also be helpful. If you are unable to continue in a normal routine, do light exercises to maintain your present conditioning level.

BIBLIOGRAPHY

Alpert, B., et al. "Blood Pressure Response to Dynamic Exercise in Healthy Children—Black vs White." *The Journal of Pediatrics* 99:4 (1981): 556–60.

Bartley, D., and F. Belgrave. "Physical Fitness and Psychological Wellbeing in college Students." *Health Education* 18:3 (1987): 57–60.

Brown, S., and D. Cundiff. "Exercise, Aging and Longevity." *Health Education* 19:2 (1988): 4–7.

Bruce, R. "Primary Intervention Against Coronary Atherosclerosis by Exercise Conditioning." *The New England Journal of Medicine* 305 (1981): 1525–26.

Dintiman, G., and Robert Ward. *Train America! Achieving Peak Performance and Fitness for Sports Competition.* Dubuque, Iowa: Kendal-Hunt 1988.

Fletcher, G. "Long-term Exercise in Coronary Artery Disease and Other Chronic Disease States." *Journal: Heart and Lung* 13:1 (1984): 28–46.

Heath, G., et al. "A Physiological Comparison of Young and Older Endurance Athletes." *Journal of Applied Physiology* 51:3 (1981): 634–40.

Holloszy, J. "Exercise, Health, and Aging: A Need for More Information." *Medicine and Science in Sports and Exercise* 15:1 (1983): 1–5.

Kaslow, R. "College Fitness Courses: What Determines Student Interest?" *Journal of Health, Physical Education, Recreation and Dance* 59:1 (1988): 28–30.

Kramsch, D., et al. "Reduction of Coronary Atherosclerosis by Moderate Conditioning Exercise in Monkeys on an Atherogenic Diet." *The New England Journal of Medicine* 305 (1981): 1483–89.

Kuntzleman, C. "Observations on Children's Health and Fitness." *Physical Fitness Council Newsletter* 4:2 (Spring 1988): 1–4.

Pate, R., and J. Ross. "Factors Associated with Health-related Fitness." *Journal of Health, Physical Education, Recreation, and Dance* 58:9 (1987): 93–95.

Ross, J., and R. Pate. "A Summary of Finding." *Journal of Health, Physical Education, Recreation, and Dance* 58:9 (1987): 51–56.

Savage, M., et al. "Exercise Training Effects on Serum Lipids of Prepubescent Boys and Adult Men." *Medicine and Science in Sports and Exercise* 18:2 (1986): 197–206.

Toufexis, A. "Older—but Coming on Strong." *Time* 131:8 (1988): 76–79.

Williams, M. *Lifetime Physical Fitness.* Dubuque: Wm. C. Brown Co., 1985.

Wood, F., ed. "Research Shows Advantages, Problems of Giving Aspirin to Stroke Victims." *American Heart News* 5:2 (1988): 11–12.

LABORATORY 1.1

Resting Heart Rate Reduction

PURPOSE: To plot resting heart rate.

SIZE OF GROUP: Alone

EQUIPMENT: Watch with second hand, or digital watch

PROCEDURE

1. Your first lab is an easy one. Lie down for 15 minutes in a comfortable place. Be sure not to eat or drink for at least three hours before doing this lab. You have, of course, given up smoking. If not, do not smoke for at least 30 minutes prior to completing this lab.

2. After the rest period and while still lying down, take your pulse at the carotid artery (either side of the neck) or use the radial pulse (thumb side of the wrist). Since your thumb has its own pulse and will cause inaccurate readings use only the fingers to find and count the pulse. Count for an entire minute. The resulting number is your resting heart rate. Record it on the chart below.

3. This lab should be repeated at least once a week.

RESULTS

By connecting the dots on the heart rate reduction chart below, you should begin to see a decline in your resting heart rate within two weeks indicating an increase in cardiovascular efficiency.

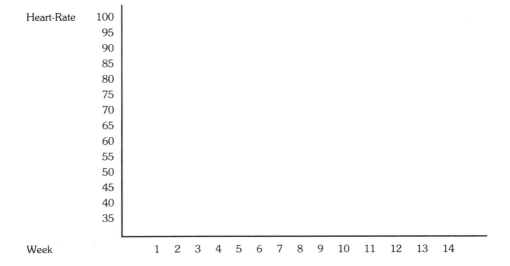

LABORATORY 1.2

Listing Reasons For Exercising

PURPOSE: To determine reasons for exercising.

SIZE OF GROUP: Five

PROCEDURE

1. Each person in group gives five reasons for participating in the class.
2. Group summarizes data and makes presentation to class. Class data is collected and summarized.

RESULTS

Class data can then be used to determine the direction of the class including what activities will be emphasized and what information will be presented.

CHAPTER TWO

Turning on to EXERCISE

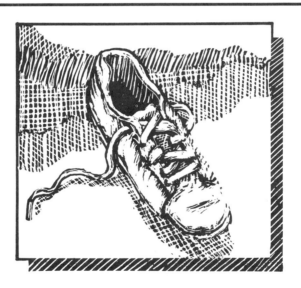

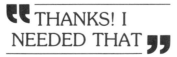 THANKS! I
NEEDED THAT

? HAVE YOU EVER WONDERED ABOUT:

How to increase your pleasure during exercise?
How to develop a new mind set about exercise?
How to use an exercise contract?
How other people can help you continue to exercise?
How to reward yourself?
How to increase activity in your daily routine?

KEY TERMS

Dropout potential
Endorphins
Enkephalins

Exercise mind set
Negative addiction
Negative exercise thoughts

The best motivator to begin and increase the exercise you do on a daily basis is pleasure. This chapter provides the information you need to help you identify the pleasurable aspects of exercise so that you can develop and maintain a moderate physical activity level for the rest of your life. You do not need to become a marathoner or a champion athlete to improve your health and increase your life span. A study at Harvard showed that people who are active and expend 2,000 calories a week in daily routine, moving about and in deliberate physical activity, live longer than others who are less active (Hales 1983). For most people, the equivalent of as little as 2½ to 3 hours of brisk walking every week in addition to normal activity will improve health and provide benefits.

By understanding more about how to find pleasure in exercise and by following the steps suggested in this chapter you can develop an exercise style that fits your particular character and taste.

You will learn to find pleasant and positive mental results in exercise. This will provide you with good feelings in the early stages of developing an exercise routine.

Mental techniques to develop positive thinking patterns will improve your chances for success. Once you gain momentum and increased motivation you can begin to improve other aspects of your lifestyle.

Getting other people to help is an important way to get going and to keep going in your new program. A contract system can help you become definite about the goals you set and the rewards you deserve for your efforts. Let's get started!

EXERCISE AND REWARD

Increasing your motivation to exercise begins when you realize immediate rewards from your efforts. Expect pleasant and positive mental results during and after your workout. The experienced exerciser already knows these pleasures. The beginner must learn them. Here is what to look for:

1. *Your mood will lift.* Mild attacks of depression and lack of energy are common among young adults and are usually self-limiting. Episodes of feeling low or hopeless can be improved through physical exercise. Natural brain hormones called neurotransmittors are probably the agents that cause the "feeling better" sensations. The mood elevation will occur immediately after your exercise bout and will continue for two hours or longer. When you begin a program, find a type of exercise such as walking or slow jogging that you can continue for at least 30 minutes or longer. You need to break a sweat and keep moving continuously for 30 minutes to feel more positive as a result of exercise. Since these lifts in mood occur everytime you exercise, learn to anticipate a positive afterglow, and use your workout to improve "blue moods."

2. *You will have a positive attitude.* Physically fit people tend to be more emotionally stable, more extroverted, and more self-assured than their inactive counterparts. When you exercise, expect to feel more happiness and joy on a day-to-day basis. It

is possible to believe, without being naive, that the pursuit of fitness can contribute to a greater sense of well-being.

3. *You will be less nervous and feel less stress.* Some estimates suggest that 10 million Americans suffer from anxiety neurosis and 70 percent of all patients seen by general practitioners are suffering from conditions aggravated by unrelieved stress. Vigorous exercise provides you with tension-relieving effects. Muscles relax after exercise with a 25 percent decrease in muscle electrical activity following aerobics and weight lifting. You should expect to feel more relaxed after your workout, with the calm feelings reaching their peak 20 to 30 minutes following your training bout.

4. *You will sleep better.* Because your muscles are relaxed after exercise and the energy used in your workout leaves you pleasantly tired, you can expect to experience deep and relaxing sleep. It is advisable to avoid aerobic exercise within 2 to 3 hours of bedtime. If you have difficulty sleeping after exercise, this may be a sign of overexertion.

Through the knowledge that you are doing something good for your body every day you exercise, and by looking for the immediate rewards listed above, you can experience constant pleasure from exercise. People who are turned on to exercise know the mental pleasures of a good workout. If you are just beginning, learn to expect a healthier mind even before your body changes by getting stronger, looking better, and having more energy. Your immediate reward is centered in the renewed self-respect that comes from your effort to improve your mind and body through exercise.

DEVELOPING A NEW MIND SET ABOUT EXERCISE

The mental rewards you can experience during and after exercise can be counterbalanced by **negative thoughts** about the prospects for changing your exercise behavior. This is normal. When people be-

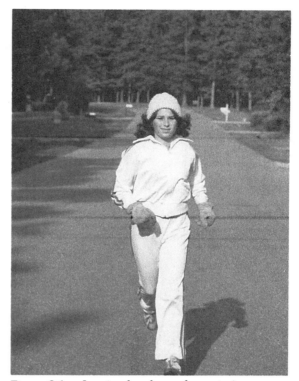

Figure 2.1   Jogging has been shown to improve one's emotional state both during and after the run.

gin developing a new habit, they are often plagued with self-doubts and thoughts of failure. During the early stages of your program, you can become your own worst enemy (see Table 2.1).

Do any of the excuses listed in Table 2.1 look familiar to you? Take a minute to prepare your own list of self-defeating thoughts about exercise as well as the logical positive argument.

Now that you have listed these positive and negative thoughts, study and memorize them. Whenever self-defeating thoughts about exercise enter your mind, counteract them immediately with your positive ones. Do not hesitate to repeat the positive ideas frequently to yourself.

You will learn to develop a more positive attitude by being conscious of these private events regarding your exercise habits. What we think, imagine, and feel is very important. Try to become conscious of what you are saying to yourself about exercise. Take time every day to go over the positive list that you have developed; soon these positive views will come to you automatically.

TABLE 2.1 POSITIVE AND NEGATIVE THOUGHTS ABOUT EXERCISE

Negative Thoughts About Exercise	Positive Thoughts That Counteract the Negative
1. I'm too busy to exercise today. I'm working too hard anyway and need a break.	1. I can find time to exercise today. I just have to think about my routine and plan carefully.
2. I'm too tired to exercise today, and if I do work out, I won't have enough energy to do the other things I must do.	2. I may feel tired today, but I'll do a light exercise routine instead of the heavy one I usually do. If I keep working out on a regular basis, I'll build my stamina so I won't feel so tired during the day.
3. I missed my workout today. I might as well forget all this fitness stuff. I don't have the self-control to keep at it.	3. Just because I missed one exercise session doesn't mean I should give up. I'm not going to let this small setback ruin everything I've accomplished all week.
4. None of my friends are fit or trim and they don't worry about it. I'm not going to either.	4. What my friends do about exercising has nothing to do with my exercise habits. I'll make additional friends who do exercise.
5. I'm already "over the hill." I should let myself go and enjoy life more.	5. I can get in shape and stay there. All I have to do is stick to my schedule. Knowing I can control my behavior is something I can enjoy every day.

Negative Exercise Thought

1. _____
_____
_____

2. _____
_____
_____

3. _____
_____
_____

4. _____
_____
_____

Positive Exercise Thought

1. _____
_____
_____

2. _____
_____
_____

3. _____
_____
_____

4. _____
_____
_____

CONCENTRATE YOUR THOUGHTS ON EXERCISE EXTREMES

Another effective thought-control method involves concentrating on the maximum or final consequences of your exercise behavior. By thinking about the extreme positive effects of exercise (I may live longer) and the extreme negative consequences of a lifetime of nonexercise (I may have a heart attack) you can achieve better results. It is unfortunate that we are more influenced by short-term positive effects of our behavior than by long-term negative effects. You rarely think of dying while you enjoy a television program instead of taking the walk you had planned. In fact, you probably ignore the final consequences of not exercising until after you have skipped the activity. You may then feel guilty and this may produce a feeling of helplessness or lack of control.

To use the final consequences of exercising to your benefit, you must examine them closely. Begin by giving careful consideration to the long-term negative effects of a life without much physical activity. Visualize yourself as feeble, infirm, weary, flaccid, and debilitated; now write the five worst consequences of a sedentary lifestyle on one side of an index card. Make sure that these negative consequences have vivid personal meaning for you. A sample list is presented below:

1. Heart attack
2. No energy
3. Weight gain
4. High blood pressure
5. Poor sex life

Turn your index card over and list the five most postive consequences of your exercise program. A sample list is presented below:

1. Longer life
2. Vigor
3. Better appearance
4. Slower aging process
5. Feeling of pride

Make a duplicate card of your list. Keep one card with you and the other in a prominent place in your office or home.

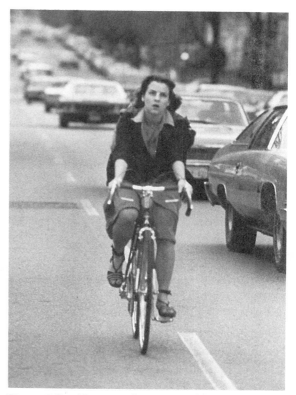

Figure 2.2   There is always time for exercise for those who plan their day.

Every time you think of skipping a planned workout, look at your index card and read it slowly. Start with the negative consequences first. Make an emotional impact on yourself by imagining what the lack of exercise will mean to you. Now, turn the card over and read the positive consequences slowly. See, feel, and actively visualize the positive effects of your exercise activities. During the first several weeks of your program, you should read these lists every day, ending on the positive results. When you practice this technique often, you will automatically consider the consequences of your actions and will no longer have to refer to the written lists.

HOW OTHER PEOPLE CAN HELP

What others do and how they respond to you will influence your behavior. If you have strong support from individuals who are important in your life, efforts to change your exercise habits have a much better chance of permanent success.

Table 2.2 is a method of identifying helpers and getting them to support your exercise endeavors. Select two important people in your life who might help you; ask people you can trust, ones with whom you feel comfortable. Write their names, and specify how you would like them to help you. Explain to them in specific terms what they can do.

Once these people have agreed to assist you, be sure you show respect and appreciation for their assistance. You might give them a gift or a thank-you note.

USING AN EXERCISE CONTRACT

Table 2.3 is a behavioral contract to make a written agreement with yourself about exercise. In section 1, set specific physical activity goals for increasing your energy use during work. In section 2, set specific goals for increasing activity during recreational periods. Section 3 is for setting the specific number of calories you intend to expend through physical activity each week. Remember to start slowly; an increase of 50 calories of activity per day may be a small amount, but it adds up to a loss in pounds and fat and an increase in stamina.

LEARNING TO REWARD YOURSELF

It is helpful to keep in mind that motivation increases when prompt rewards are realized as a result of your efforts. When you reach the final stages of skill development in exercise activities and the habit of regular physical activity becomes integrated into your life, the intrinsic values of exercise serve to motivate. The pleasant anticipation of "working up a good sweat," the trouble-free interlude, a renewed capacity to think creatively during the workout, and the mood lift and relaxation during the exercise afterglow combine to make exercise its own reward. This degree of develop-

---

TABLE 2.2　EXERCISE HELP

How Others Can Help Me

Examples:

Sue
1. Go for a walk with me every morning before work.
2. Praise me regularly for changing my exercise habits.

Bill
1. Jog with me after work three times a week for 20 minutes.

Yours:

---

ment in positive exercise mind set takes time to reach.

During the early stages in developing your exercise habits, you will learn to use mental rewards to motivate yourself. In addition, section 4 of the exercise contract asks you to list specific daily and weekly rewards for meeting exercise goals. Consider the list of possible concrete rewards that you can give yourself for a productive workout or a successful exercise week. Self payments can range from eating special foods, to treating yourself to a night out, to simply allowing an extra hour of rest

TABLE 2.3 CONTRACT TO INCREASE MY PHYSICAL ACTIVITY LEVEL

During this week _____ 19 _____ , I hereby agree to work as hard as possible at achieving the following:

1. Physical activity goals for increasing my energy use during occupational time:
   A. I will park my car or leave public transportation and walk _____ additional minutes per day.
   B. I will spend _____ minutes daily standing instead of sitting while I work.
   C. I will walk up _____ flights of stairs each working day.
   D. I will walk around my work area _____ minutes every day.
   E. I will spend _____ minutes during each coffee break standing instead of sitting.
   F. I will spend _____ minutes during each lunch break walking outside in the open air.

2. Physical activity goals for increasing my energy use during recreational time:
   A. I will spend _____ minutes daily doing stretching activities to increase my flexibility.
   B. I will spend _____ minutes at least three times per week doing aerobic activities to improve my endurance.
   C. I will spend _____ minutes at least three times per week doing strength activities.
   D. I will spend _____ minutes Saturday and Sunday in active recreational activities.

3. By increasing my activity levels in the work and recreational periods listed above I will use up _____ more calories per week (see Appendix F).

4. My rewards and consequences:
   A. I will reward myself daily with one of the following pleasures when I achieve my daily goals in increased activity:
      1) _____   4) _____
      2) _____   5) _____
      3) _____   6) _____
   B. When I do *not* make my daily goals I agree to do the following:
      1) _____   2) _____
   C. I will reward myself every week with one of the following pleasures when I achieve my weekly exercise goals:
      1) _____   4) _____
      2) _____   5) _____
      3) _____   6) _____
   D. When I do *not* make my weekly goals I agree to do the following:
      1) _____   2) _____

I now agree to the above contract and with the goals and consequences. I also agree to follow this contract until my goals are reached.
Signed _____ Date _____ Witnessed _____

in a day. Choose rewards that aren't destructive to your overall fitness program; a bowl of ice cream is a great reward for devotion to your schedule, but is something that is wise to avoid in excessive amounts.

You can use the behavioral contract as a systematic approach to achieving exercise goals. This approach works best when you make a game out of its use. The contract and rewards are artificial and contrived. You do not *have* to meet your own agreements and you can have the rewards you select without meeting any goals. The rules and rewards are simple, artificial limits that you set for yourself to help produce results. Your task is to play the contract game—set goals, select rewards, stick to your contract, have fun, and get results.

SETTING GOALS

One certain way to lose interest in exercise is to begin your program with unrealistic goals. In order to become a champion athlete, a marathon runner, or a model, you need an unlimited devotion to fitness. Such goals are too high or unrealistic for the beginning exerciser and set the stage for failure. Goals that are set too high demand a standard of perfection that leaves little room for success. Unless you can spend several hours daily developing your physical potential, do not aim for physical perfection. Choose to improve your physical shape a little bit at a time, regardless of how far out of condition you are when you begin. Remember the adage: "Inch by inch, anything's a cinch."

The goals you set should be small, immediate behaviors that move you in the direction of your final goals. Immediate goals might include walking for 30 minutes during lunch. Your final goal might be to run for 5 miles without stopping. To accomplish the final goal, you begin with walking, then jogging, and then finally running over a period of months. Select your end goal, but do not set that as your immediate goal. Rather, devise small, challenging steps that will lead you to your final goals.

It is important to recognize that immediate goals need to be flexible. You may find that a goal seemed reasonable but proved too difficult to achieve. In that case, reevaluate and lower the goal or postpone it for awhile. A reasonable goal is one that is slightly more difficult than one you have actually achieved.

INCREASING ACTIVITY IN YOUR DAILY ROUTINE

The modern American is under the impression that all labor-saving devices are desirable and that saving steps is a goal to aim for in *every* aspect of life. The telephone company sells extension phones with the claim that the use of one extension will save the customer 70 miles of walking per year; it also *deprives* you of valuable muscular effort, improved muscle tone, and the opportunity to lose weight. One extension phone can prevent you from burning approximately 10,500 calories and losing three pounds of fat per year. Other modern conveniences are even worse.

After thinking about the many ways in which mechanization results in reducing physical exertion, you may be thankful for these tools. You are absolutely not going to return to a life of drudgery regardless of your desire to become fit or lose weight. But remember, you have become less efficient! The more energy you save using mechanical conveniences, the more you lose in physical conditioning. Degenerative processes, such as lost muscular strength and endurance, poor blood supply to vital organs, atherosclerosis, poor digestion, increased chance of a fatal heart attack, and weight gain, all come with easy living.

Included below is a list of suggestions for weaving more exercise into your routine. Read this list and choose two activities that you will start this week.

1. Walking is the most common form of exercise for Americans. Do not save steps, but consciously increase the steps necessary to carry out your daily duties.

2. Climb stairs; do not use the elevator or escalator. Stair climbing is excellent exercise.

3. If you drive to work, park half a mile away and walk.

4. If you ride the bus, train, or taxi, get off several stops early and walk the remaining distance.

5. Do a stretching routine while watching television. There are 10 minutes of advertising every hour. If you watch TV for 3 hours, that's 30 minutes of potential exercise without missing a thing.

INCREASING ACTIVITY DURING RECREATIONAL TIME

Because most Americans have a sedentary occupation and shorter working hours, the type of exercise performed during leisure hours has the most important impact on daily energy expenditure. Table 2.4 rates the intensity and energy expenditure of sport-recreational activities. A more complete list is provided in Appendix F.

Plan your recreational time so that during the early stages of your fitness program you spend a minimum of 15 minutes per day, four days per week in active exercise that demands at least 5 kilocalories per minute. Those in fair physical condition should engage in activities costing 5 to 10 kcal/minute, four days per week for 20 minutes

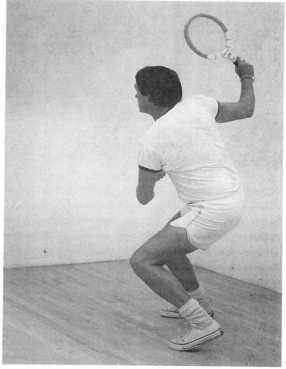

Figure 2.3 Racquetball is an excellent choice for both fun, fitness, and weight control.

TABLE 2.4 EXERCISE INTENSITY CLASSIFICATION OF SPORT-RECREATIONAL PHYSICAL ACTIVITIES

Selected Sport-Recreational Activities	Exercise Intensity Level	Energy Expenditure kcal/minute
Playing cards, listening to music, watching T.V., eating	very light	2.0 to 2.5
Archery, baseball, billiards, leisurely dancing, horseback riding (walking)	light	2.6 to 4.6
Recreational bicycling, golf, gymnastics, recreational skating, table tennis, badminton, American football	moderate	5.2 to 7.2
Energetic dancing, horseback riding (trotting), mountaineering, jogging, recreational skiing (downhill, cross-country), soccer, softball, recreational swimming, tennis (singles, doubles), volleyball, recreational bicycling, racquetball	heavy to very heavy	7.5 to 12.4

Values are based on low and high extremes in each level of intensity for both men and women and depend on efficiency and body size. Add 10 percent for each 15 pounds above 150, subtract 10 percent for each 15 pounds under 150. A complete caloric list is included in Appendix F.

per workout. For people in good physical condition, spending 20 minutes per day, four days per week doing activities demanding 10 kcal/minute or more is sufficient. Once you have formed a regular exercise habit, you can begin to increase the time or the intensity of your exercise session.

OVERCOMING THE BARRIERS

It is important that you start and progress slowly in your exercise program. In the early stages of the program, the temptations to quit are great. The following suggestions will help your new program become an important part of your daily routine:

1. Keep track of your progress as you shift from using your body as a passive receptacle to an active machine. Use your fitness profile sheet in Appendix B to periodically check your progress.

2. View yourself as taking an active role to improve the condition and health of your body. With this thought you will feel new self-respect and a sense of real triumph. This choice will provide you with good feelings and rewards in the early stages of developing an exercise routine.

3. Use the mental techniques offered to deal with self-doubts and negative thoughts about exercise. The more positive your thinking patterns, the better the chances for success.

4. Once you develop some momentum from regular exercise, use the self-discipline you have gained to improve other aspects of your lifestyle.

5. Tell other people about your new exercise program. Get your family or roommates involved. This is probably the most important way to get going and keep going. If possible, find a friend to exercise with. If you cannot find a workout partner, do not use this as an excuse.

6. Through the contract system, be more definite about goals and rewards.

7. Avoid trying to be perfect. Do not think in terms of workout hours per week. Assume that progress will be slow, but that minutes every day will add up. Simple improvement should be your goal.

FREQUENTLY ASKED QUESTIONS

What are the most important factors that keep a person involved in an exercise program once they have begun to exercise?

Business executives who continue in an exercise program seem to do so because there are exercise facilities close to their jobs or houses. Those who live or work near a gym or workout area seem to have a definite advantage over those who do not. Another important factor is choosing an exercise approach that provides enjoyment and success. Skill improvement in any phase of a sport is a strong motivation to continue in the future.

Can exercise benefits be stored?

No. When you stop exercising for more than a few days, muscle strength begins to diminish. Both the size of the muscle and muscle tone decline. An immobilized limb, for example, shows a tremendous decrease in size, tone, and strength after a few weeks. Muscular strength and muscular endurance can be maintained with one strenuous workout weekly. The maintenance of aerobic endurance requires two to three workouts per week.

How can I avoid temptations not to exercise?

Plan your next day's exercise routine each night as you are getting ready for bed. Take a few minutes to think of tomorrow's time demands and carefully fit exercise into your schedule. Set aside that particular time and stick to your plan. You can also leave your workout clothes in a conspicuous place as a reminder. Take your exercise gear with you when you leave for a trip and try to stay at lodgings that have exercise facilities.

How fast will I see results?

Do not expect instant results in terms of body fat or weight loss, improved muscle firmness, or improved aerobic conditioning level. However, although it may not be noticeable to you, your body is carefully responding to each exercise workout with computerlike precision: reduced caloric intake and increased caloric expenditure is producing weight and fat loss, muscles are becoming stronger and larger, cardiovascular efficiency is improving, muscular endurance and flexibility are improving, and a number of additional beneficial changes are occurring. You will begin to notice some results in four to six weeks. These changes will be minimal, however, compared to bodily changes and health benefits likely to accrue after one year or more of regular exercise and sensible eating.

Doesn't exercise bring about a natural tranquilizer effect to mask pain and stress?

The pituitary gland produces two types of hormones (**endorphins** and **enkephalins**) very similar in chemical composition to morphine to assist the body in handling pain and stress. Abnormally high amounts of these morphinelike substances have been found in the blood plasma of exercising subjects. Researchers have been investigating the relationship between blood levels of endorphins and enkephalins and so-called "runner's high" (if one does indeed exist), pain threshold (an athlete's ability to ignore injuries and continue exercise), and mood. While it is well-established that exercise significantly increases the immediate plasma beta-endorphin level, the true function of these secretions and their true effect upon the human body is still relatively unknown.

How much exercise is enough?

How long and how often should college students exercise? Is 30 minutes per week really enough? Can you become fit with 2 to 5 minutes per day? Some people suggest that 30 minutes of exercise per week (4½ minutes per day) is sufficient for the average American adult. A combination of aerobic and calisthenic exercises is recommended. Three 30-second isometric contractions daily have been advocated by others as a means of improving total body strength and decreasing the waistline. These are examples of hundreds of short-cut approaches to fitness that have been used by adults in the past. Each program has the obvious advantages of convenience of time, minimal equipment (do it in a business suit in your office or do it in the kitchen), and little pain or suffering (after all, you can endure almost anything for 2 to 4 minutes). Unfortunately, such short-cut approaches are quite ineffective in meeting any but the most feeble exercise objectives. There is little hope of improving heart/lung endurance, firming body parts, or losing weight through caloric expenditure. There just are not any quick approaches that will turn you into a well-conditioned individual.

How much exercise is enough? The answer depends upon your training objectives. If you seek cardiovascular development (heart/lung) and protection from early heart disease, you must reach your target heart rate and maintain this level of intensity for 20 to 30 minutes at least three times weekly. If weight loss is your goal, a minimum of 30 to 60 minutes of less intense exercise is recommended. Ideally, this level of intensity would also elicit your target heart rate, but the key to weight loss is volume, not intensity (distance, not speed; increased exercise time at a slower pace). If strength improvement is your goal, three workouts of 30 minutes duration weekly may be sufficient, providing you move quickly from one exercise set to another. If you are training for competition in a team or individual sport, daily workouts of one to three hours may be needed, alternating light and heavy days. Since it is our recommendation that college students select an aerobic program as their foundation, four workouts weekly of 30 minutes duration at the target heart rate should be considered the minimum level.

Negative addiction: *is too much of a good thing harmful?*

Although the affected person may ignore them, the physiological signs of overindulgence are usually easy to recognize. Resting pulse rates usually rise, joints become stiff and sore, fatigue is common, and sleeping, eating, and elimination habits are disturbed. Although the telltale signs of physiological overindulgence appear common, it is unlikely that any one person will experience all of them. Factors such as age, conditioning level, rest habits, diet, and health factors such as anemia, illness, and mental stress determine when and if symptoms appear.

Competition seems to be a common denominator for most exercise addicts. With the inclusion of age group categories in nearly all sports, special olympics for the aged, and continued emphasis on exercise beyond the college years, there is more motivation to seek higher levels of fitness than are necessary for health alone. There are, therefore, many who are seeking to capture past glories or seeking glories never received.

You can usually tell when you're addicted by your behavior. You are compulsive about exercise; not a day can be missed; daily schedules are made around exercise; and workouts often receive priority over everything. Whether such behavior is a result of the exercise or of personality is unknown. It is generally agreed, however, that negative addiction is unhealthy and, as the name implies, should be avoided. The longterm results would seem to be harmful, both physiologically and psychologically.

MYTHS AND FALLACIES

There are no special problems for women who exercise.

Moderate activity is beneficial for both sexes. For women, a lifelong plan of regular exercise is found to strengthen bones and help prevent osteoporosis. But with high levels of exercise, hormonal changes may occur. Up to 50 percent of competitive female runners fail to have regular menstrual cycles. As a result, some women experience temporary infertility and spinal bone loss associated with lower levels of estrogen and calcium.

For women who do aerobic dance (85 percent of participants in exercise classes are women) involving jumping and hopping, injuries to the lower legs are common. The American College of Obstetricians and Gynecologists has suggested a three-day-a-week limit on aerobic dancing and jogging, with limits on jumping.

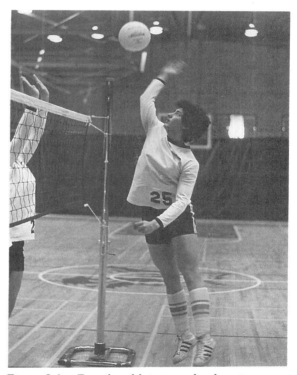

Figure 2.4   Female athletes can do almost anything male athletes can do with no restrictions or dangers.

Pregnant women should not engage in regular exercise.

Guidelines have been developed for pregnant women for exercise during pregnancy and the postnatal period. They are listed below.

American College of Obstetricians and Gynecologists Guidelines for Exercise During Pregnancy and Postpartum

1. Regular exercise (at least three times per week) is preferable to intermittent activity. Competitive activities should be discouraged.
2. Vigorous exercise should not be performed in hot, humid weather or during a period of febrile illness.
3. Ballistic movements (jerky, bouncy motions) should be avoided. Exercise should be done on a wooden floor or a tightly carpeted surface to reduce shock and provide a sure footing.
4. Deep flexion or extension of joints should be avoided because of connective tissue laxity. Activities that require jumping, jarring motions, or rapid changes in direction should be avoided because of joint instability.
5. Vigorous exercise should be preceded by a five-minute period of muscle warm-up. This can be accomplished by slow walking or stationary cycling with low resistance.
6. Vigorous exercise should be followed by a period of gradually declining activity that includes gentle stationary stretching. Because connective tissue laxity increases the risk of joint injury, stretches should not be taken to the point of maximum resistance.
7. Heart rate should be measured at times of peak activity. Target heart rates and limits established in consultation with the physician should not be exceeded.
8. Care should be taken to gradually rise from the floor to avoid orthostatic hypotension. Some form of activity involving the legs shold be continued for a brief period.
9. Liquids should be taken liberally before and after exercise to prevent dehydration. If necessary, activity should be interrupted to replenish fluids.
10. Women who have led sedentary life-styles should begin with physical activity of very low intensity and advance activity levels very gradually.
11. Activity should be stopped and the physician consulted if any unusual symptoms appear.

Pregnancy only

1. Maternal heart rate should not exceed 140 beats per min.
2. Strenous activities should not exceed 15 minutes in duration.
3. No exercise should be performed in the supine position after the fourth month of gestation is completed.
4. Calorie intake should be adequate to meet not only the extra energy needs of pregnancy, but also of the exercise performed.
5. Maternal core temperature should not exceed 38°C.

Reprinted with permission from the American College of Obstetricians and Gynecologists: "Exercise During Pregnancy and the Postnatal Period (ACOG Home Exercise Programs)." Washington, D.C.: ACOG, 1985.

Vigorous exercise is safe for everyone.

Exercise is advocated not only for normal, healthy individuals but for patients with known underlying ailments such as heart disease. Most of these individuals feel good, have better endurance than those who do not exercise, weigh less, have lower blood pressure and lower blood fats, and may even live longer. According to some experts, however, exercise may be dangerous and even fatal to some individuals, including the highly conditioned young person under the age of 25.

Sudden death in young athletes and exercising individuals during physical activity has occurred in many sports to both the poorly and highly conditioned individual. The causes of instantaneous death are usually cardiac related, particularly in the 25 and under age group. In the 25 to 50 age group, coronary artery disease due to undiagnosed atherosclerosis is usually the cause of sudden death. The third major cause of collapse and occasional death during extreme exertion is heat injury (see Chapter 8). Although a heart attack is generally cited in the sudden death of exercising individuals, it can be documented only about 20 percent of the time. Most victims show atherosclerosis without coronary thrombosis (blockage). Death appears to be caused by lack of oxygen to the heart muscle, producing irregular heart beat.

Orthopedic surgeons have also voiced their concerns about the hazards of jogging (back injuries, knee deterioration, feet and ankle problems) and the potential danger for exercising females. Others argue that exercise is potentially dangerous for everyone in the early stages of a newly started program and almost always results in numerous injuries in the later stages from too much volume (overuse) and overtraining. Each of these concerns are discussed in Chapter 8, Injury Prevention and Emergency Treatment.

Exercising proponents argue that the dangers of injury or death are grossly exaggerated and often represent isolated, well-publicized cases of celebrities who died during exercise. Newspapers often fail to reveal significant facts such as previous heart and other health conditions, drugs found in the body, congenital disorders, or heat and humidity conditions. Exercise gets the blame and reinforces the sedentary living habits of millions of Americans. The chances of injury can be minimized by following the suggestions in this book. Overtraining, avoiding a preconditioning or starter program if you have been previously inactive, exercising too much too soon, attempting to get in condition in one day after months or years of inactivity, and neglecting a physical examination from your physician before starting a program all increase the danger of injury or illness. Rarely does a properly conceived exercise program result in serious injury or illness. It must be understood, however, that the potential does exist for injury and serious illness or death and it is important for high risk individuals (obese, those with signs of heart disease, and individuals with hypertension) to receive the "green light" from their physicians, start and progress slowly, and follow the suggestions in this book.

Exercise can be misused, and incorrect practices may lead to serious injury or illness. Whether this is also the case with properly conceived programs is another matter.

BIBLIOGRAPHY

Cooper, Kenneth H. *The Aerobics Program for Total Well-Being.* New York: M. Evans and Co. 1982.

Dintiman, George B., and Robert Ward. *Train America! Achieving Peak Performance and Fitness for Sports Competition.* Dubuque, Iowa: Kendal Hunt Publishing Co. 1988.

Hales, Dianne, and Robert E. Hales. "How Much is Enough?" *American Health Magazine.* (July–August, 1983): 120–125.

Jerome, John. "Getting It All Back." *American Health Magazine.* (April 1982): 36–38.

Office of Disease Prevention and Health Promotion. *The 1990 Health Objectives of the Nation: A Midcourse Review.* Washington, D.C.: U.S. Department of Health and Human Services 1986.

Reid, J. Gavin, and John M. Thompson. *Exercise Prescription for Fitness.* Englewood Cliffs, New Jersey: Prentice-Hall 1985.

LABORATORY 2.1

Do You Have Dropout Potential?

PURPOSE: To determine if you will stick with your exercise program.

SIZE OF GROUP: Alone

PROCEDURE

Place a checkmark in front of the statements that are true for you now.

_____ Exercise is not very important to me.
_____ I would exercise primarily to change my appearance.
_____ I find I have little time to exercise.
_____ I'm not very good at committing myself to doing things.
_____ I get discouraged easily.
_____ Whenever I get bored with projects, I drop them to do something else.
_____ I never force myself to do things I don't feel like doing.
_____ If something gets to be too much of an effort to do, I'm likely to just forget it.
_____ I avoid stressful situations.
_____ I'm not very patient.

If you checked any of these statements, you are likely to drop out of an exercise program. To increase motivation, you need to do one, some, or all of the following:

1. Find an activity you love
2. Set reasonable goals
3. Think positively
4. Arrange for rewards

RESULTS

Data will help class members avoid dropping out.

LABORATORY 2.2

Finding Exercise Forms That Will Give You Pleasure

PURPOSE: To determine what type of exercise fits your personality.

SIZE OF GROUP: Alone

PROCEDURE

Read the items below and underline the areas that apply to your tastes in exercise.

If you are a team player, try: badminton, baseball/softball, basketball, bowling, rowing, tennis, touch football, volleyball.

If you prefer to go solo, try: bicycling, cross-country skiing, gymnastics, martial arts, rowing, running/jogging, skating, swimming, walking.

If you like strenuous aerobic exercise, try: aerobic dance, basketball, bicycling, brisk walking, cross-country skiing, racquetball/squash, rowing, running/jogging, swimming.

If you prefer an easier pace, try: badminton, baseball/softball, bowling, downhill skiing, golf, gymnastics, martial arts, skating, touch football, tennis, volleyball.

If you like to exercise and socialize, try: aerobic dance, badminton, baseball/softball, basketball, bowling, downhill skiing, golf, racquetball/squash, tennis, touch football, volleyball, walking.

If you like to compete, try: just about any sport. You can even compete at walking/racewalking.

RESULTS

Data will aid class members in selecting an activity that is right for them.

CHAPTER THREE

GETTING STARTED

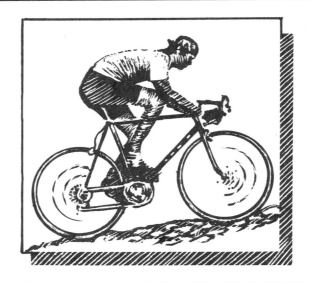

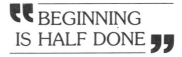 BEGINNING
IS HALF DONE

? HAVE YOU EVER WONDERED ABOUT:

Fitness concepts?

How to begin an exercise program?

How to progress safely and efficiently?

The value of a medical exam?

How to determine your present aerobic fitness level?

How to find your target heart rate?

Warm-up and cool-down?

How fast you will see results?

How much exercise is enough?

Exercise dangers?

KEY TERMS

Cool-down	1.5-mile test
Daily log	Preconditioning period
Frequency	Progressive overload
Intensity	Target heart-rate
Interval training	Time
Medical exam	Warm-up

Starting a fitness program is the hardest part. With that decision made, you need information on how to progress safely. After reading Chapters 1 and 2, you are hopefully motivated to begin your program. This chapter will focus on those fitness concepts you will need to start a program, as well as provide information on how to test and improve aerobic capacity.

A CAUTIOUS BEGINNING

You must begin cautiously. Depending upon your age and physical condition, it may be necessary to have a medical exam. While exercising, you will need to apply basic fitness concepts. The following information will help you get started as well as keep you going safely.

MEDICAL EXAM

A **medical exam** may or may not be necessary prior to beginning an exercise program. The standard medical examination performed in a doctor's office usually includes: blood pressure; ear, nose, and throat scan; hernia check; height and weight; and a stethoscope examination of heart and lungs. Of what value is such an examination? Is a physician likely to uncover any meaningful data on an asymptomatic individual? Does such an exam really provide meaningful diagnostic data? These and other questions are being raised about the time-honored practice of annual or semiannual physical exams. Even some physicians have indicated that the annual examination may be both unnecessary and expensive. The annual physical has, however, been just as vigorously defended by others in the medical field.

Opponents argue that the traditional approach to an annual physical is useless, expensive, and a wasteful way to spend valuable medical time. Some have even suggested that there is a strong monetary motivation for the practice. An individual who has no history of high blood pressure or any other symptoms will not, it is felt, discover much useful knowledge from the standard examination given in a doctor's office. There is also the chance of exposure in the waiting room to sick individuals seeking treatment.

Proponents feel there is value in routine examinations. They feel it makes people more health conscious, gives the doctor a chance to communicate with patients about health concerns, and may offer the opportunity to detect a health problem.

The major problem seems to lie with the examination rather than with its frequency. The main objective of an annual physical is to acquire important medical data on a regular basis. These data should include present health habits; an exercise EKG for those over 40; exercise evaluation including body fat, abdominal strength, aerobic capacity, and flexibility of back and hamstring muscles; blood pressure and pulse; blood work; rectal exam; skin inspection; ear, nose, and throat; lymph nodes; chest x-ray; pap smear and breast exam for women; and urinalysis.

For the college-age individual, such tests should be performed every two years. Guidelines for frequency are presented by Dintiman and Greenberg (1989):

Age	Frequency
6 to 15 years	Every 2 or 3 years
16 to 35 years	Every 2 years
35 to 59 years	Annually
60 years and up	Twice a year

If you want to enter a fitness program, you are faced with the decision of whether to secure a stress test. Many cardiologists recommend a stress electrocardiogram prior to aerobic activity for anyone over 40 and for those in a high-risk group. The fact that a resting EKG does not detect potential exercise abnormalities has long been recognized. The exercise EKG, although much more effective, is also not without its problems. Often, normal individuals and particularly those who have good to excellent cardiovascular fitness are diagnosed as having heart problems. These false positive readings are more common than the medical community is often willing to admit. The stress test in combination with an analysis of the patient's heart disease risk profile (family history of heart disease, blood pressure, body fat, smoking and exercise habits, presence of diabetes, blood serum cholesterol analysis, personality type), provide a much more accurate diagnosis.

FITNESS CONCEPTS

Participation in an exercise program or sport is no guarantee that you will improve. By applying a few basic concepts, however, you can make significant gains with little risk of injury or illness.

TO PREVENT INJURY, BEGIN GRADUALLY AND PROGRESS SLOWLY

It takes at least two to three months to get into even fair condition, particularly in the aerobic area. Attempting to progress any faster can cause problems. Too much too soon can produce muscle soreness, increase the chance for a soft-tissue injury, and cause you to quit long before results are noticeable.

Preconditioning The first three weeks should be considered a **preconditioning period** to prepare you for testing. By gradually conditioning your body, the testing is less likely to cause injury or significant soreness. Preconditioning activities should be as identical as possible to the actual test (do sit-ups to prepare for the muscular endurance test that uses sit-ups).

The preparation for the **1.5-mile test** could include a combination of running and walking interspaced with rest periods. Over the preconditioning period, the rest periods are gradually reduced while the time running is increased. The preconditioning goal should be the ability to run 1.5 miles without stopping (see Laboratory 3.2 for instructions on taking the test). This goal can be accomplished by practicing the interval schedule shown in Table 3.2, page 61.

Residual Soreness Although preconditioning will help reduce residual soreness, you can expect some delayed soreness following an exercise bout that involves unconditioned muscles. The time between the exercise and the highest soreness level is dependent upon your age. There is a direct relationship between exercise soreness and age: the older you are, the longer it will take to experience the muscle soreness. As a rule of thumb, the soreness is delayed about 24 hours for each 10 years above age 20. It is not unusual, for example, for a 50-year-old to experience the greatest discomfort 72 hours after physical activity.

No matter how gradually you pre-condition, there is likely to be some residual soreness following testing. Muscle soreness is not a common exercise problem, but the maximum testing effort may result in temporary discomfort.

APPLY THE PROGRESSIVE OVERLOAD PRINCIPLE TO PRODUCE THE BEST RESULTS

The **progressive overload** principle is simple to understand and has fascinating implications when correctly applied. If you gradually overload one of the body systems (muscular, circulatory, and so on), it will develop additional capacity. When you repeatedly perform more strenuous exercise each workout, the body repairs itself through elaborate cellular changes to prepare for more challenging future demands. Application of the progressive overload concept produces dramatic changes in the heart and circulatory system. Regular exercise stresses the heart, causing it to become larger and stronger and pump more blood each beat (improved stroke volume). A trained heart muscle can pump considerably more blood per beat, allowing it to slow down (beat fewer times per minute) and rest longer between beats. As the heart muscle adapts to the stress of exercise, the arteries that supply it enlarge and become more numerous.

The progressive overload concept also applies to the skeletal system. Gradual stress to the bones stimulates the laying down of calcium and other minerals. When bones are not stressed, such nutrients are not added to the bone structure. In the adult years, osteoporosis—loss of bone density due to lack of exercise—occurs. This process happens to astronauts freed from the stress of resisting gravity. It is also common in aging men and women. When you walk, jog, run, or perform other aerobic exercise, the force of your feet hitting the ground sends an important signal to your body to maintain bone density.

Everyone begins an exercise program at a different conditioning level. Your first exercise bout actually lowers this level at the workout's end. At this point, however, nature regenerates tissue and rebuilds the body to a point higher than it was before the initial workout began. It is similar to nature's reaction to your hands after you have shoveled the first winter snow. Calluses form within a short time to toughen the hands in preparation for more vigorous shoveling. On the second workout day you are equipped to perform more exercise than before, and in order to continue to apply the progressive resistance concept, you must do more each workout so that nature again rebuilds the body beyond the level of the previous workout.

There are only a few points to remember in applying the concept of progressive overload:

1. Exercise must be intense enough to injure tissue—nature's rebuilding process is somewhat in proportion to this intensity.
2. The second, third, and subsequent workouts must take place without too much recovery time between them (no more than 24 to 48 hours). Allowing more time than this will result in a lower conditioning level.
3. Enough recovery time—24 to 48 hours—must be allowed for rebuilding to take place.
4. Each workout should be progressively more strenuous than the previous one. (Note: an increase in strenuous activity means an increase in intensity, which is not necessarily an increase in distance or time per workout.)

EXERCISE A MINIMUM OF FOUR TIMES WEEKLY FOR 30 MINUTES OR MORE

Now that you know your heart rate will increase during exercise, you are ready to stress regularity and duration—two additional keys to weight loss and aerobic fitness. Daily or every-other-day exercise sessions are necessary to improve cardiovascular fitness, change the way your body handles fats, and decrease body fat.

If weight loss is your objective, it is important to keep in mind that walking three miles and running three miles burn up about the same number of calories. The longer you walk or run, the more calories you burn. It may be good advice to slow down your walking, pedaling, running, rope jumping, and so on and exercise longer. Providing your target heart rate (see Laboratory 3.1) is reached, you are not only burning a high number of calories but improving the cardiovascular system as well. Running or walking three miles on Monday and three miles on Tuesday also burns more calories than one six-mile run. This occurs because of the extra 60 to 150 calories burned from metabolic rate increases (calories burned while the body is at rest) during the two to four hours following each exercise session (this process is called afterburn). If you walk or run too far in one day and are unable to exercise the next day, you lose the benefit of these 60 to 150 calories. Late afternoon, when metabolic rates begin to slow considerably in most people, may be one of the best times to exercise. You then burn calories while exercising and activate a faster metabolic rate for two to four hours at a time in the day when metabolic rate normally slows down.

As previously mentioned, researchers have also found that target heart-rates should be maintained for 20 to 30 minutes for optimum results. In the early stages of your program, you will need to slowly work up to 30 minutes of continuous exercise in four to six weeks. The starter programs in Chapter 9 show you how to gradually increase the duration of the workout.

ALTERNATING LIGHT AND HEAVY WORKOUTS WILL REDUCE INJURIES

The body responds best to training programs that alternate light and heavy workouts. This approach reduces the risk of injury, provides several emotionally relaxing workouts each week, and allows the body time to repair fully between workouts.

In other words, it helps you receive maximum benefit from your fitness program. Consider these suggestions:

1. Do some stretching exercises at the beginning of your workout, but save most of your stretching for the end of the exercise session.
2. Alternate hard and easy days; never train extremely hard on consecutive days.
3. Train hard no more than three times weekly.
4. Schedule one extra-hard, all-out workout once weekly.
5. Know your body and allow it to direct you; if pain continues or worsens or if you get heavy-legged, stop, regardless of whether it is a light or heavy day.

A WARM-UP BEFORE EACH EXERCISE SESSION IS IMPORTANT

Warm-up is almost universally used in all activities to improve performance and prevent injury. The theory behind warm-up is the dependency of muscle contractions upon temperature. Since increased muscle temperature improves work capacity, and warm-up increases muscle temperature, it is assumed that it is a necessary practice. The amount of knee fluid is also increased with warm-up, oxygen intake is improved, and the amount of oxygen needed for exercise is reduced following warm-up. Nerve messages also travel faster at higher temperatures.

The following suggestions are drawn from the findings of well-controlled studies on warm-up:

1. Warm-up should be done for 10 to 15 minutes prior to activity.
2. Only a few minutes should elapse from completion of the warm-up until the start of activity.
3. More warm-up is needed in a cold environment to cause the body to reach the desired temperature prior to activity.
4. Warm-up will not bring about early fatigue and hinder performance. You probably have a slightly greater chance of injury without warm-up. Experiment with different types of warm-up exercises and determine the best method for you and your activity. It should also be pointed out that groups with a favorable attitude toward warm-up perform better with it, whereas groups with an unfavorable attitude do not.

Warm-up methods fall into four categories:

1. *Formal*—The skill or act that will be used in competition such as running before a 100-yard dash or shooting and jumping before a basketball game.
2. *Informal*—General warm-up involving calisthenics or other unrelated exercises.
3. *Passive*—Applying heat to various body parts.
4. *Overload*—Simulating the activity for which warm-up is being used by increasing the load or resistance, such as swinging two bats prior to hitting in baseball.

Each of the above methods has been shown by some researchers to be helpful. Each has also been shown by others to be of no value. Formal warm-up appears to be superior to informal procedures.

As important as the type of warm-up is its length. Muscle temperature rises in 5 minutes and continues to rise for 25 to 30 minutes. With inactivity, the effects drop rapidly until, after 45 minutes, additional warm-up is needed. It would seem advisable to use 10 to 15 minutes of warm-up that cause perspiration and are a progressive procedure leading to all-out effort. Warm-up should end about 5 or 10 minutes before the contest begins and be initiated again just prior to the contest. Find the magic combination for you and your activity— then stay with it.

A COOL-DOWN SHOULD FOLLOW EACH EXERCISE SESSION

The explanation for a **cool-down** period following a rigorous workout is quite simple: blood returns to the heart through a system of vessels called veins. The blood is pushed along by heart contractions and the veins' "milking" action. The veins contract or squeeze and move the blood forward against gravity while valves prevent the blood from backing up. If you stop exercising suddenly, the veins' milking action, which occurs only through muscle contraction, will stop; the blood return will drop quickly and may cause blood pooling in the legs (blood remains in the same area), leading to shock or deep breathing. The deep breathing then lowers carbon dioxide levels and muscle cramps develop. These cramps may last for 24 to 48 hours.

You should cool down following a long aerobic exercise session. A general cool-down routine might consist of walking or jogging a quarter mile to a mile at a pace of 2 to 3 minutes per quarter mile, each one slower than the previous one. The ideal cool-down routine should take place in the same environment as the workout, last at least 10 minutes, and be followed by stretching.

WHAT YOU WEAR CAN MAKE A DIFFERENCE

What you wear is dependent upon your program and the weather. The general rule is to have good shoes and to wear as little clothing as the weather permits.

Shoes To avoid injuries, quality shoes are essential for most aerobic activities. Cost often—but not always—indicates quality. The primary criteria are fit, comfort, and quality. Most aerobic activities require a specialized shoe, and although they often look identical, the various construction styles affect individuals differently. By purchasing your shoes from a specialty, not just sporting good store, you should be able to get advice regarding the best shoe for your aerobic goals. Since fit is so important, when selecting a new shoe be sure to wear the same style socks you use for exercising.

Clothes What you wear can make a substantial difference in your aerobic activity. For indoor activities and warm-weather, outdoor exercise, the general rule is to wear the least clothing possible. The cooling process requires air to pass over the skin and evaporate sweat; clothing must allow this process to take place. Some individuals mistakenly feel they will lose weight by wearing multiple layers

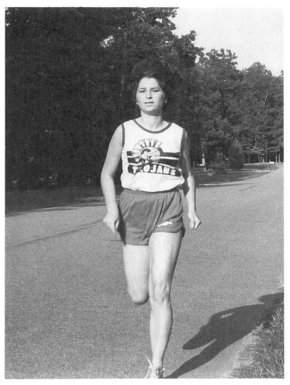

Figure 3.1   Proper dress in warm, humid weather helps keep the body cool.

of clothes to increase fluid loss. Since weight lost through sweating can lead to heat stroke or heat exhaustion, it is weight that must be maintained.

When exercising outside during the winter, extreme caution must be taken not to either overdress or underdress. Like summer clothing, winter attire must allow the skin to breathe. Windbreakers and other nylon garments are therefore not recommended. There are several expensive materials on the market specifically designed to allow for the necessary air exchange, but less costly materials such as wool can also be effective. Combining a T-shirt with a wool sweater, hat, and gloves (mittens are recommended) is usually sufficient for protection down to the freezing level. Under extremely cold conditions, however, frostbite is a real danger, particularly to exposed skin. The skin can be protected to a certain degree with creams and jellies, but even protected areas can be affected. Males, for example, must protect the penis and testicles from frostbite; nylon shorts just do not provide the needed protection, and frostbite can occur without warning.

HOT, HUMID WEATHER CAN BE DANGEROUS

As indicated above, the skin must breathe during exercise. As the body's core temperature rises with exercise, sweat is produced which is then evaporated by air passing over the skin. This evaporation cools the blood, which is then transported to the body core to cool the internal organs. During hot, humid conditions, the sweat cannot evaporate and cooling cannot take place. The core temperature will rise and additional fluid will be lost through sweating. Without any cooling, considerable fluid can be quickly lost, and heat stroke or death is possible.

EXERCISING OUTSIDE CAN BE DANGEROUS

Besides the weather, there are other problems associated with exercising outside.

Pollution Lack of clean air is a national tragedy that is being dealt with slowly, and it will be some time, if ever, before we will be able to exercise in a pollution-free environment. The benefits of exercise tend to overshadow the dangers, but exercising during smog alerts common to some areas should be avoided.

Vehicles Motor vehicles and even bicycles can present life-threatening situations, to runners as well as to others who choose to exercise outside. Rules of the road are as follows:

1. Give cars the right-of-way no matter what you or the law says.
2. Run or walk toward traffic.
3. Use reflective gear at night.
4. Expect the unexpected and watch out for objects thrown from vehicles.
5. Avoid antagonizing drivers with the famous one-finger salute—better to ignore and live.

Dogs Most dogs have considerable bark and little bite, but the exceptions can be most detrimental to unprotected runners and walkers. Dogs are generally territorial, so avoiding property lines is a must. For the occasional dog that comes after you, the best action is to stop and face the dog and then slowly back away, trying not to antagonize it.

The Human Animal The two-legged animal is far more dangerous than the four-legged variety. Female exercisers in particular must be alert to dangerous situations. Recommendations for avoiding attacks include exercising with others, not exercising outside at night, ignoring taunts, and being alert.

A SOFT SURFACE IS USUALLY BEST

The surface upon which you exercise can help to reduce injuries. Generally speaking, the harder the surface the greater the injury potential. Exercise does carry an injury risk (see Chapter 8), but you can usually reduce this risk by exercising on a soft surface. A surface that is too soft, however, actually increases risk of injuries. A soft, uneven surface such as a beach can cause ankle and knee injuries. Dirt and gravel paths and paths covered with wood chips seem to be best for walking and running, but the isolated nature of most trails increases the chances of assault. Public park vitae courses usually provide a relatively safe, soft place to exercise. Exercising on concrete floors or sidewalks should be avoided whenever possible, except for city running, where it is safer to run on the sidewalks than on the slightly softer road. Golf courses are great places to run in the winter, but most runners are not welcome during the season.

MONITORING YOUR PROGRESS CAN REDUCE INJURIES AND INCREASE MOTIVATION

Records can be a source of motivation and can aid in injury prevention. Keeping records of resting heart rate, the number of miles run, laps swum, weight lifted, and number of workouts completed can provide the needed incentive to continue an exercise program.

By keeping records you can also vary the intensity of daily workouts to avoid injuries. If an injury from overuse should occur, a perusal of your records could aid in determining its cause and help you in setting a course toward recovery. Unfortunately, records can lead to compulsive behavior known as negative addiction. To the addicted, records are made to be broken; more is better; and the record rather than the fitness benefits becomes the goal. Such individuals experience frequent injury intermixed with emotional stress in attempting to maintain or break records.

Daily Log A **daily log** can help you apply the concept of alternating light and heavy days as well as monitor your progress. The log information should include the number of minutes spent in aerobic activity or the distance covered. This information can be used to control the stress level during the initial training sessions. A log can also contain weather conditions; water temperature if swimming; how you felt; any particular problem that might indicate the possibility of future injury;

the number and type of activities completed; and, for weight training, the weight and number of repetitions for each exercise. Table 3.1 is an example of a daily log for running.

TESTING YOUR PRESENT FITNESS LEVEL

Observing the precautions mentioned earlier, and keeping the fitness concepts in mind, you need to test your present fitness level. Your goals will determine those areas you wish to evaluate, but a comprehensive program will include your aerobic fitness (this chapter), muscular strength and endurance (Chapter 4), flexibility (Chapter 5), and body composition (Chapter 7). Laboratory 3.2 details the procedures for testing your aerobic capacity.

TABLE 3.1   DAILY LOG FOR RUNNING

Date _____   Time of Day _____
Distance Covered _____   Total Exercise Time _____
Weather Conditions _____
Terrain (flat, hills, etc.) _____
Intensity (heart rate):   Heavy Day _____ Light Day _____
Positive Impressions of Workout:

Unusual Feelings or Problems During Workout:

Overall Rating on a Scale from 1–10 _____
(10 = Excellent and 1 = Horrible)

DEVELOPING AEROBIC FITNESS

The acronym FIT will help you remember the three criteria for developing aerobic fitness: frequency, intensity, and time. You will also want to know something about interval training to help you during the early stages of your program.

FREQUENCY

Frequency is how many times a week you exercise. The recommendation is at least every other day, but many find that a three-times-a-week schedule fits them best. It is not harmful to exercise daily, as long as you remember the light/heavy concept discussed earlier.

INTENSITY

The aerobic exercise you choose must involve at least 50 percent of the body's large muscles, and its **intensity** must raise the heart rate to the "target" level. The **target heart rate** is the desired beats per minute sustained throughout a workout. The procedure for calculating your target heart rate is presented in Laboratory 3.1. To improve your aerobic capacity, a heart rate between 60 and 75 percent of your prediction maximum is necessary. Although the 60-percent-intensity heart rate level is sufficient to improve the cardiovascular system, better results are achieved by moving to a 70 to 75-percent level as you gradually improve your aerobic capacity. These higher percentages make more efficient use of your exercise time. Levels beyond 75 percent are for those who desire aerobic capacity beyond the health fitness level (see Chapter 11).

One nice thing about aerobic exercise is the ease with which you can monitor the workload. Since there is a direct relationship between heart rate and the amount of work you are doing, all you need is a watch with a second hand, or a digital watch. By periodically taking your pulse, you will know how hard you are working. With practice, you will be able to estimate your heart rate without having to take it. The heart rate should

be taken about every five minutes during the early phase of your program. As you learn to monitor your body through feel, you will be able to maintain the proper exercise intensity without the need to constantly check your pulse.

The purpose of high-intensity workouts is to condition the cardiovascular system by making the heart beat faster for short time periods. With conditioning, the heart becomes a more efficient pump and requires fewer beats to get the job done. By conditioning the heart for two to three hours a week, the resting heart rate can be reduced 10 to 20 or more beats per minute, thus saving thousands of beats per week.

Several activities meet the aerobic development criteria, including running, lap swimming, stationary cycling, aerobic dance, aerobic calisthenics, and even walking. Each of these activities is discussed later.

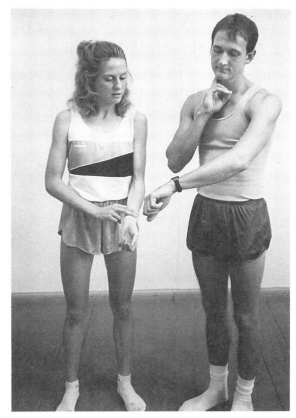

Figure 3.2   Both the radial and carotid pulse can be used to monitor heart rate.

TIME

The exercise heart rate must be maintained for at least 20 minutes. With a 5-minute warm-up to gradually raise the heart rate, 20 minutes at the target level, and a 10-minute cool-down, the total exercise **time** would be around 35 minutes. Figure 3.3 is a presentation of the minimum workout time and intensity necessary to improve cardiovascular efficiency.

High-intensity workouts lasting more than about 40 minutes do not seem to produce any additional health benefits and often lead to overuse injuries. There is even evidence that those who go well beyond the 40-minute fitness level may actually be adversely effecting their health. Many would argue the benefits of longer workouts, but the important point to consider is that more is not always better.

INTERVAL TRAINING

Interval training is a technique that can be used at all fitness levels and is highly recommended during the initial stages of conditioning. Interval training helps you develop the endurance required to last the entire 20 minutes at your target heart rate. Although the training principles can be applied to all aerobic activities, a running example will be used for illustration (see Table 3.2 for a

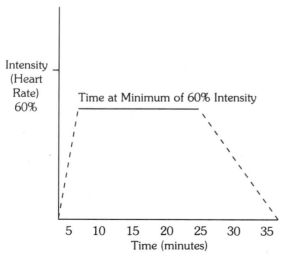

Figure 3.3   A minimum cardiovascular workout includes 20 minutes of activity at 60% intensity.

sample schedule). The four interval training factors are:

1. Heart rate (determined by running speed)
2. Total training time
3. Repetitions (number of times you run per exercise period)
4. Rest intervals (walking)

These factors are varied as fitness increases. Assuming you can run continuously for one minute before resting, you should begin with a warm-up of slow running, followed by a 1-minute run at your target heart rate, followed by walking until the heart rate is below 120 beats per minute. You should try to increase the number of repetitions as you gradually increase total workout time to about 40 minutes, including warm-up and cool-down. The time between rest periods should be increased until no rest is required during the entire workout. This can usually be achieved in about six to eight weeks. An every-other-day or four-times-a-week schedule is highly recommended during the initial three months of training. See Chapter 9 for individual programs.

AEROBIC DEVELOPMENT ACTIVITIES

Several activities meet the aerobic development criteria of frequency, intensity, and time (FIT). The more popular ones are discussed below.

WALKING

The most popular exercise among Americans is walking, which, if done properly, can improve aerobic capacity. For those who have not been exercising, brisk walking may raise the heart rate to the conditioning level. As fitness level improves, however, most people will find it necessary to increase the workload in order to reach an exercise heart rate.

Weights and Walking   A way to increase the workload is to use weights. These weights are normally carried in the hands, but can be attached

TABLE 3.2 SAMPLE INTERVAL WORKOUTS FOR DEVELOPING ENDURANCE

Week 1

Monday: Walk 1 minute, run 1 minute; walk 1 minute, run 2 minutes; walk 1 minute, run 1 minute; walk until recovered.

Tuesday: Rest.

Wednesday: Walk 1 minute, run 1 minute; walk 1 minute, run 2 minutes; walk 1 minute, run 2 minutes; walk until recovered.

Thursday: Rest.

Friday: Walk 1 minute, run 2 minutes; walk 1 minute, run 2 minutes; walk 1 minute, run 2 minutes; walk until recovered.

Week 2

Monday: Walk 1 minute, run 2 minutes; walk 1 minute, run 3 minutes; walk 1 minute, run 3 minutes; walk until recovered.

Tuesday: Rest.

Wednesday: Walk 1 minute, run 3 minutes; walk 1 minute, run 3 minutes; walk 1 minute, run 3 minutes; walk until recovered.

Thursday: Rest.

Friday: Walk 1 minute, run 3 minutes; walk 1 minute, run 4 minutes; walk 1 minute, run 4 minutes; walk until recovered.

Week 3

Monday: Walk 1 minute, run 4 minutes; walk 1 minute, run 4 minutes; walk 1 minute, run 5 minutes; walk until recovered.

Tuesday: Rest.

Wednesday: Walk 1 minute, run 4 minutes; walk 1 minute, run 5 minutes; walk 1 minute, run 6 minutes; walk until recovered.

Thursday: Rest.

Friday: Walk 1 minute, run 4 minutes; walk 1 minute, run 6 minutes; walk 1 minute, run 7 minutes; walk until recovered.

Week 4

Monday: Walk 1 minute, run 6 minutes; walk 1 minute, run 7 minutes; walk 1 minute, run 8 minutes; walk until recovered.

Tuesday: Rest.

Week 4 (Cont.)

Wednesday: Walk 1 minute, run 6 minutes; walk 1 minute, run 7 minutes; walk 1 minute, run 9 minutes; walk until recovered.

Thursday: Rest.

Friday: Walk 1 minute, run 6 minutes; walk 1 minute, run 8 minutes; walk 1 minute, run 10 minutes; walk until recovered.

Week 5

Monday: Take the 1.5 mile test.

This schedule is designed for a beginning runner. The interval principle, however, can be applied to any endurance activity.

All walking should be done briskly except during the cool-down period following the workout. Initial running should be as slow as necessary to complete the entire workout. The intensity should be gradually increased until the target heart rate is reached.

to the wrists. Merely carrying the weights is not enough; they must be lifted; and the workload will be increased by how far they are lifted. The minimum workload should include bending alternate arms to about 90 degrees with each step. A higher intensity is achieved by raising one weight at a time to the shoulder level.

Walking Speed The faster you walk, the greater the workload. By monitoring the heart rate, you can adjust your pace to achieve the appropriate intensity.

JOGGING/RUNNING

Ever since jogging became a popular word indicative of the boom in exercise, there has been confusion as to how jogging and running differ. Jogging seems to be reserved for exercise designed to improve your health, while running is associated with road and track racing. *Running,* according to *The American Heritage Dictionary,* is "to move rapidly, to move on foot at a pace faster than a walk and in such a manner that both feet leave the ground during each stride." *Jogging* is "to run . . . at a steady slow trot." Rather than confuse the issue, the focus here will be on exercising, either by jogging or running, to raise the heart rate to the target level. For purposes of discussion, we will use the word *running* synonymously with *jogging.* Running as a form of exercise is not new, just more popular. This popularity is based on low cost, safety, minimum hassle (no special equipment or partner is required), and high fitness value (physical and mental).

Warm-up Most runners begin with stretching exercises, although these may not be as necessary as some people believe. There is mounting concern that some running injuries are caused by overstretching and that existing problems can be aggravated by unnecessary stretching. For good advice on stretching carefully and properly, follow the guidelines established in Chapter 5. There seems to be general agreement regarding the need to begin running at a speed slower than you desire to achieve four to five minutes into the run.

On the Run To achieve fitness, the intensity and duration must meet the fitness guidelines of

heart rate and time established earlier. Remember to keep the heart rate at or slightly above your target level. With experience, keeping the heart rate in the target zone is not difficult to do; until sufficient endurance is developed, however, it can be a problem.

The interval training principles discussed previously can be applied to the early stages of a running program. A combination of running, brisk walking, and then running again is recommended. More detailed model programs for running are given in Chapter 9.

Cool-down The cool-down begins during the last four to five minutes of the run through a gradual slowing to a walk, followed by stretching.

Problems Joint injuries are a major problem for nearly all runners. The constant pounding from hard surface running, particularly at a slow rate, normally has an adverse effect on the ankle, knee, and hip joints as well as on the lower back. The slower you run, the more vertical force is applied to joints. Faster runners tend to dissipate the downward force through linear (forward) motion. The swift runner glides along the ground while the jogger seems to heavily plod along. Running on softer surfaces helps all runners, although very spongy terrain can also cause joint and muscle problems in the ankle and knee areas. Although there are no guarantees, warm-up, cool-down, proper shoes, running surface, and common sense all help to alleviate running problems.

SWIMMING

Swimming is one of the best overall exercise programs. The combination of cardiovascular development, muscular strength and endurance, and freedom from injury make it superior in many ways to other forms of exercise.

Equipment/Facilities Unless you live in a place where you can swim in the ocean or in an outside pool year-round, or belong to a club or community center, swimming as a form of exercise may be impractical.

Warm-up Although many people stretch prior to swimming, it is probably not necessary unless you desire to begin with a racing dive. As with running, you should begin slowly and gradually increase speed.

In the Swim
Initially, you may find any stroke difficult to sustain, but you should try using either a front or back crawl stroke. Other strokes such as the side, breast, and elementary back can be used as resting strokes so movement can be continuous. These easier strokes, however, are not usually sufficient to raise the heart rate to the target level. Particular attention must be paid to heart rate since swimming does not provide the same environmental factors as running. The major difference other than water environment is gravity. With the body in a horizontal position, the heart does not have to work against gravity. This means you will have to work harder to reach your target heart rate.

Interval training can be applied by alternating difficult strokes with easier ones. To be safe, it is best to rest in the shallow end of the pool.

Cool-down
As with other forms of exercise, a cool-down is necessary. With swimming, it could be a very slow side or back stroke, walking on the pool deck, or stretching.

ROPE JUMPING

Jumping rope is an inexpensive way to develop cardiovascular fitness and is frequently used in combination with other exercises in an overall fitness program. It is not, however, as effective as running. At one time it was believed that 10 minutes of rope jumping was as effective as 20 minutes of jogging. Researchers have now given the fitness edge to running.

Equipment
With an inexpensive rope and clothing allowing free movement, you are ready to begin.

Warm-up
Because stress is placed on the Achilles tendon during rope jumping, stretching prior to a workout is required (see Chapter 5). Rope jumping tends to cause more tightness in the leg area than most exercise programs. Warm-up can also include slow running in place and slow rope jumping.

Turning On
Although there is some opportunity for variety, the primary purpose of rope jumping is to elevate and maintain heart rate at the target level to develop cardiovascular fitness. Variety comes with the type of jump used or through the manipulation of the rope. You can do a regular two-foot jump, run in place, hop on one foot, move around the room, turn in a circle, turn the rope backward, and cross the rope in front or back.

Cool-down
Cooling down should consist of walking and stretching. Since the legs have done the work, continued muscle action is needed to assist in recovery. Slow static stretching of the lower leg muscles is essential.

Problems
It is difficult for most people to maintain a one-dimensional exercise program. Most people use rope jumping in a fitness program that includes weight training, calisthenics, and running or cycling.

Some people have also experienced stress to the orthopedic system from rope jumping. Because of the vertical force that is applied, injuries to the ankles, knees, and back may occur. Correct jumping technique helps reduce the risk. The correct method is to stay up on the toes and absorb shock by a slight lowering of the heels and through knee flexion on impact.

CYCLING

Cycling is a popular form of exercise. It can be done on the road or on a stationary bike, with the latter being usually most effective for developing cardiovascular (CV) fitness. A good stationary exercise bike allows you to carefully control the intensity of the workout; there is little stress on the orthopedic system; and no expense for special clothes. It is particularly good for those who are rehabilitating injured areas such as the back, feet, or arms.

Equipment
A regular road bike is expensive and requires special protective gear. Unlike exercising with the stationary bike, the passing scenery is generally more interesting. To get wherever you are going, however, requires clothes such as those used in running in addition to protective head gear. Unfortunately, cycling along the road

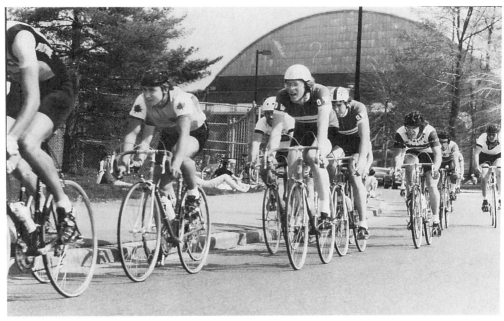

Figure 3.4   Cycling is an excellent exercise choice.

is seldom sufficient to develop cardiovascular fitness unless target heart rates are reached and maintained. For those willing to work at it, it can improve aerobic conditioning.

Warm-up   The warm-up can include stretching followed by a gradual buildup of riding speed. If you use the stationary bike, the workload can be carefully controlled. If you are on a regular bike, you should avoid hills during warm-up and try to ride with the wind.

On the Bike   The object is to get the heart rate up and keep it up continuously; this is easy to do with the stationary bike but a problem on the road. When riding a regular bike, the heart rate tends to rise and fall according to the terrain. With the body weight supported by the bike, the heart rate is determined primarily by a combination of speed and hills. Most people tend to relax downhill and the heart rate falls. The multispeed bike can be used to reduce the load, which also affects heart rate. You must keep up the intensity both uphill and downhill to maintain your target heart rate.

On the stationary bike, gradually increasing the workload will elevate the heart rate to the target

level. The rate will remain at the target level until fatigue begins to set in. As fatigue increases, the level can be gradually reduced to keep the heart rate at the appropriate level.

Cool-down   Walking, stretching, and gradually reduced speeds for 5 to 10 minutes provide an excellent, relaxing cool-down.

Problems   The major problems with road biking are traffic, and the difficulty in maintaining target heart rate. Conversely, the stationary bike is safe but often boring.

AEROBICS

Aerobic dance and aerobic exercise are two forms of exercise designed to develop aerobic fitness. Aerobic dance is a series of choreographed dance routines done to music. The routines are designed to produce 20 to 30 minutes of exercise in the target heart range. Aerobic exercise is nothing more than vigorous activities, usually in the form of calisthenics, that are designed to elevate heart rate. Low impact aerobics are growing in popularity. By eliminating hopping and jumping actions which lift the body off the ground, stress is reduced, thereby lowering the risk of injury.

Warm-up   Warm-up consists of stretching and gradually increasing the exercise intensity.

Workout   The workout is a series of continuous dance routines or exercises suffcient to reach and maintain the target heart rate.

Cool-down   The cool-down is done by gradually decreasing the intensity of activity, followed by walking and stretching.

FREQUENTLY ASKED QUESTIONS

Why do people die during road races?

Mainly because more people are participating, many who probably should not be. As numbers increase, the statistical probability of death also increases. Most deaths, however, have been related to heat and would be preventable if runners and race directors were more careful. Race directors must be willing to start races earlier and to provide more water. Racers must know their abilities and be willing to stop at the first sign of heat stroke.

Some doctors say running is not good for you. Why?

Running is not for everyone. The medical concern is for joint problems and for those who overdo it. Good shoes and sensible approaches to training make running a good form of exercise for most, but not all, individuals.

Why is weight training not highly recommended as an aerobic activity?

It is difficult to develop the cardiovascular system through weight training. Seldom are you able to maintain a sufficient heart rate to bring about a conditioning effect. Changing weights on the bar or crowded conditions in a weight room usually slow the routine.

What is the proper way to breathe during vigorous exercise?

Through the mouth. Since there is less resistance to overcome, mouth breathing allows air to enter and exit much faster. During exercise, nose breathing cannot keep up with oxygen demand.

What is the side pain I get while exercising?

This is probably the common "side stitch," which occurs most frequently among unconditioned individuals. The exact cause is unknown, but it is theorized that the pain is caused by insufficient oxygen to the diaphragm. Most people get relief by lowering the workload and breathing from the abdomen rather than with the chest muscles allowing the diaphragm to drop down and the lungs to fill. It is not usually necessary to stop exercising. As your conditioning level improves, side stitches seldom occur.

What is a heat stroke?

A heat stroke occurs when the body's heat regulating mechanism ceases to function properly and the core temperature reaches 104–106 degrees. When 10 percent or more of the body's fluid weight is lost in a matter of hours, the heat regulator is in danger of failing. Weight losses exceeding 10 percent are not uncommon during hot, humid conditions. You should never try to accelerate sweating by wearing rubber suits or excess clothing during the winter or summer. Clothing must allow for air exchange between the skin and outside air. While exercising, you should wear the least amount of clothing possible, and whether you feel the need or not, drink plenty of water.

What are the signs of a heat stroke?

Anyone exercising under hot, humid conditions should be aware of the signs of heat stroke. The victim's skin will be hot, red, and dry; the heart rate will be rapid but weak; slurred speech and inability to do simple calculations are common. Unconsciousness indicates an advanced stage of the problem.

What is first aid for heat stroke?

Rapidly cooling the body is paramount. Get the person out of the conditions that caused the stroke and get the core temperature down by having the person drink ice cold water. If unconscious, pack the victim in ice. Be careful not to lower the temperature too much since hypothermia could result. *Get immediate medical assistance.*

How can I avoid muscle cramps?

Cramps seem to be caused by a low potassium level and/or low fluid level. To avoid cramps, increase your fruit intake, particularly bananas, and be sure to drink plenty of fluid before, during, and after exercising.

Are ankle weights and weighted vests of any value?

Adding weight to the body will increase the workload, but it can also increase injuries. Any additional weight can add stress to ankles, knees, and hip joints, and will usually alter your walking and running stride, which almost always leads to joint problems.

MYTHS AND FALLACIES

Aerobic development can be achieved in half the time by doubling the workout intensity.

Short, high-intensity workouts will not achieve aerobic conditioning and may lead to excessive fatigue and injury. There is no evidence to suggest that there are any shortcuts to aerobic development.

More of a good thing results in added health.

Health levels for life can be achieved by following the concepts described in this text. Going beyond the FIT limits increases the risk of injury. Those that exercise beyond the health fitness level are usually seeking conditioning for athletic competition rather than health (see Chapter 11).

Ice water will cause stomach cramps.

There is no evidence that cold water causes stomach cramps. In fact, ice water is recommended as the best replenishment fluid during hot, humid periods because it exits the stomach more rapidly than warm water. To be effective as a replenishment fluid, a substance must quickly leave the stomach, where no absorption takes place, and enter the intestines, where it is absorbed and transported to the cells.

You should not drink water while exercising.

Not drinking fluids during exercise can lead to cramps and heat stroke. Some coaches still believe athletes can build up a tolerance for low fluid levels by not drinking during practice, and each year several young athletes lose their lives to this insanity. Whether you feel thirsty or not, you should force yourself to drink cold water when exercising under hot, humid conditions.

During exercise, sugar drinks are good for replenishing fluids

Any fluid containing even a trace of sugar is not a good replenishment fluid during exercise. When a sugar drink enters the stomach it triggers the digestive process and delays movement of the fluid into the intestines, where absorption can take place. Cold water is the best replenishment fluid during exercise.

Salt tablets should be taken during hot, humid conditions.

Under no circumstances should salt tablets be taken before or during exercise. Such high salt concentrations rob the cells of fluid and increase the chances of cramps and a heat stroke. Even though salt is lost through sweat, the body retains plenty of the substance. Cramps and heat stroke are caused by low fluid levels, not by a salt shortage.

BIBLIOGRAPHY

Cooper, K. *The Aerobics Program for Total Well-Being.* New York: M. Evans and Co., 1982.

Denis, C., et al. "Endurance Training, V02 Max and OBLA: A Longitudinal Study of Two Different Age Groups." *International Journal of Sports Medicine* 5 (1984): 167–73.

Dintiman, G., and J. Greenberg. *Health Through Discovery.* 4th ed. Reading, Mass.: Addison-Wesley, 1989.

Dintiman, G., and Robert Ward. *Train America! Achieving Peak Performance and Fitness for Sports Competition.* Dubuque, Iowa: Kendal-Hunt 1988.

Francesconi, R. "Endocrinological Responses to Exercise in Stressful Environments." In *Exercise and Sport Sciences Reviews.* Vol. 16, American College of Sports Medicine Series, K. Pandolf. editor, New York: MacMillan, 1988.

Greer, N., and F. Katch. "Validity of Palpation Recovery Pulse Rate to Estimate Heart Rate Following Four Intensities of Bench Step Exercise." *Research Quarterly* 53:4 (1982): 340–43.

Hickson, R., et al. "Time Course of the Adaptive Responses of Aerobic Power and Heart Rate to Training." *Medicine and Science in Sports and Exercise* 13:1 (1981): 17–20.

Kenney, W. and C. Armstrong. "The effect of Aerobic Conditioning on Venous Pooling in the Foot." *Medicine and Science in Sports and Exercise* 19:5 (1987): 474–9.

Markoff, R., et al. "Endorphins and Mood Changes in Long-Distance Running." *Medicine and Science in Sports and Exercise* 14:1 (1982): 11–15.

Morris, W., ed. *The American Heritage Dictionary of the English Language.* Boston: Houghton Mifflin Co., 1971.

O'Shea, M. "Guide to Better Fitness." *Parade Magazine* (5 June 1988):15.

Quirk, J., and W. Sinning. "Anaerobic and Aerobic Responses of Males and Females to Rope Skipping." *Medicine and Science in Sports and Exercise* 14:1 (1982): 26–29.

Rahkila, P., et al. "Response of Plasma Endorphins to Running Exercises in Male and Female Endurance Athletes." *Medicine and Science in Sports and Exercise* 19:5 (1987): 451–5.

Ricci, G., et al., "Left Ventricular Size Following Endurance, Sprint and Strength Training." *Medicine and Science in Sports and Exercise* 14:5 (1982): 344–7.

Riddle, P., "Attitudes, Beliefs, Behavioral Intentions, and Behaviors of Women and Men toward Regular Jogging." *Research Quarterly* 51:4 (1980): 663–74.

Rubal, B., et al. "Effects of Physical Conditioning on the Heart Size and Wall Thickness of College Women." *Medicine and Science in Sports and Exercise* 19:5 (1987): 423–9.

Vaccaro, P., and M. Clinton. "The Effects of Aerobic Dance Conditioning on the Body Composition and Maximal Oxygen Uptake of College Women." *Journal of Sports Medicine* 21 (1981): 291–4.

Washburn, R., and R. LaPorte. "Assessment of Walking Behavior: Effect of Speed and Monitor Position on Two Objective Physical Activity Monitors." *Research Quarterly* 59:1 (1988): 83–85.

Wilmore, J., et al. "Physiological Alterations Consequent to 20-Week Conditioning Programs of Bicycling, Tennis, and Jogging." *Medicine and Science in Sports and Exercise* 12:1 (1980): 1–8.

LABORATORY 3.1

Maximum and Exercise Heart Rates

PURPOSE: To determine your maximum and exercise heart rates.

SIZE OF GROUP: Alone

PROCEDURE

1. To find your predicted maximum heart rate, subtract your age from 220:
   220
   −Age
   _____

   (Maximum heart rate)

2. To determine your target heart rate for exercise, calculate the percentage difference between resting heart rate and maximum heart rate, and add base resting rate to obtain desired exercise rate.
   a. Use the resting heart rate you determined in Laboratory 1.1
   b. Subtract your resting heart rate from your maximum heart rate.
   c. Multiply the figure from *b* by 60%.
   d. Add your resting heart rate from *a* to the figure from *c*.
   e. The resulting number is your 60% exercise heart rate.

3. To determine your exercise heart rate for any other percentage, substitute the desired percentage in *c* while following all the other steps.

4. An *example* for the 60% level for a *20-year-old* with a resting heart rate of 75 follows:

Sept 1	220	**Step 2**	200	**Step 3**	125	**Step 4**	75
	− 20		− 75		× .60		+ 75
	= 200		125		75		150

   The maximum heart rate = 200 and the exercise rate = 150.

LABORATORY 3.2

Testing Aerobic Capacity

PURPOSE: To determine your present aerobic capacity.

SIZE OF GROUP: Can be done individually or in groups

EQUIPMENT: Measured course and a stopwatch

PROCEDURE

You can easily determine your aerobic fitness level by completing this lab and comparing your score with others of your age and sex. If you have been aerobically inactive for more than six months, however, it is advisable to avoid this test until you have gone through a preconditioning period of at least three weeks. For planning purposes, you could forget the test for now and merely assume that you fall in the "very poor" category.

This lab can be completed periodically throughout your fitness program to determine your progress.

1. Before doing any testing, be sure to read this entire chapter, paying particular attention to the precautions regarding testing.

2. Go to a 400-meter or quarter-mile track. If no track is available, measure 1.5 miles on the road or other flat area such as a golf course.

3. Warm up with 3 to 5 minutes of stretching and 5 to 8 minutes of light jogging.

4. Using a stopwatch, time yourself over the course (6 laps around the quarter-mile or the 400-meter track; you must, however, go 13.5 yards beyond the 6 laps on the metered track to make the 1.5 miles). Depending upon your conditioning level, you may have to walk part of the distance.

5. Stop exercising immediately if you experience pain or pressure in the left or midchest area, pain in the shoulder or arm, extreme breathlessness, or dizziness.

Continued on next page

Testing Aerobic Capacity

RESULTS

Check your performance using Table 3.3.

TABLE 3.3   AEROBIC FITNESS GUIDELINES FOR THE 1.5 MILE TEST (TIMES IN MINUTES)

Fitness Category		Age (years)					
		13–19	20–29	30–39	40–49	50–59	60+
I. Very poor	(men)	>15:31*	>16:01	>16:31	>17:31	>19:01	>20:01
	(women)	>18:31	>19:01	>19:31	>20:01	>20:31	>21:01
II. Poor	(men)	12:11–15:30	14:01–16:00	14:44–16:30	15:36–17:30	17:01–19:00	19:01–20:00
	(women)	16:55–18:30	18:31–19:00	19:01–19:30	19:31–20:00	20:01–20:30	21:00–21:31
III. Fair	(men)	10:49–12:10	12:01–14:00	12:31–14:45	13:01–15:35	14:31–17:00	16:16–19:00
	(women)	14:31–16:54	15:55–18:30	16:31–19:00	17:31–19:30	19:01–20:00	19:31–20:30
IV. Good	(men)	9:41–10:48	10:46–12:00	11:01–12:30	11:31–13:00	12:31–14:30	14:00–16:15
	(women)	12:30–14:30	13:31–15:54	14:31–16:30	15:56–17:30	16:31–19:00	17:31–19:30
V. Excellent	(men)	8:37– 9:40	9:45–10:45	10:00–11:00	10:30–11:30	11:00–12:30	11:15–13:59
	(women)	11:50–12:29	12:30–13:30	13:00–14:30	13:45–15:55	14:30–16:30	16:30–17:30
VI. Superior	(men)	< 8:37	< 9:45	<10:00	<10:30	<11:00	<11:15
	(women)	<11:50	<12:30	<13:00	<13:45	<14:30	<16:30

*< Means "less than"; > means "more than."

Reprinted with permission of Bantam Books FROM *The Aerobics Program for Total Well-Being* by Dr. Kenneth H. Cooper. (New York: Bantam 1982).

CHAPTER FOUR

MUSCULAR STRENGTH and ENDURANCE TRAINING

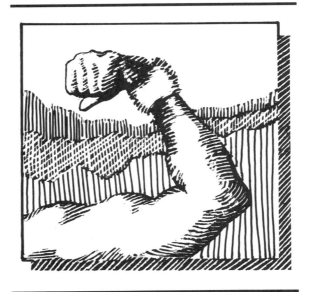

"LOOKING GOOD "

? HAVE YOU EVER WONDERED ABOUT:

The difference between muscular strength and muscular endurance?

How muscles get stronger?

The value of weight training for women?

Whether young children should train with weights?

How to place weight training exercises in the proper sequence?

How to breathe properly when you are training with weights?

How to keep your body looking good?

KEY TERMS

Cocooning

Isokinetics

Isometrics

Isotonics

Negative phase

Positive phase

Repetition maximum (RM)

Resistance

Rest interval

Sets

Muscular strength and endurance are closely related. However, it is important to differentiate between the two. Strength is merely the amount of force (weight) a muscle or group of muscles can exert for one repetition. It is generally measured by a single maximal contraction such as in using heavy weights in pressing a barbell overhead. Endurance is the capacity of the same muscle or group of muscles to sustain a series of repetitive contractions such as in pressing a barbell overhead, with light weights, and as often as possible in a series of uninterrupted contractions. Depending upon your preference and how you manipulate the variables discussed in this chapter, weight training can be strength-oriented, endurance-oriented, or both.

This chapter will address the various factors involved in training for the development of muscular strength and muscular endurance. Basic training principles and variables will be presented in addition to assessment testing, specific exercises, training suggestions, equipment, and other related concerns.

TRAINING PRINCIPLES

Before starting your strength program, certain factors need to be understood in order to maximize benefits and minimize risks. To avoid possible injury to muscles and joints, a 10 to 15 minute warm-up period of stretching and calisthenic movements is suggested (see Chapter 5). The use of light to moderate barbell weights for the first set of each exercise will also help reduce the risk of injury from muscle strain.

PROPER BREATHING

Breath should not be held during muscular contraction. The recommended breathing procedure is to inhale as the weight is lowered and to exhale as the weight is raised or pushed away from the body. You should attempt to blow the weight away from the body. This procedure will improve your efficiency and reduce the risk of blacking out during a demanding exertion. Until the correct technique is mastered, correct inhaling and exhaling should be practiced using light weights.

SEQUENCE OF EXERCISES

The large muscle groups should be exercised before the smaller muscles. It is difficult to exhaust large muscle groups when the smaller muscles that serve as connections between the resistance and the large muscle groups have been prematurely fatigued. It is also important for the abdominal muscles, used in most exercises to stabilize the rib cage, to remain relatively unfatigued until the latter phase of the workout. A typical sequence applying the concept of moving from large to small muscle groups is:

1. Hips and lower back
2. Legs: quadriceps, hamstrings, and calves
3. Torso: back, shoulders, chest
4. Arms: triceps, biceps, and forearms
5. Abdominals
6. Neck

POSITIVE AND NEGATIVE PERFORMANCE

There are two distinct phases of a weight training exercise. The weight is raised (**positive phase**) and, after a brief pause, it is lowered (**negative phase**). The muscle contracts and shortens during the positive phase and relaxes and lengthens during the negative phase. For each repetition, the same muscles are used for both the positive and negative phases of the exercise and each phase contributes to strength and endurance development. Weight should be raised and lowered slowly to maximize benefits. Arching the back, jerking the weight, or deviating from accepted technique in any manner to secure better leverage merely lessens the benefits and increases the possibility of injury.

Although momentary muscular fatigue is reached more quickly during the positive phase, muscles can continue in the negative phase with more weight than they can raise. If the negative phase is done correctly, the workout will be much more productive. Lowering the resistance is more important for strength development than raising the resistance. If you take two seconds to raise the weight, it should take four seconds or twice as long to lower the weight. A complete set of 10 repetitions using correct technique should consume no less than one minute.

FULL RANGE OF MOVEMENT

Each exercise should start from a fully extended, prestretched position and continue to a fully contracted position. It is important to carry each repetition to the full range of movement to exercise the entire range of the muscle and to improve joint flexibility.

HIGH INTENSITY MUSCLE RECRUITMENT

High intensity exercise involves continuous repetitions designed to momentarily exhaust a muscle group. This can be accomplished by performing 8 to 10 repetitions of each exercise. On the eighth or tenth repetition, you should be physically incapable of performing even the start of one more movement. Be aware that the selected weight needs to be adjusted accordingly.

COOL-DOWN

An aspect of weight training that is generally neglected is the cool-down phase. Proper cool-down alleviates muscle tightening and lessens the tendency for immediate or delayed soreness. Approximately 10 minutes should be allowed for cool-down (see Chapter 3 for related information on cool-down techniques).

TRAINING VARIABLES

In a sound weight training program, muscles are gradually placed under increased **resistance** (weight). The muscle group must be taxed above and beyond its normal limits. Muscular strength and endurance gains will not occur unless this overload principle is applied and certain training variables are manipulated correctly.

REPETITIONS

The number of consecutive times an exercise is performed through the complete range of motion without rest is called repetitions. A high number of repetitions (9 to 20) with lighter weights tends to produce greater endurance changes; whereas a low number (1 to 8) with heavier weights tends to favor strength development. For a combination of strength and endurance, approximately 6 to 10 repetitions are recommended.

For the 6 to 10 cycle, a starting weight is chosen that permits 6 repetitions only. On each subsequent workout (every other day) an attempt is made to perform one additional repetition. When you can perform 10 repetitions with a particular weight, the weight is increased (5 pounds for upper body and 10 pounds for lower body exercises) and you return to 6 repetitions. For example, on workout I you may be capable of doing 6 arm curls with 30 pounds. On workout II you perform 7 curls, 8 on workout III, 9 on workout IV, and 10 on workout V. On the next workout you increase the weight to 35 pounds and return to 6 repetitions. The process is then repeated over and over again as you become stronger.

SETS

One group of repetitions for a particular exercise is referred to as a **set**. When using conventional free weights, two to three sets of each exercise are recommended. Sets should be performed consecutively (three sets of one exercise before going on to another muscle group) with approximately one to two minutes of rest or until breathlessness is not an interfering factor for the next set. The two to three set approach may also be used on training apparatus such as the Universal Gym, isokinetic, and isometric units.

WEIGHT (RESISTANCE)

The weight with which you can perform a specific number of repetitions is termed the **RM (repetitions maximum).** The 10 RM, then, is the amount of weight with which you can perform only 10 repetitions. After you decide on the range of repetitions for your training objectives, your starting weight for the first workout is the RM for the lower repetition. For example, with the 6 to 10 cycle, your starting weight is the 6 RM.

REST INTERVAL (BETWEEN SETS)

The time between sets is called the **rest interval.** Muscle fibers will recover to within 50 percent of their innate capacity within 3 to 5 seconds after a set. The recovery rate will continue to increase in proportion to the rest time allotted. A rest interval may range from 30 seconds to a maximum of one minute. The first set usually tires the muscle, while the next are conditioning. If the rest is too long between sets, you would only be tiring the muscle again. Any rest period longer than two minutes usually results in pooled blood draining from the exercised area. The rest interval should diminish as conditioning levels improve.

In a program designed to increase strength only, the length of the rest interval is less important. For muscular endurance training, however, the rest interval should gradually decrease from two minutes to 15 to 20 seconds over several months. Research on the effects of short rest intervals on cardiovascular development is underway and inconclusive at this time. It has been determined that heart rates do remain significantly elevated throughout the workout when rest intervals are reduced to 30 seconds or less.

REST INTERVAL (BETWEEN WORKOUTS)

Best results occur when there are at least 48 hours and no more than 96 hours between workouts. Training on an alternate day basis seems best for most individuals. Advanced weight trainers who use heavier resistance and train with a higher level of intensity may need to work out less frequently.

Table 4.1 serves as a guide to the manipulation of the training variables just discussed, and should aid you in reaching your training objectives.

WEIGHT TRAINING

The adage "use it or lose it" is applicable to strength and endurance training. Muscles that are exercised regularly increase in size and efficiency; those that are neglected become atrophied and weak. The most effective means of increasing muscle size and strength is through weight training. A properly developed program is capable of producing strength gains, power gains, muscle definition (making each small muscle group visible), endurance gains, or muscle bulk, none of which occur automatically.

Weight training will not necessarily produce oversized, bulgy muscles unless you specifically design your program for this purpose. Individuals involved in the art of body building spend long, laborious hours carving out their physiques by carefully planning a program to increase muscle size and muscle definition. Contrary to popular belief, those who choose weight training for the purposes of improving general fitness and strength, or for skill improvement in sports, will not observe dramatic changes in muscle size. Weight training is also unlikely to cause "muscle boundness" or to limit joint flexibility. For instance, John Grimek, once a world class weight lifting champion, could easily perform a scissors split on either side.

There is also no reason for females to fear loss of femininity from involvement in weight training. It will not happen. Researchers have concluded that such concerns are unfounded—women, due to low levels of the androgenic hormones that enlarge muscles, can increase strength 50 to 70 percent with no increase in muscle bulk. Strength, endurance, and body appearance will improve without a transformation to the Hulk. Unfortunately, the myth of developing masculinelike features causes many misinformed females to avoid any type of strength training.

THE IMPORTANCE OF STRENGTH

Strength is a key prerequisite to other fitness qualities. Improved strength in the musculature surrounding the joints aids in the prevention of certain injuries. Strength training also causes the bones and connective tissue (tendons and ligaments) to become more dense and stronger. In addition, strength training is critical to recovery following certain muscle, bone, and joint injuries. Strength

TABLE 4.1 WEIGHT TRAINING OBJECTIVES AND VARIABLE CONTROL

Desired Physical Outcomes	Variable Control
Cardiovascular endurance	Moderate to heavy weight, rapid contractions, the use of repeated power exercises, 6 to 10 repetitions for 3 sets, 5 to 15 seconds rest between each set and exercise.
Local muscular endurance	Light weight, 10 to 15 repetitions, 3 sets, moderate contractions, and minimum rest interval.
Explosive power/speed	Moderate weight, 1 to 5 repetitions, rapid contractions, decreasing rest interval, 1 to 5 sets, and use of power exercises.
Flexibility	Moderate weight, slow contractions, 6 to 10 repetitions, 1 to 3 sets, carrying each exercise to the extreme range of motion and applying static pressure for several seconds before returning to the starting position. Avoid ballistic movements that force the joints quickly beyond the normal range of movement.
Muscle mass or bulk	Heavy weight, maximum number of repetitions, 2 sets, slow contractions, repeated heavy or maximum lifts, use of "flushing," or activation of the same muscle groups repeatedly to provide a prolonged flow of blood to a specific area.
Rehabilitation of injured muscles and joints	Light weights, slow contractions, 6 to 10 repetitions after initial training sessions involving no weight and 3 to 5 contractions, 3 sets, utilizing exercises that activate the supporting muscles of a joint such as those of the ankle, knee, and shoulder. Also helpful for prevention of injury to these areas.
Strength	Heavy weights (2 to 5 RM), low repetitions, slow contractions, minimum rest between sets and exercises, maximum lifts, Groves' Super-Overload Method.
Strength and endurance (general body development)	Moderate weight (8 RM), 6 to 10 repetitions, moderate contractions, decreasing rest interval, 3 sets, varied exercises to activate all major muscle groups.

training is beneficial for improving muscle tone and physical appearance and for aiding performance in practically all fitness activities and sports. It is the one fitness component that can be quickly improved through training.

EXPECTATIONS FROM WEIGHT TRAINING

Identical weight training programs have varying effects on individuals. Although nearly everyone experiences strength and endurance gains, some improve more than others. Even various muscle groups within the same individual respond differently to training. One factor causing these discrepancies is the individual's initial strength level.

Those who have not previously been involved in a strength development program can anticipate rapid improvement; whereas those with a high level of strength improve at a much slower rate.

STRENGTH TESTING

A convenient method for testing muscular strength in males and females is the determination of the one repetition maximum (1 RM). The specific muscle group to be tested is selected, and individuals are given a series of trials to determine the maximal weight they can lift one time. Since most people are inexperienced in weight training, the test is conducted largely through trial and error.

For each test, a weight is selected that can be lifted comfortably. Additional weight is then added in subsequent trials until the weight is found that can be lifted correctly just one time. If the weight can be lifted more than once, more weight needs to be added until a true 1 RM is determined. Approximately three trials, with a two to three minute rest between each, are needed to locate the 1 RM for each exercise.

One RM can be obtained for any basic weight training exercise (see Table 4.2). Since the resistances to be overcome in 1-RM testing are heavy, it is advisable to follow proper safety procedures. Subjects should exhale during the resistance phase of the exercise (i.e., when the weight is lifted) to avoid breath holding and working with a closed glottis. A partner serves as a spotter with the responsibility of protecting the lifter.

GRIP STRENGTH

The hand dynamometer is used to measure the muscular strength of the fingers, hand, and forearm (see Figure 4.1). This instrument has a reported reliability coefficient of .98.

The gripping part of the hand grip dynamometer can be adjusted to fit any hand size. This

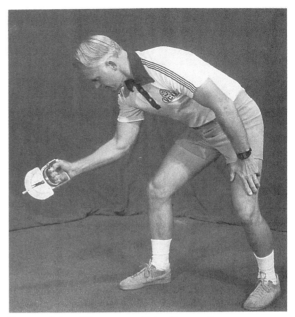

Figure 4.1   Measuring Grip Strength

feature makes the device feasible for testing both males and females. The needle indicator and the scoring dial are marked off in kilograms for ease of scoring. Once the proper grip has been established for the dominant hand, the dynamometer

TABLE 4.2   OPTIMAL STRENGTH VALUES FOR VARIOUS BODY WEIGHTS (BASED ON THE 1-RM TEST)

Body Weight (lb)	Bench Press		Shoulder Press		Biceps Curl		Leg Press	
	Male	Female	Male	Female	Male	Female	Male	Female
80	70	60	55	40	40	30	160	120
100	85	70	70	50	50	35	200	150
120	105	85	80	60	60	40	240	180
140	125	100	95	65	70	50	280	210
160	145	115	110	75	80	60	320	240
180	160	125	120	85	90	65	360	270
200	180	140	135	95	100	70	400	300
220	200	155	150	105	110	75	440	330
240	225	170	160	115	120	85	480	360

Data in pounds; obtained on Universal Gym apparatus; applicable ages 17 to 30.

Reprinted with permission of Macmillan Publishing Company from *Health and Fitness Through Physical Activity* by M. L. Pollock, J. H. Wilmore, and S. M. Fox (New York: Macmillan 1978).

is held overhead and the arm is steadily dropped downward and to the side as you continue to tighten your grip. The indicator needle will hold at your maximum grip squeeze to provide a reading in kilograms (2.2 kg = 1 lb). The best of two trials is recorded (see Table 4.3). Avoid letting the hand, arm, or elbow touch the body or any other object while drawing the arm down.

MUSCULAR ENDURANCE TESTING

The pull-up (males), modified pull-ups (females) and bar dips (males) are popular tests for determining upper arm muscular strength and endurance. These tests are easy to administer and provide a fairly valid strength assessment (see Table 4.4).

PULL-UP

For the pull-up, grasp an adjustable horizontal bar with the palms facing away from the body (see Figure 4.2). Raise your body weight until the chin clears the top of the bar. Then, slowly lower your body weight to a full hang without any pause. Repeat this action as many times as possible. The body must return to a stretch position (elbows locked) each time. Deliberate swinging, resting, or leg kicking is not permitted.

MODIFIED PULL-UP

The modified pull-up closely resembles the regular pull-up discussed above (see Figure 4.3). Using an adjustable horizontal bar, grasp the bar (palms away) at a level just even with the base of the sternum (breastbone) before placing the body under the bar until a 90-degree angle is formed at the point where the arms and chest join. Only the heels will support the weight of the lower body. One point is scored each time the chin is pulled over the bar and the body returns to the support position with the arms fully extended.

BAR DIP

The bar dip test is frequently used as a valid measure for determining muscular strength and endurance of the triceps (extensors of the arms) and shoulder girdle (see Figure 4.4). Using parallel bars, begin in a straight arm support position close to the bar ends. The idea is to lower your body slowly until the arms form a 90-degree bent arm position. After reaching right angles, attempt to straighten

TABLE 4.3 GRIP STRENGTH SCORING TABLE IN KILOGRAMS[1]

College Females, Dominant Grip	Performance Standards	College Males, Dominant Grip
37 or above	Excellent	62 or above
32 to 36	Good	56 to 61
25 to 31	Average	45 to 55
15 to 24	Poor	29 to 44

[1]Multiply by 2.2 to determine the equivalent grip scores in pounds.

TABLE 4.4 SCORING OF PULL-UPS, MODIFIED PULL-UPS, AND DIPS

Performance Standards	Pull-Ups (No.)	Modified Pull-Ups (No.)	Bar Dips (No.)
Excellent	13 or above	30 or above	20 or above
Good	10 to 12	25 to 29	15 to 19
Average	5 to 9	16 to 24	7 to 14
Poor	0 to 4	0 to 15	0 to 6

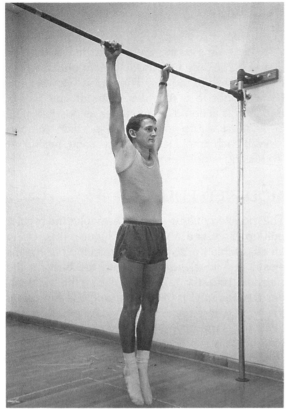

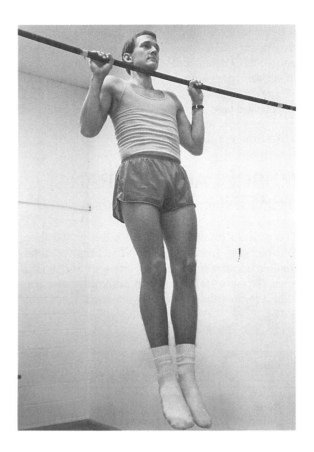

Figure 4.2 Pull-ups

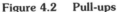

the arms until the starting position is obtained. This action is repeated as many times as possible. Swinging or kicking movements are not permitted. Partial dips or otherwise incomplete dips are not counted.

ABDOMINAL STRENGTH AND ENDURANCE TESTING

It is difficult to obtain a pure isolated measurement of the abdominal region. The bent-knee sit-up, however, is one of the best tests available (see Figure 4.5). In the 60-second bent-knee sit-up test, subjects attempt to move as rapidly as possible from the supine position with knees bent to a sitting position and continue to repeat this action for 60 seconds (see Table 4.5). To start, assume a supine position with arms folded across the chest. The

TABLE 4.5 NORMS FOR THE 60-SECOND TIMED BENT-KNEE SIT-UP

College Females	Performance Standards	College Males
51 or above	Excellent	60 or above
46 to 50	Good	50 to 59
33 to 45	Average	34 to 49
21 to 32	Low	26 to 33
0 to 20	Poor	0 to 25

knees should be bent at about a 90-degree angle with both feet flat and in front of the buttocks. The feet are anchored or held stationary by a partner who grasps your ankles while kneeling between your feet. You may do several practice sit-ups prior

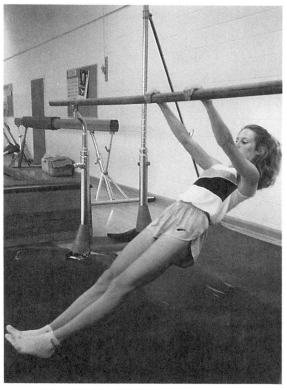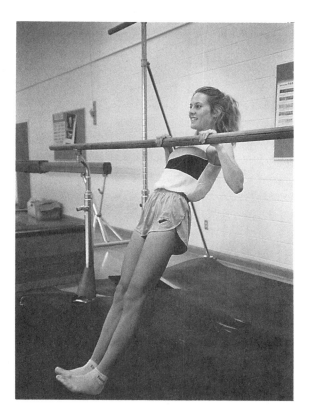

Figure 4.3   Modified Pull-ups

to the official testing session if you wish. At the command *go*, begin a series of rapidly executed bent-knee sit-ups and try to continue for 60 seconds.

Procedural infractions that eliminate a bent-knee sit-up from your score include:

1. Failing to reach the vertical sitting position.
2. Neglecting to keep the feet flat and approximately 18 inches in front of the buttocks.
3. Not returning each time to the starting position where the middle of the back touches the mat.

SPECIAL WEIGHT TRAINING METHODS AND DEVICES

There are three acceptable strength training methods: isotonics, isokinetics, and isometrics. Each approach requires special equipment and yields significant results.

During an **isotonic** contraction the muscle shortens (positive phase) and lengthens (negative phase) with each repetition. **Isokinetic** movements require special equipment designed to provide maximal resistance for a muscle throughout the full range of movement. In an **isometric** contraction (applying force against an immovable object), the muscle contracts; its overall length, however, remains unchanged (it does not shorten).

ISOTONICS (FREE WEIGHTS, UNIVERSAL GYM, NAUTILUS, CAM II, POLARIS)

Free Weights   Free weights (barbells, dumbbells) are probably best in that their use for strength development can simulate specific muscular movements in practically any sport, improve general bodily development, and increase muscular strength and endurance in practically any muscle group. Free weight exercises can also be per-

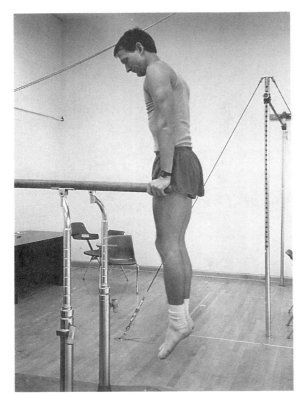 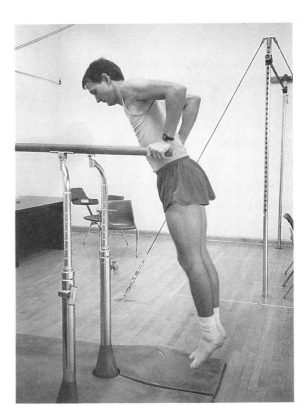

Figure 4.4   Bar Dips

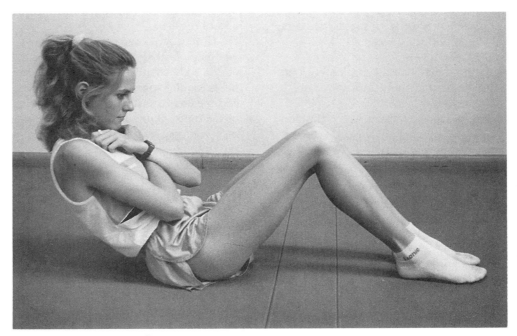

Figure 4.5   Bent-Knee Sit-up

formed in a small area with minimum equipment. The amount of weight needed depends upon the training objectives. For a young adult male, 175 pounds of disc weights is generally adequate. A young female may find 125 pounds sufficient. Sample barbell and dumbbell equipment is shown in Figure 4.6.

Universal Gym The Universal Gym provides variable resistance. Muscular development can be acquired through both the positive and negative phases of muscular contraction. The device consists of various exercise stations and can accommodate up to 16 individuals simultaneously. It is designed to duplicate most barbell exercises. Stacked weights travel up and down on fixed tracks, and weight adjustments are conveniently made by simply removing and inserting a metal pin at each desired weight increment. This arrangement eliminates many of the safety hazards so prevalent with free weights. The Universal Gym is a versatile piece of equipment; it is easy to operate, and can be repositioned by one person (see Figure 4.7).

Nautilus Most Nautilus equipment is designed to work a single muscle group through a full range of movement. The name *Nautilus* comes from the resistance pulley, which is shaped like a nautilus

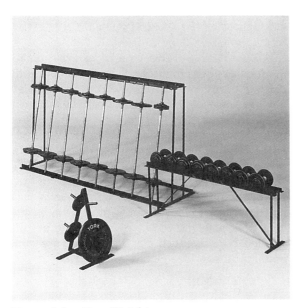

Figure 4.6   Free Weights

shell. The counter-weight is timed like an automobile ignition system to provide variable resistance throughout the full range of movement. Strict emphasis is placed on proper form for one set of each exercise. Some disadvantages of the Nautilus system are the cost, the need for many different machines to accomplish a complete workout, and the large space needed to house the equipment (see Figure 4.8).

CAM II—Weightless Machines The latest pieces of exercise equipment to infiltrate the nation's health parlors and professional training facilities are compressed air machines (cams). There are no cables, chains, pulleys, or iron plates. Instead, the CAM II provides variable resistance from air pressure generated by a compressor. Each machine is capable of working one specific muscle group. The machines weigh approximately 180 pounds each and are easily moved. Although expensive, they are easy to adjust, quiet, and extremely safe (see Figure 4.9).

Polaris This type of variable-resistance exercise system is fashioned after the cam principle. A cable rolls over an oval-shaped plate during the exercise movement. The individually designed cams assure the most effective resistance ratio in every movement involved. There are over 25 different machines designed for developing the upper and lower body areas with this system.

ISOKINETICS (MINI-GYM)

Mini-Gym This device utilizes the isokinetic or "accommodating resistance" principle. Resistance increases as the force increases—the harder you pull, the harder the Mini-Gym resists your pull (see Figure 4.10). Unlike with free weights, resistance during isokinetics is not greatly dissipated by acceleration; rather, resistance is always directly related to your applied force. Variable resistance is provided throughout the entire range of movement while force is being applied. Warm-up is not as crucial as with other devices since the apparatus merely adjusts to the force of your pull. Advocaters of this program prefer its simplicity, its safety, and the accessibility of dials and graphs that allow you to monitor your progress during each exercise ef-

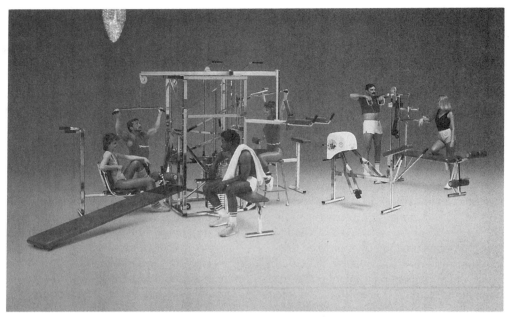

Figure 4.7   The Universal Gym

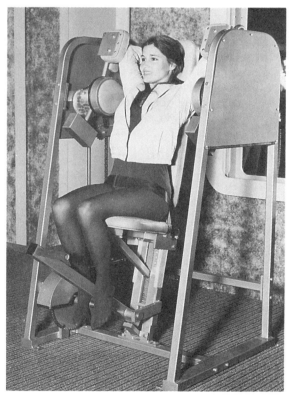

Figure 4.8   Nautilus Equipment

fort. Since there is no negative phase, very little muscle soreness or joint discomfort occurs with isokinetics.

COMBINATIONS: ISOTONIC AND ISOKINETIC (HYDRA-FITNESS, EAGLE PERFORMANCE SYSTEMS)

Hydra-Fitness   This type of exercise equipment utilizes both the isotonic and isokinetic principles and is referred to as "powernetic resistance." Hydra-Fitness equipment automatically and continuously adjusts to the strength and the speed output of the individual. It is built around a patented cylinder which accommodates the power output of the user. There are no cables, pulleys, pins, or weights to manipulate. This system does not depend on gravity to pull weight down once it is lifted; instead the individual must replace gravity's work with his or her own, thereby accomplishing twice as much positive work in the same amount of time (see Figure 4.11).

Eagle Performance Systems   This is a line of variable-resistance exercise machines and free

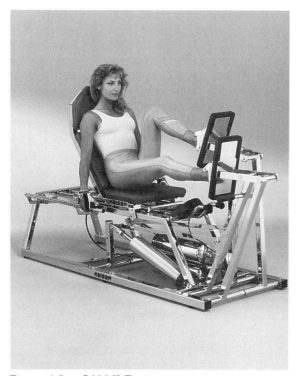

Figure 4.9   CAM II Equipment

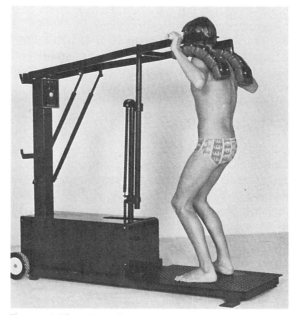

Figure 4.10   Mini-Gym Equipment

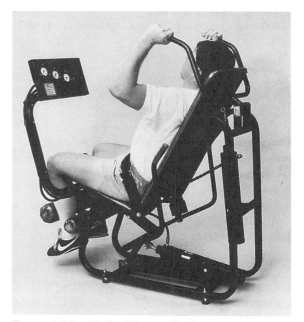

Figure 4.11   Hydra-Fitness Equipment

weights combining the isokinetic and isotonic concept for strength training. Currently, there are 16 machines designed for developing the upper body, lower body, and trunk areas.

ISOMETRICS

Isometric exercises can be compared to weight training movements in which the weight is so heavy that it cannot be moved. It involves a steady muscle contraction against an immovable resistance object. This may be a wall, the bleachers, a door jam, or a partner. Researchers recommend that the duration of the isometric hold be from six to eight seconds with one to three sets of each exercise performed daily using about 75 percent of a maximum effort. Although many researchers have found that strength can be increased through isometric training, the effect on sports performance and general fitness is questionable. The strength gains appear to be limited primarily to that specific joint angle at which the isometric contraction occurred. Such gains, therefore, do not transfer to

increased strength throughout the full range of motion.

Most physicians discourage isometric training for individuals over 30 years of age. There is evidence that the isometric hold tends to occlude blood flow through the contracting muscles, significantly elevating blood pressure and hindering the return of venous blood to the heart. This effect is particularly dangerous to those with atherosclerosis, high blood pressure, or other known vascular abnormalities.

CALISTHENICS

Calisthenics include a series of formal exercises using the body as the resistance or training device. They represent a practical, safe, and effective method of developing muscular strength and endurance. Since the resistance is low, exercises such as sit-ups, toe-touchers, trunk rotation, jumping jacks, push-ups, and a wide variety of others must be performed in a high number of repetitions. Since resistance (body weight) also remains constant, the number of repetitions must be gradually increased, the rest interval between exercises decreased, the speed or rate of execution increased, and the duration of the workout increased. Calisthenics are generally recommended over weights for developing muscular strength and endurance in children.

THE EFFECTIVENESS OF EACH METHOD—WHAT RESEARCHERS SAY

The following represents a brief summary of findings to date on the effectiveness of various devices in producing strength and endurance gains:

1. Calisthenics produce only slight strength gains and are considered more valuable for warm-up and flexibility improvement. Use of weighted vests (ankles, back) or a partner can alter the resistance variable, of course, and produce significant gains in strength.

2. Isometrics, performed to near maximum effort for 6 to 10 seconds, will provide rapid strength gains. Strength gains are equal to those produced through free weights and consume less than one-third the time. Unfortunately, there is limited carry-over to sports performance since

strength is improved only at the angle used, while at other angles strength remains unchanged. Motivation, boredom, and the inability to control force application are other limitations of isometrics. Following muscle and joint injuries, isometrics is a sound rehabilitation choice until the injured area is pain-free at which time weight training is recommended.

3. Free weights, using three sets of 6 to 10 repetitions, three times weekly, will produce significant improvement in muscular strength and endurance. One vigorous workout weekly will maintain already acquired strength.

4. The Universal Gym offers variable resistance and is capable of duplicating most barbell exercises. Significant strength and endurance gains occur after only 4 to 6 weeks of regular training.

5. Isokinetics provides accommodating resistance throughout the entire range of movement. The muscles exert maximum effort each repetition. The machine automatically adjusts to fatigue or pain, which is conducive to rehabilitative causes. There are no bulky weights to change, and muscle and joint soreness is negligible because the negative phase is absent (no weight to lower).

6. Nautilus machines provide resistance in both the positive and negative phase. They incorporate rotary movement, direct resistance, variable resistance, and balanced resistance. In addition, the Nautilus provides for a full range of motion with all exercises. Promoters of these machines advocate only one quality set. It is believed that performing multiple sets encourages "pacing" or saving oneself for subsequent sets.

STRENGTH TRAINING TECHNIQUES

Exercises discussed in this chapter represent a wide variety of possible movements using the various methods and machines—free weights, isometrics, isokinetics, and the Nautilus system. The following techniques apply to practically all movements:

1. For the basic stance, place the feet slightly wider than shoulder width with the toes parallel. Primary considerations are balance (maintaining the weight directly above the medial plane of the body) and agility. The stronger leg is sometimes placed back in a heel-toe alignment (left heel is even with the right toe), depending upon individual preference.

2. Toes should be placed just under the bar in the starting phase of exercises in which the barbell is resting on the floor.

3. Maintain an erect back (unless this is the muscle group being exercised) with the head up and eyes looking straight ahead.

4. Grasp the bar using the appropriate grip (see Figure 4.12) with hands approximately shoulder width apart and with the weight equally distributed on each hand. Utilize the mixed grip described below when heavy weights must be supported by the arms, as in the dead and straddle lifts:

   Overhand Grip: In this most common grip, the bar is grasped until the thumb wraps around and meets the index finger. The thumb may be placed next to the index finger without wrapping around the bar if so desired in a particular lift.

   Underhand Grip: For this grip the bar is grasped with the palms turned upward away from the body. The fingers and thumb are wrapped around as indicated above.

   Mixed Grip: The mixed grip is a combination of the above two styles, with one hand assuming an overhand and the other an underhand grip in order to reduce finger strain in heavy lifts.

5. Avoid leaning backward to assist the completion of a repetition designed to strengthen the arm muscles.

6. In early training sessions, choose realistic starting weights that provide little strain,

Figure 4.12   Basic Grips

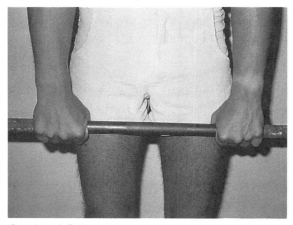

Overhand Grip

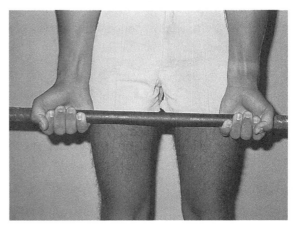

Underhand Grip

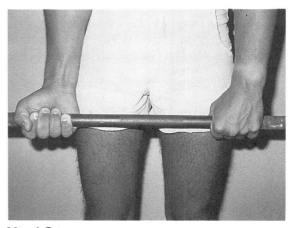

Mixed Grip

adjusting them rapidly within three to four workouts.

7. Days lifting the maximum weight possible should be built into the program for variation.

8. Overcome training plateaus or sticking points by altering the exercises and the variables.

9. Practice adequate safety precautions at all times and use a partner to spot on exercises involving heavy weight:

Avoid attempting to move more resistance than you can safely handle.

Secure collars and engage pins before attempting any type of lift.

Stay clear of an individual engaging in a lift.

Avoid distractions while another person is concentrating on a lift.

Avoid holding your breath while lifting heavy weights.

Practice returning all weights to the floor or rack in a controlled manner.

Bend the knees when attempting to move heavy weights from one place to another for storage.

Protect the back by developing strong abdominal muscles.

A wide variety of exercises to strengthen various muscle groups is discussed later in this chapter. Select your routine from this list.

Sample programs for various fitness objectives are shown in Table 4.6. Perform one to three sets of repetitions for each exercise and rest for 30 seconds to 1 minute between sets.

BARBELL AND DUMBBELL EXERCISES

There are many barbell and dumbbell exercises and several variations of each exercise. Table 4.7 includes some of the more common exercises for you to try. Caution: practice safety at all times and always try to work out with a buddy.

HOME FITNESS EQUIPMENT

Cocooning. Are you doing it, contemplating it, or maybe just curious about what it is? **Cocooning** is a new national trend toward improved home exercise environments. Primary cocooning considerations are style, convenience, privacy, and price.

Before setting up your home/office fitness center, consult with your physician or health professional to discuss your particular needs. It is especially important that you evaluate your fitness capabilities before investing in any equipment. Then ask yourself the following questions:

1. *What are my physical goals?* Balance is the key. It is important that you develop all the physical components (flexibility, strength, and cardio-respiratory efficiency) in proportion for best results. If you wish to specialize in any one fitness component keep in mind that the end result will be greatly affected by your overall level of efficiency.

2. *What equipment do I need to achieve specific goals?* The equipment you choose should affect your flexibility, strength, and cardio-respiratory efficiency. If you have a low budget, you might consider equipment that works several fitness components simultaneously. Ideally, a combination of machines will prevent boredom by offering several alternatives to meet your training goals.

3. *How often will I use my home gym?* In order to attain noticeable results, a concentrated effort for self-betterment must be applied on a regular basis over a period of time. You must develop a training strategy or the chances are that the equipment, no matter how sophisticated or interesting, will end up merely collecting dust.

The following fitness equipment/devices are gaining much popularity and usage in the home setting. They are designed for either strength or aerobic conditioning, with some machines providing multifitness features.

TABLE 4.6 BASIC AND ALTERNATE PROGRAMS FOR GENERAL BODILY DEVELOPMENT

Exercises	Repetitions	Starting Weight	Speed of Contraction
Basic Program			
Two-arm curl	6–10	8 RM	Moderate
Military press	6–10	8 RM	Moderate
Sit-ups (bent-knee)	25–50	30 RM	Rapid
Rowing (upright)	6–10	8 RM	Moderate
Bench press	6–10	8 RM	Moderate
Squat	6–10	8 RM	Rapid
Heel raise	15–25	20 RM	Rapid
Dead lift (bent-knee)	6–10	8 RM	Rapid
Alternate I			
Reverse curl	6–10	8 RM	Moderate
Triceps press	6–10	8 RM	Moderate
Sit-ups (bent-knee)	25–50	30 RM	Rapid
Shoulder shrug	6–10	8 RM	Moderate
Squat jump	15–25	20 RM	Rapid
Knee flexor	6–10	8 RM	Rapid
Knee extensor	6–10	8 RM	Rapid
Pull-over (bent-arm)	6–10	8 RM	Moderate
Alternate II			
Wrist curl	6–10	8 RM	Moderate
Side bender	6–10	8 RM	Moderate
Lateral raise	6–10	8 RM	Moderate
Straddle lift	6–10	8 RM	Rapid
Supine leg lift	6–10	8 RM	Rapid
Hip flexor	6–10	8 RM	Rapid
Leg abductor	6–10	8 RM	Rapid
Forward raise	6–10	8 RM	Moderate

Stationary cycle The more sophisticated cycles provide instrumentation to measure speed, distance, time, and energy expended. The rider pedals against a variable resistance that will improve aerobic conditioning.

Rower This piece of equipment is designed to work the arms and legs simultaneously while seated. Some of the more expensive units provide extensive energy feedback.

Ski trainer This machine is designed to simulate cross-country skiing movements. Some types offer variable resistances that are separately adjustable for arms and legs. They are considered the best overall aerobic conditioning devices on the market today.

Treadmill This equipment resembles a miniconveyor belt with mounted front and side safety bars. Some of the less expensive treadmills are driven by the exercisor. The more sophisticated units are motorized, provide instrumentation for energy expended, and have variable inclines and belt speeds.

Rebound joggers This is simply a very small trampoline upon which a person performs a stationary run. Speed and duration of the run are governed entirely by the individual. It is designed primarily for aerobic conditioning.

TABLE 4.7 BARBELL AND DUMBBELL EXERCISES

Exercise	Equipment	Basic Movement	Helpful Hints	Muscle Groups
Bench press	Barbell, bench rack, spotter	Using an overhand grip, slowly lower the bar to the chest, then press back to the starting position.	Bend knees at 90° and keep feet off the bench and the floor.	Shoulder extensors

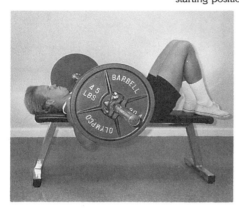 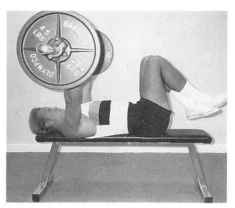

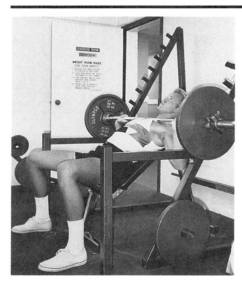 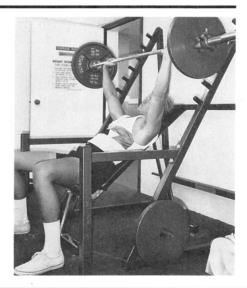

Exercise	Equipment	Basic Movement	Helpful Hints	Muscle Groups
Incline bench press	Incline bench, squat rack, spotter	Using an overhand grip, slowly raise and lower the bar to the chest (both feet flat on the floor).	Use a weight rack to support the weight above the bench. Avoid lifting the buttock or arching the back while lifting.	Upper pectoralis major Anterios deltoid Tricep

TABLE 4.7 BARBELL AND DUMBBELL EXERCISES

Exercise	Equipment	Basic Movement	Helpful Hints	Muscle Groups
Power cleans	Barbell	Using an overhand grip, pull the bar explosively to the highest point of your chest. Rotate hands under the bar and bend your knees. Straighten to standing position. Bend the arms, legs, and hips to return the bar to the thighs, then slowly bend the knees and hips to lower to the floor.	Grasp the bar at shoulder width. Start with knees bent so hips are knee level. Keep head up and back straight.	Trapezius Erector spinae Gluteus Quadriceps

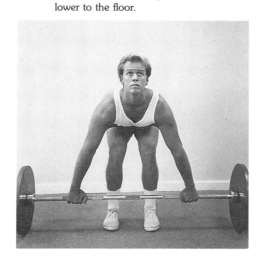

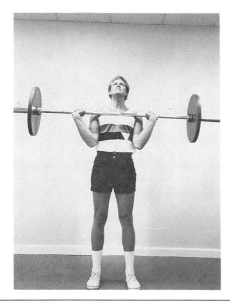

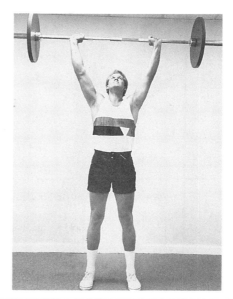

TABLE 4.7   BARBELL AND DUMBBELL EXERCISES

Exercise	Equipment	Basic Movement	Helpful Hints	Muscle Groups
Deadlift	Barbell	Using a mixed grip, bend knees so hips are close to knee level. Straighten knees and hips to standing position. Bend at knees and hips to return.	Keep head up and back flat. Grasp bar at shoulder width.	Erector spinae Gluteus Quadriceps

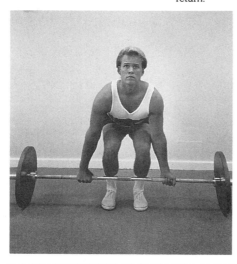 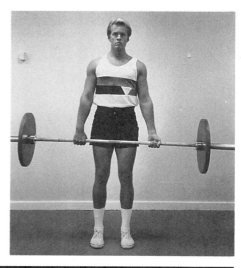

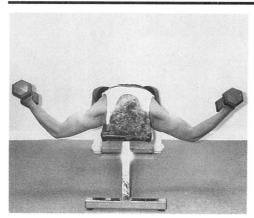 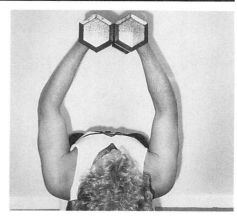

Exercise	Equipment	Basic Movement	Helpful Hints	Muscle Groups
Bent arm flyes	Dumbbells	Using an underhand grip, hold a dumbbell in each hand above the shoulders with the elbows slightly bent.	Keep elbows slightly bent at all times.	Pectoralis major

TABLE 4.7 BARBELL AND DUMBBELL EXERCISES

Exercise	Equipment	Basic Movement	Helpful Hints	Muscle Groups
Barbell rowing	Barbell	Using an overhand grip, hold the barbell directly below your shoulders. With elbows leading, pull the barbell to chest and hold momentarily, then slowly return to the starting position.	Grasp bar slightly wider than shoulder width. Refrain from swinging or jerking the weights upward to the chest region.	Latissimos dorsi Rear deltoid Trapezius

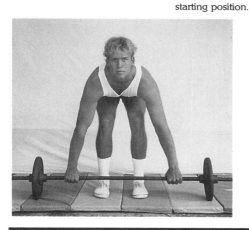 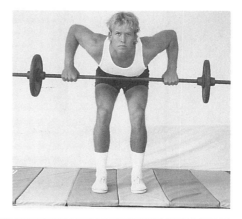

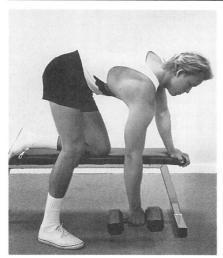 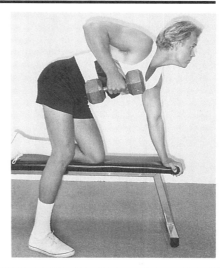

Exercise	Equipment	Basic Movement	Helpful Hints	Muscle Groups
One dumbbell rowing	Dumbbells	Using an underhand grip, kneel with one hand and one knee on exercise mat. Pull weight on support side upward to chest.	Hold dumbbell briefly at chest before returning.	Latissimus dorsi

TABLE 4.7   BARBELL AND DUMBBELL EXERCISES

Exercise	Equipment	Basic Movement	Helpful Hints	Muscle Groups
Shoulder shrug	Barbell	Using an overhand grip, elevate both shoulders until they nearly touch the earlobes, then relax and return bar to the thighs.	Keep the extremities fully extended. Heavy weights (within limitations) will bring more rapid strength gains.	Shoulder girdle elevators

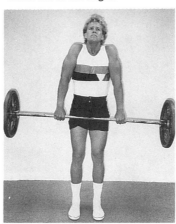

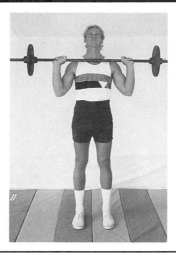 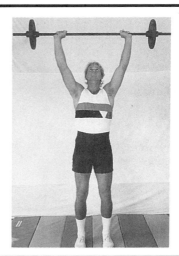

Exercise	Equipment	Basic Movement	Helpful Hints	Muscle Groups
Military press	Barbell	Using an overhead grip, slowly push bar overhead from chest until both arms are fully extended.	Keep neck and back erect, and knees extended and locked. Avoid jerky movements and leaning.	Abductors Flexors Arm extensors Deltoid Triceps

TABLE 4.7   BARBELL AND DUMBBELL EXERCISES

Exercise	Equipment	Basic Movement	Helpful Hints	Muscle Groups
Upright rowing	Barbell	Using an overhand grip, raise bar to the chin, and then return to thighs.	Grasp bar 6 to 8 inches apart. Keep elbows higher than the hands. Maintain an erect, stationary position.	Abductors Arm flexors Deltoid Trapezius

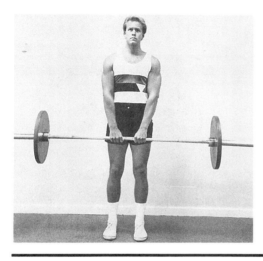 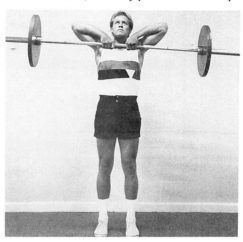

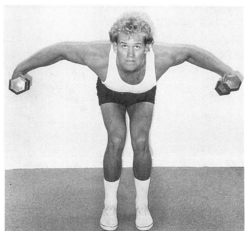

Exercise	Equipment	Basic Movement	Helpful Hints	Muscle Groups
Bent-over lateral raise.	Dumbbells	Using an overhand grip, grasp dumbbell in each hand and draw arms to shoulder level. Slowly return to hanging position.	Keep knees and elbows slightly bent. Hold weights for 1–2 seconds before returning to hanging position.	Rear deltoid

TABLE 4.7   BARBELL AND DUMBBELL EXERCISES

Exercise	Equipment	Basic Movement	Helpful Hints	Muscle Groups
Two-arm curl	Barbell	Using overhand grip, raise bar from thighs to chest level, and return.	Keep body erect and motionless throughout	Upper arm flexors Wrist flexors Long finger flexors

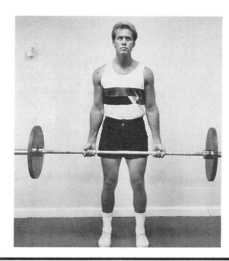 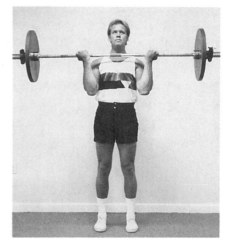

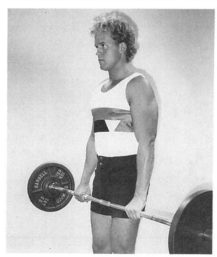 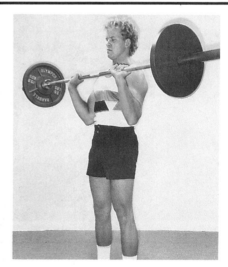

Exercise	Equipment	Basic Movement	Helpful Hints	Muscle Groups
Reverse curl	Barbell	Using overhand grip, raise bar from thighs to chest level, and return.	Use less weight than in two-arm curl.	Upper arm flexors Hand extensors Finger extensors

TABLE 4.7   BARBELL AND DUMBBELL EXERCISES

Exercise	Equipment	Basic Movement	Helpful Hints	Muscle Groups
Seated dumbbell curl	Dumbbells	Using an underhand grip, curl one or both dumbbells to the shoulder, then slowly return the weight to the sides of the body.	Keep the back straight throughout the entire movement.	Biceps

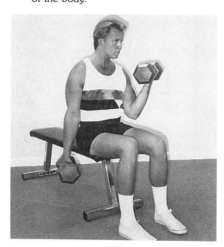

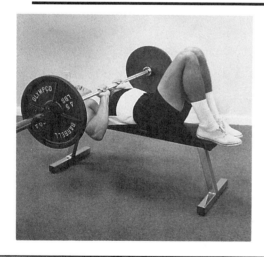 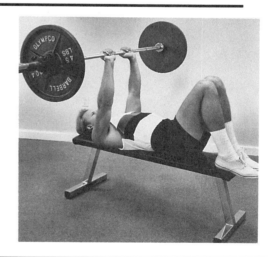

Exercise	Equipment	Basic Movement	Helpful Hints	Muscle Groups
Close grip bench press	Barbell, squat rack, spotter	Using an overhand grip, slowly lower the barbell to the chest and press back to the starting position.	Grasp center of bar (hands 2 to 4 inches apart). Bend knees at 90°; keep feet off the bench/floor so as to avoid arching the back. Keep elbows in; extend arms fully.	Triceps Anterior deltoid Pectoralis major

TABLE 4.7 BARBELL AND DUMBBELL EXERCISES

Exercise	Equipment	Basic Movement	Helpful Hints	Muscle Groups
Standing or seated tricep extension	Dumbbell	With both hands grasped around the inner side of one dumbbell overhead, lower the weight behind your head, then return.	Keep the elbows close together throughout the maneuver.	Triceps

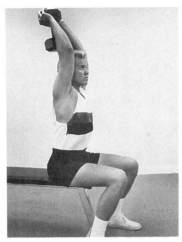 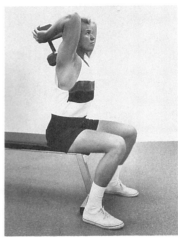

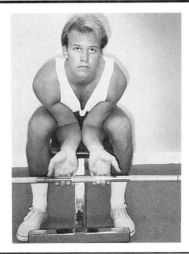 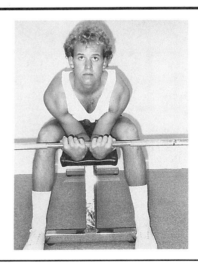

Exercise	Equipment	Basic Movement	Helpful Hints	Muscle Groups
Barbell wrist curl	Barbell	Using an underhand grip, let the bar hang down toward the floor and then curl toward you.	Grasp center of bar (hands 2 to 4 inches apart). Keep forearms in steady contact with the bench while moving the weight.	Forearm flexors

TABLE 4.7   BARBELL AND DUMBBELL EXERCISES

Exercise	Equipment	Basic Movement	Helpful Hints	Muscle Groups
Reverse wrist curl	Barbell	Using an overhand grip, and moving the wrists only, raise bar as high as possible, and then return to the starting position.	Grasp barbell at shoulder width. Movement should only be at the wrist joint.	Forearm extensors

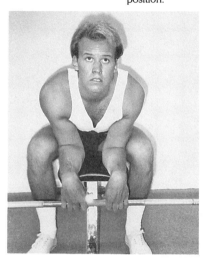 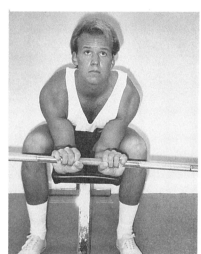

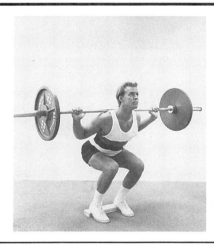 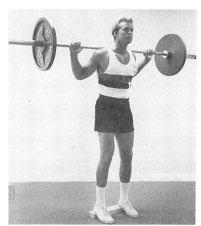

Exercise	Equipment	Basic Movement	Helpful Hints	Muscle Groups
Front squat	Barbell, squat rack, chair or bench, 2 to 3-inch board, spotters	Using an overhand grip, flex legs to a 90° angle. Return to standing position.	Keep the toes up, and point the chin outward slightly. A chair or bench can be placed below the body (touch buttocks slightly to surface).	Thigh extensors Lower leg extensors

TABLE 4.7   BARBELL AND DUMBBELL EXERCISES

Exercise	Equipment	Basic Movement	Helpful Hints	Muscle Groups
Lunge with dumbbells	Dumbbells	Overhand grip; alternate stepping forward with each leg, bending the knee of the lead leg, and lowering your body until thigh of the front leg is level to the floor. Barely touch the knee of rear leg before returning to the starting position.	Keep your head up and the upper body erect throughout the exercise. Avoid bending front knee more than 90°.	Quadriceps Gluteus

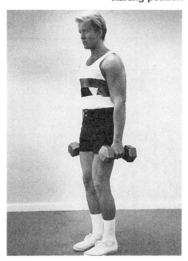 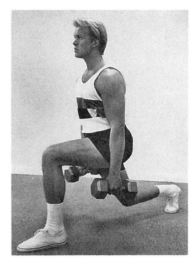

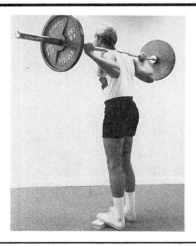 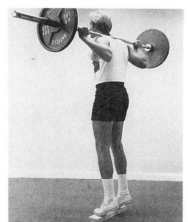

Exercise	Equipment	Basic Movement	Helpful Hints	Muscle Groups
Heel raise	Barbell, squat rack, spotters, 2 to 3-inch board	Using an overhand grip, the body is raised upward to the maximum height of the toes.	Alter the position from straight ahead to pointed in and out. Keep the body erect.	Foot plantar flexors

TABLE 4.7 BARBELL AND DUMBBELL EXERCISES

Exercise	Equipment	Basic Movement	Helpful Hints	Muscle Groups
One dumbbell heel raise	Dumbbell, 2 to 3-inch board	Using an overhand grip, shift entire body weight on the leg next to the dumbbell, and raise the foot off the floor behind. Raise the heel of the support foot upward as high as possible and hold momentarily.	A wall is useful for balance, but avoid using free hand for assistance.	Gastrocnemius Soleus

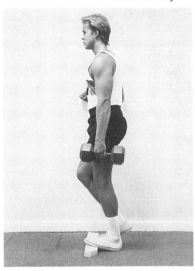 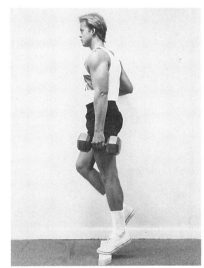

Jump rope This inexpensive device is used mainly for aerobic conditioning. The individual simply swings the rope and jumps over it. Rope speed and jumping styles can be regulated.

Heavy jump rope This specially designed jump rope is weighted with 1 to 10 pounds to employ the overload principle. Jumping the heavy rope can be beneficial either aerobically or anaerobically, depending on the jumping emphasis.

Chinning bar This device can be either a permanent or a portable bar. It is designed for strength development of the upper arm muscles, primarily biceps.

Slantboard This is a padded board with or without a padded shelf for keeping the knees bent while doing sit-ups. The end piece provides an anchor strap for the feet as well as an attachment for raising the board to an inclined position. It is used primarily for strength and muscular-endurance development of the abdominals.

FREQUENTLY ASKED QUESTIONS

Should women train with weights?

At this time there is no scientific evidence to suggest restricting the normal woman from weight training. There is little reason to advocate different training or conditioning regimes on the basis of sex. Both male and female athletes need the additional strength that can be acquired through weight training. According to Dr. Jack Wilmore, University of Arizona physiologist, a woman who trains with weights does not face the prospect of turning into the Hulk. Because of their naturally low level of the hormone testosterone, women can't possibly take on the physical dimensions of Mr. America. It has been demonstrated that in a 10-week weight training program the mean upper body strength of young, nonathletic women can be improved by an average of 30 percent with only a slight increase in muscle size (Hanc 1985). Practicing weight training is one of the fastest approaches to firming the body and looking good, and should not be avoided.

Is it safe for children to weight train?

For many years it was feared that the stresses of weight-training on the bones and ligaments of a young child could hinder the growth process, but contemporary research has shown that children beyond the age of 10 can weight train without harm to their growth pattern. In fact, with proper supervision and guidance, weight training can actually strengthen the supporting structures around a child's bones and actually facilitate growth. A parent must be sure that the trainer or coach follows the guidelines for prepubescent strength training issued by the National Strength and Conditioning Association.

What is the benefit of negative repetitions in weight-training?

The negatives phase is at least as effective as the positives in building strength. Because muscles are 30–40 percent stronger in the negative direction, heavier weights must be used, requiring a spotter to assist with the positive part of the movement.

Can breath holding during weight-lifting be dangerous?

It is dangerous to hold your breath during any form of exercise, especially weight lifting. The pressure in your chest increases and decreases as you inhale and exhale. When you exercise and are breathing more heavily, these pressure changes are even greater. When you hold your breath the additional stress placed on the heart will raise the blood pressure two to three times above normal, which in extreme cases could lead to a rupturing of arteries or even a heart attack. Always breathe as you exercise, and develop a rhythm of inhaling and exhaling to coincide with the expanding and contracting movements of the exercise.

Next to being genetically well endowed, what is the next most important body building factor we can control?

Intensity of exercise is the most important element in muscle development. Intensity means doing an exercise to the point where one more repetition would be physically impossible (Repetition Maximum). Intensity varies; what is intense for one person may be easy for another. For this reason, when we mention intensity in the weight room we mean percent of the individual RM. Using percentage as the guide in regulating intensity makes the workouts more accurate. Most workout percentages are based on the person's 1 RM (the most weight he or she can do for one repetition). For improvement to take place, workouts must impose a demand on the body system. It has been shown that the athlete has to train with loads greater than 80 percent of maximum for strength and power to be optimally increased.

Which method of strength development is best: isotonic, isometric, or isokinetic?

In isotonic exercise, the muscle must shorten as it contracts. The most popular sources of resistance in isotonic exercise are weights (barbells, dumbbells, weighted pulleys, etc.—and the exerciser's body in such exercises as push-ups and pull-ups). Isometric exercise calls for contraction against immovable resistance. The contractions are executed mainly by pushing or pulling one body part against another with sufficient force to cause a stalemate (no movement). With isokinetics there is a constant speed of contraction regardless of the amount of resistance. In effect, variable friction controls both the amount of resistance and the speed at which the exercise is performed. You either push or pull against the mechanism; by exerting more force you increase the resistance.

Isotonic and isokinetic strength training are superior to isometric training. Numerous studies indicate that isometric training tends to produce strength gains at certain angles and not at others. For spots participation, it is strength through the range of motion that is important. All three methods will, however, result in increased muscle strength if the principles described in this chapter are applied.

What causes a muscle to grow?

A muscle will only grow when it is stimulated to do so by some form of high-intensity exercise. High-intensity muscular contraction, such as the exercises in weight training, trigger the formation of a chemical called creatine. The presence of creatine stimulates the muscle unit to form myosin, a contraction-producing protein discharged within the muscle fiber. The release of creatine results in the production of still more myosin, which in turn stimulates it to produce more contractions. This process continues and, with each cycle, the muscle increases in size.

Why is it that the older we get, the greater the midsection becomes?

In a recent study, young and old men were grouped according to the amount of exercise they did. When percentages of body fat were measured for each group, no difference was found between the young and the old. It was concluded that inactivity, not aging, was responsible for the midsection paunch (Donahue 1988).

MYTHS AND FALLACIES

If stomach exercises don't hurt, they won't work.

"Pain isn't necessary to improve fitness," says James Skinner, director of the Exercise and Sports Research Institute at Arizona State University, "It is a warning that the body has been over-stimulated," (Fain 1988). When you start getting that burning sensation, ease off. Otherwise you'll slow yourself down as well as become more susceptible to injury and soreness.

Sit-ups are the best stomach-flattening exercise.

According to Gary Skrinar, professor of exercise science at Boston University, sit-ups are not the cure-all for bulging stomachs because most people do them incorrectly, often predisposing themselves to back problems. "A better exercise would be the curl-up, where the knees are bent and you just curl your head, shoulders and a little of your upper back off the floor." But it really takes a combination of waist and stomach exercises to completely tone the abdominal muscles.

If I keep lifting weights, I'm going to end up looking like one of those muscled body builders.

Highly unlikely—not unless you're the one in a million with the genes of an Arnold Schwarzenegger. Even then, you'd have to endure the same kind of grueling, high-intensity workouts that most body builders do. "The average person who works out three times a week for a half-hour will never get this look," notes Dr. Robert J. Murphy, head team physician and clinical associate professor of medicine at Ohio State University (Hanc 1985).

I don't want to start building muscle, because if I stop working out my muscle will turn to fat.

Muscle can't turn into fat and fat can't turn into muscle, although a muscle might atrophy with disuse and its place be taken by fat. "The reason many retired athletes often appear overweight is simple," says Joshua Simon, assistant professor of applied physiology and education at Teachers College, Columbia University. "They don't use their muscles as much as they did in competitive days. Thus their muscles get smaller. But they're still eating about the amount they used to, so they gain fat," (Hanc 1985).

BIBLIOGRAPHY

Astrand, P. O., and K. Rodahl. *Textbook of Work Physiology: Physiological Basis of Exercise.* 3d ed. New York: McGraw-Hill, 1986.

Dintiman, George B., and Robert Ward. *Train America! Achieving Peak Performance and Fitness for Sports Competition.* Dubuque, Iowa: Kendal Hunt, 1988.

Dintiman, George B., and Robert Ward. *Sportspeed: Speed Improvement for Football, Basketball, and Baseball.* Champaign, Ill.: Human Kinetics, 1988.

Donahue, Paul G. "Good Health." *Richmond News Leader.* Irving, CA, April 1988.

Fain, Jean. "Stomach Flattening Myths Abound." *Los Angeles Times,* March 1988.

Hanc, John. "Ten Great Myths of Physical Fitness." *Newsday,* November 10, 1985.

Hatfield, Frederick C., and March Krotee. *Personalized Weight Training for Fitness and Athletics.* Dubuque, Iowa: Kendal Hunt, 1984.

Hatfield, Frederic C. *Aerobic Weight Training: The Athlete's Guide to Improved Sports Performance.* Chicago: Contemporary Books, 1983.

Hay, James G., and J. Gavin Reid. *The Anatomical and Mechanical Bases of Human Motion.* Englewood Cliffs, N.J.: Prentice-Hall, 1982.

Katch, Frank I., and William McArdle. *Nutrition, Weight Con-* *trol and Exercise.* 3d ed. Philadelphia: Lea & Febiger, 1988.

Luthi, J. M., et al. "Structural Changes in Skeletal Muscle Tissue with Heavy-Resistance Exercise." *International Journal of Sports Medicine* 7:123 (1986).

Frank D. Rosato, *Fitness and Wellness.* St. Paul: West, 1986.

LABORATORY 4.1

Evaluating Your Muscular Endurance

PURPOSE: To determine whether you possess adequate muscular endurance in the arms, shoulders, and abdominal area.

PROCEDURE

Complete the pull-up or bar dip test (men), modified pull-up (women), and 60-second bent-knee sit-up. Give your best effort on each test.

RESULTS

Use Tables 4.4 and 4.5 to evaluate your muscular endurance in these key areas.

1. Did your score fall in the average or above category in the pull-up, modified pull-up or bar dip test?

   If the answer is no: Describe a weight training or calisthenic program that will increase the muscular endurance in your arms and shoulders. Include the specific exercise, and the number of sets and repetitions you plan to perform.

2. Did your score fall in the average or above category in the sit-up test?

   If the answer is no: Develop an abdominal exercise program (see Appendix J) that will improve your endurance in this important area. Include the specific exercise, and the number of sets and repetitions you plan to perform.

LABORATORY 4.2

Evaluating Your Muscular Strength

PURPOSE: To determine whether you possess adequate muscular strength in the arms, shoulders, and legs.

PROCEDURE

Complete the bench press, shoulder press, biceps curl, and leg press test in your weight room. Your task is to find your 1RM (the maximum amount of weight you can move through a complete range of motion for one repetition). Give your best effort on each test.

RESULTS

Use Table 4.2 to evaluate your scores.

1. Did you meet the minimum standard for your weight in both the bench press and shoulder press?
   If the answer is no: describe a weight training program that will increase the muscular strength in your arms and shoulders. Include the specific exercises and the number of sets and repetitions you plan to perform.

2. Did you meet the minimum standard for your weight in the biceps curl test?
   If the answer is no: describe a weight training program that will increase the strength of the bicep muscles. Include the specific exercises, and the number of sets and repetitions you plan to perform.

3. Did you meet the minimum standard for your weight in the leg press?
   If the answer is no: describe a weight training program that will increase the strength of your quadricep muscles. Include the specific exercises, and the number of sets and repetitions you plan to perform.

CHAPTER FIVE

FLEXIBILITY

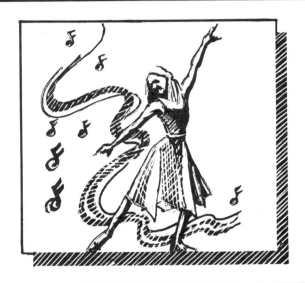

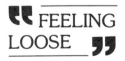 FEELING
LOOSE

? HAVE YOU EVER WONDERED ABOUT:

The importance of flexibility?
Factors that affect flexibility?
How much flexibility you need?
How to measure flexibility?
How to improve your flexibility?
What are some good flexibility exercises?
When you should do flexibility exercises?
Which exercises to avoid?

KEY TERMS

Antagonistic muscle
Ballistic stretch
Flexibility
Passive stretch

Range of motion
Reciprocal stretch (RS)
Sit-and-reach
Static stretch

Flexibility is a health fitness component, and is defined as the range of motion around a joint as determined by the elasticity of the muscles, ligaments, and tendons associated with the joint. Flexibility is specific to each body area, for instance having good hip flexibility does not ensure high shoulder flexibility (it is also possible for one shoulder joint to be more flexible than the other). Although it is not known precisely how much flexibility is enough, it is important that everyone strive to maintain minimum levels of flexibility throughout the aging process. Retaining this fitness component will allow more freedom of movement, coordination will be enhanced, movements will require less work, and your body will be able to handle stress with less chance of injury.

This chapter is a presentation of all aspects of flexibility: assessment, development and maintenance, and injury prevention. In addition to providing flexibility exercises for all body areas, it includes a section on exercises to avoid.

FACTORS AFFECTING FLEXIBILITY

Several factors may influence flexibility, including body type, sex, age, lifestyle, and injuries. Excess fat associated with the endomorphic body type (heavy, rounded body build) may decrease flexibility. Females generally are more flexible than males, and tend to maintain this advantage throughout life. Young children have more flexibility than adults but seem to lose it more quickly than did their more-active counterparts of twenty years ago; the tendency to become inflexible with age is closely associated with inactivity. Many fitness buffs think flexibility is a by-product of aerobic activities such as jogging, swimming, and cycling, but training for these activities is specific. A complete aerobic fitness program will also include flexibility exercises.

The formation of scar tissue following a muscle or connective tissue injury can decrease flexibility. Arthritis and calcium deposits can damage a joint by causing inflammation, chronic pain, and restriction of movement. Failure to regularly exercise the major joints may lead to shortening of muscles and ligaments. Poor posture, long periods of sitting or standing, or immobilization of a limb can have a similar effect. Exercise that over-develops one muscle group while neglecting the opposing group produces an imbalance that also restricts flexibility.

MEASURING FLEXIBILITY

In order to determine the effectiveness of your flexibility routine, it is important to measure your present flexibility level prior to starting a program. Your goals will help you select the appropriate tests. Since there is no such thing as a test of general flexibility, you will need to individually measure those areas you wish to improve. The most commonly used test is the **sit-and-reach**, which is used to measure back and hamstring flexibility. With inactivity and aging, most people lose flexibility in the back and hamstring muscles; this loss may be associated with lower back pain. Laboratory 1 shows how to perform this test. Laboratory 2 provides information on how to evaluate ten additional areas.

DEVELOPING AND MAINTAINING FLEXIBILITY

Flexibility can be improved more rapidly and retained longer than other fitness components. There are three methods used for developing and maintaining flexibility: ballistic, static, and reciprocal stretch (RS). Ballistic and static stretching are the more commonly practiced flexibility methods. **Ballistic** refers to the bouncing style of stretching, such as bobbing up and down in an attempt to touch your toes. Ballistic stretching can activate a reflex in the muscle, which may result in an injury. The safer **static** method refers to holding a stretched position for 10 to 30 seconds. Static stretching may be performed alone or with a partner. Partners must be careful to avoid causing an injury by applying too much pressure. It is important to stretch the muscles only to the point of mild discomfort; pain should not be associated with flexibility exercises.

Another flexibility development method that has gained acceptance is the **reciprocal stretch** or **RS** method. This method can also be performed with a partner. The RS method involves an isometric muscle contraction for five seconds followed immediately by a passive stretch of the **antagonistic** (opposing) **muscle** for five seconds. The following exercise is an example of the RS method for increasing lower back and hamstring flexibility: While lying on your back, raise your leg and grasp it behind the calf. Keeping the leg straight, forcefully press it against your hands in an attempting to lower it. Hold this isometric contraction for 5 seconds and then pull the leg gently toward your head, holding this next stretch position for five seconds.

All three stretching methods will increase the range of motion in 2 to 3 weeks. These increases can be maintained for 8 to 16 weeks with minimal effort, and almost indefinitely with a regular flexibility routine.

FLEXIBILITY CONCEPTS

When developing and conducting a flexibility routine, be sure to apply the following concepts in order to avoid injuries and get the most out of the exercises.

Slow, Gradual Stretching is Favored Over a Jerking Motion. The emphasis should be on stretching slowly, over a 30-second period while gradually increasing the range of motion. When you reach the point of mild discomfort, you will be able to increase the range of motion by gently continuing to apply pressure.

Flexibility Exercises Should Not Produce Pain. The muscle should be stretched to the point of mild discomfort but not pain. Pain indicates a problem and should be avoided.

Flexibility Exercises Should Be Held for 10 to 30 Seconds. When first beginning a flexibility program, the exercises should be held for only about 10 seconds. The time should be increased to 30 seconds as you gradually increase your flexibility.

Flexibility Exercises Should Not be Performed During the Initial Phase of the Warm-up Routine. You should warm up to stretch, not stretch to warm-up. By doing five to ten minutes of calisthenics and other exercises to raise the body's core temperature about 2 degrees Celsius (you should sweat), stretching exercises will be less likely to injure the muscles.

Some Flexibility Activities Should Precede an Aerobic Workout. After elevating your core temperature, but prior to doing your aerobic activity, about five minutes should be devoted to flexibility exercises.

The Majority of Flexibility Exercises Should Follow the Aerobic Activity. The aerobic workout should end with about ten minutes of flexibility exercises, performed during the cool-down period.

Do Not hold Your Breath While Stretching. During any stretching routine, you should not hold your breath. Breathe normally and strive for complete relaxation. Always relax the muscle being stretched and avoid the urge to bounce.

Apply Flexibility Exercises Equally to Both Sides of the Body. In order to maintain good posture as well as increase flexibility uniformly, your routine should include equal time for each side of the body.

EASY WARM-UP EXERCISES

Prior to any stretching, muscles must be made pliable through adequate warm-up exercises. A proper warm-up followed by stretching can improve performance in daily activities and prevent muscle injuries. Any activity that makes you perspire can be considered a warm-up. Gross muscle exercise involving the large muscles is preferred. Keep in mind that the warm-up period is intended solely to increase circulation and elevate the body's core temperature; it is NOT a competition. You should therefore set your own pace, and enter this facet of the workout in a leisurely, upbeat manner.

The warm-up session should last anywhere from five to ten minutes. Choose activities from the following exercises that use mainly the large muscle groups:

1. *General warm-up* (gross motor exercises). Perform a stationary run, vertical or lateral jumps, jump/hop variations, jumping jack variations, rope skipping, light jogging, bench step-ups, etc.
2. *Circle movements.* Do easy circular movements with arms and legs, in both directions.
3. *Agility moves* (shuttle run). Execute short, easy runs involving directional changes between two points 15 to 20 yards apart.
4. *Sport skill mimicking.* Without equipment, demonstrate throwing, kicking, swinging, etc.
5. *Sports participation.* Play the actual sport, but at a much slower pace and reduced intensity.

6. *Isometric exercising.* Contract muscles so that force is exerted against an immovable object. No visible movement takes place during the muscle action. Hold the steady state position for a brief period (6 to 10 seconds) for each position.

A FLEXIBILITY ROUTINE

The eleven exercise general flexibility routine (Table 5.1) is designed to develop flexibility in the major body areas. Before doing any of the exercises, be sure to read the concepts discussed earlier. After completing a warm-up, hold each static position in the routine a minimum of 10 seconds. The stretching process should be done gradually and slowly, adding perhaps two seconds to your hold time each subsequent workout until you can comfortably perform each exercise a maximum of 30 seconds.

FLEXIBILITY EXERCISES TO AVOID

Some flexibility exercises that have been used for years have recently been shown to cause or aggravate rather than prevent injuries. Table 5.2 shows these exercises, along with an alternate, safer exercise that will produce the desired results.

TABLE 5.1   GENERAL FLEXIBILITY ROUTINE

Exercise	Description
Neck	
Head Pull-down	Interlace the fingers and place them behind the neck. Gently pull your head forward, being careful not to exceed the discomfort zone.

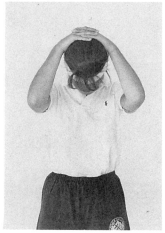

Exercise	Description
Shoulders	
Shoulder Shrug	Raise both shoulders upward simultaneously in an attempt to touch the ear lobes.

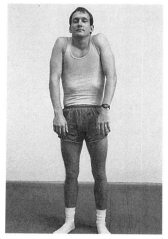

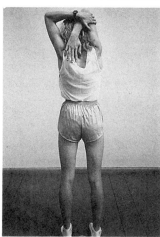

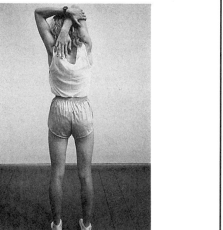

Exercise	Description
Shoulders	
Shoulder Blade Reach	With the right arm, reach behind your head for the opposite shoulder blade. The other hand can be used to assist. Repeat on the other side.

Exercise	Description
Chest	
Shoulder Pull	With the upper arms at shoulder height, steadily move the elbows backward and hold.

TABLE 5.1 GENERAL FLEXIBILITY ROUTINE

Exercise	Description
Lower Back, Hamstrings	
Upper Torso Dangle	Standing; bend forward at the waist with slightly bent knees. Dangle upper torso loosely.

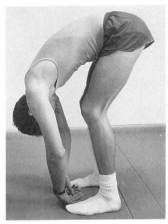

Exercise	Description
Hamstrings	
Toe Touch	Sitting; place right foot on left, lean forward, and grasp upper foot. Repeat.

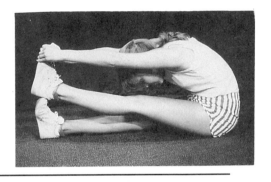

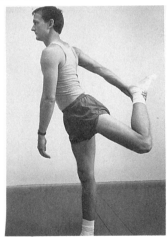

Exercise	Description
Quadriceps,	
Opposite Toe Pull	Balancing on right leg, reach right arm behind back and grasp left ankle. Slowly lean forward, stretching quadriceps and lower back. Alternate legs.

Exercise	Description
Lower Back	
Knee Hug	Lying on your back, keep the leg extended, slightly bent, with heel on the floor. Grasp hands behind right knee, round the back, and attempt to kiss the knee by raising your head.

TABLE 5.1   GENERAL FLEXIBILITY ROUTINE

Exercise	Description
Side Abdominals	
Side Benders	Stand with your feet spread comfortably apart and your arms extended overhead with hands interclasped. Alternate bending and holding to the right side, then the left side.

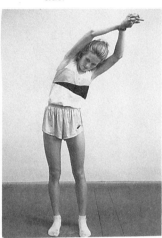

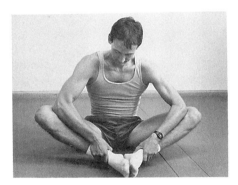

Exercise	Description
Groin	From a sitting position, bend the knees and place the soles of the feet together. Pull the ankles up and push the knees down with the elbows.
Modified Lotus	

Exercise	Description
Calf Stretch	
Lower Leg Calf Stretch	Stand about 3 feet from a wall with your back in a neutral position. Place one foot about six to fourteen inches in front of the other; the back leg should remain straight and the front leg be bent at the knee. Slowly lean forward, keeping both heels on the floor and using your arms to support yourself against the wall. By bending the knee of the back leg you can stretch the Achilles tendon (heel cord). Alternate legs.

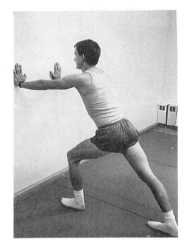

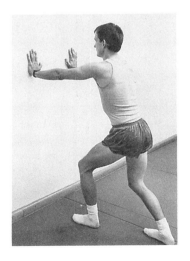

TABLE 5.2   DANGEROUS AND APPROVED FLEXIBILITY EXERCISES

Old Method	**Danger**	**New Method**	**Description**
Neck Roll (circling)	Drawing the head backward could damage the disks in the neck area, and may even precipitate arthritis.	Forward Neck Roll	Bend forward at the waist with the hands on the knees. Gently roll the head.

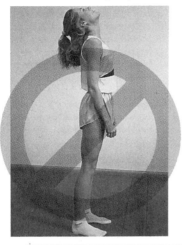
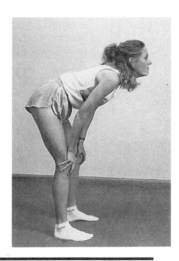

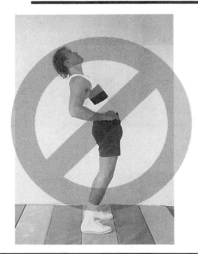
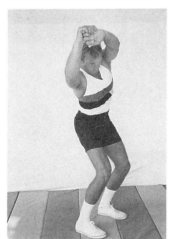

Old Method	**Danger**	**New Method**	**Description**
Trunk Roll (circling)	Undue pressure is placed on the lower back and the sciatic nerve when the knees are straight.	Bent Knee Trunk Roll	Pull the abdomen in and draw the pelvis under, keeping the knees slightly bent. Pretend you are forming a pocket with your midsection and hold.

TABLE 5.2 DANGEROUS AND APPROVED FLEXIBILITY EXERCISES

Old Method	Danger	New Method	Description
Upright Toe Toucher (with knees locked)	Undue strain is placed on the main supporting ligaments in the spine. Excess strain is also placed on the sciatic nerve, and there is danger of undoing a disk.	Sitting Toe Toucher with the knees slightly bent, or Standing Toe Toucher with knees slightly bent.	Bent knee relieves lower back pressure, and still stretches the hamstring muscle group.

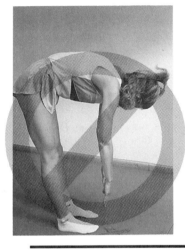
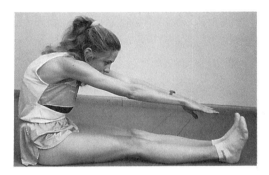

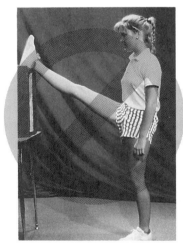

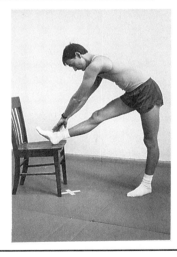

Old Method	Danger	New Method	Description
Ballistic Ballet Bar Stretch	Produces an unnaturally elongated sciatic nerve from excessive stretching of the back of the knee, lower back ligaments, muscles, joints, and disks.	Upright Bent Knee Stretch.	Place the lead leg on a chair with the knee slightly bent. Bend forward slowly as far as possible and hold.

TABLE 5.2 DANGEROUS AND APPROVED FLEXIBILITY EXERCISES

Old Method	Danger	New Method	Description
Quadricep Stretch	If the ankle is pulled too hard, muscle, ligament, and cartilage damage may occur.	Opposite Leg Pull	Grasp one ankle with your opposite hand. Instead of pulling, attempt to straighten the right leg.

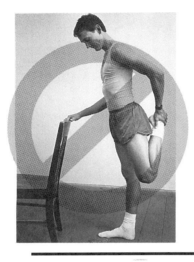 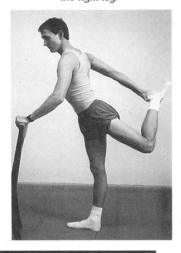

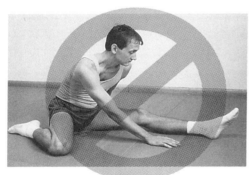 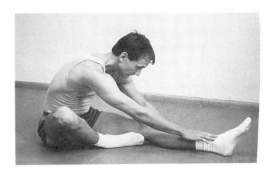

Old Method	Danger	New Method	Description
Hurdler's Stretch	Hip, knee, and ankle are subjected to abnormal stress.	Everted Hurdler's Stretch	Bend the right leg at the knee and slide the left foot underneath. Pull yourself forward slowly by using a towel, or by grasping the toe.

TABLE 5.2 DANGEROUS AND APPROVED FLEXIBILITY EXERCISES

Old Method	Danger	New Method	Description
Deep Knee Bend (or any exercise that bends the knee beyond a right angle)	Excessive stress is placed on ligament, tendon, and cartilage tissue.	Single Knee Lunge	Place one leg in front of your body and extend the other behind. Bend forward at the trunk as you bend the lead leg to right angles.

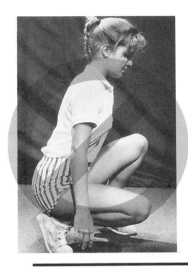

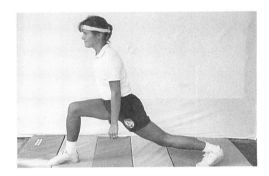

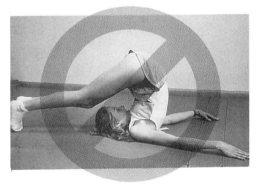

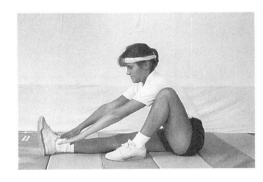

Old Method	Danger	New Method	Description
Yoga Plow	This exercise could overstretch muscles and ligaments, injure spinal disks, or cause fainting.	Extended One-Leg Stretcher	Lead leg extended and slightly bent at the knee; With your foot on the floor, draw the knee of the other leg toward your chest. Bend forward at the trunk as far as possible.

TABLE 5.2　DANGEROUS AND APPROVED FLEXIBILITY EXERCISES

Old Method	Danger	New Method	Description
Inverted Neck/Shoulder Stand	Pressure on the neck could cause a disk injury, or reduce blood flow to the brain	Neck Stretch	Gently pull the head diagonally forward.

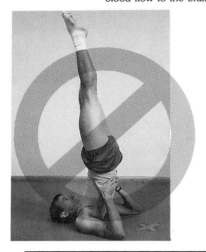

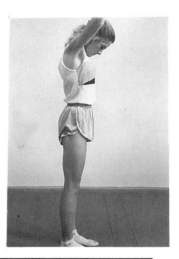

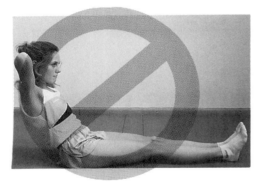

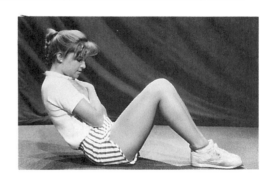

Old Method	Danger	New Method	Description
Straight-leg Sit-up	Produces back strain and sciatic nerve elongation. It also moves the hip flexor muscles, and does not flatten the abdomen.	Bent-knee Sit-up	Cross both hands on your chest, with the knees slightly bent. Raise the upper body slightly to about 25° on each repetition.

TABLE 5.2   DANGEROUS AND APPROVED FLEXIBILITY EXERCISES

Old Method	Danger	New Method	Description
Double Leg Raise	Stretches the sciatic nerve beyond its normal limits, and places too much stress on ligaments, muscles, and disks.	Knee-to-Chest Stretch	Clasp both your hands behind the neck. Draw the knee toward the chest, and hold that position of maximum stretch for 15–30 seconds.

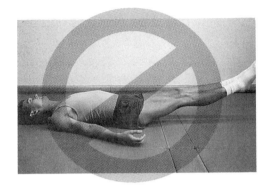 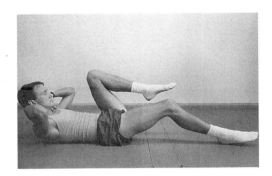

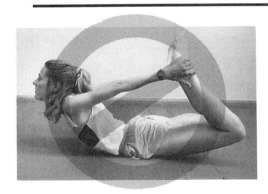 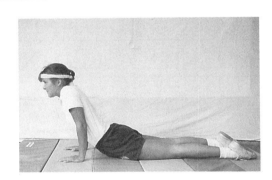

Old Method	Danger	New Method	Description
Prone Arch	Hyperextension of the lower back places extreme pressure on spinal disks.	Stomach Push-up	Lie flat on your stomach, rest on your elbows. Push slowly to raise the upper body as the lower torso remains pressured against the surface.

TABLE 5.2   DANGEROUS AND APPROVED FLEXIBILITY EXERCISES

Old Method	Danger	New Method	Description
Back Bends	Spinal disks can easily be damaged.	No exercise has been approved.	

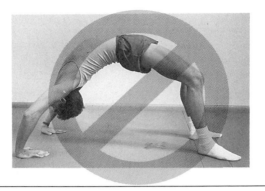

FREQUENTLY ASKED QUESTIONS

Can you have too much flexibility?

It is important to note that too much flexibility can be undesirable. For example, when a ligament is unduly stretched, it can lose elasticity and remain in a lengthened state. When this occurs, the joint becomes unstable and is prone to injury. In a weight-bearing area such as the knee joint, loose ligaments can allow the knee to twist or move laterally, tearing the cartilage and damaging surrounding tissue.

When is the best time to stretch?

There is no sacred time to do stretching activities. If you are involved in high-intensity exercises or competition, it would be beneficial to stretch before each event. For the average exerciser, stretching should follow the aerobic phase of the workout.

What should you do if you experience pain during one of the "common" stretch exercises?

Stop doing it. If you adjust the body or limb position again and the pain does not subside, have the instructor show you another exercise to work the same muscle group. If pain continues, stop all activity until you have seen a physician.

If you have an injured joint or muscle, how soon do you start stretching that area again?

Check with a doctor first to make sure the bones and ligaments will support movement without causing more injury. Allow the area to heal for several days (four to five) until severe pain is gone. Then begin gentle stretches of the injured area to relieve stiffness. It is important not to rush into any exercise that may aggravate the injury.

How do you know if you have stretched enough?

Be aware of your body and how it feels. Can you bend and stretch with ease and without pain? Do the muscles feel loose? DO YOU FEEL GOOD?

MYTHS AND FALLACIES

Muscular individuals have poor flexibility.

Body builders and weight lifters understand the need to include flexibility exercises in their workouts. They are probably more flexible than most, and certainly more flexible than inactive individuals. Without the flexibility exercises, anyone building muscle bulk unevenly could lose range of motion at a particular joint.

Children are naturally flexible.

Although active children will usually maintain flexibility, inactive children will suffer the same fate as their inactive parents—loss of flexibility. The declining fitness of children is demonstrated by poor flexibility scores on national tests.

Lost flexibility is an inevitable part of the aging process.

Aging is not the problem, inactivity is. Most of the research done on aging and flexibility has used inactive subjects. Now that more of the graying population are remaining active, many of the findings regarding aging are being reconsidered.

BIBLIOGRAPHY

Abraham, W. "Exercise-Induced Muscle Soreness." *Sportsmedicine* 7 (1979): 57–60.

Alter, J. *Stretch and Strengthen*. Boston: Houghton Mifflin Co., 1986.

Alter, M. *Science of Stretching*. Human Kinetics (1988): 3–11.

Anderson, R. *Stretching*. Bolinas, California: Shelter Publications, 1980.

Beaulieu, J. *Stretching for All Sports*. Pasadena, California: Athletic Press, 1982.

Corbin, C. "Profiling for Athletics." In *Clinics in Sports Medicine: Profiling*, ed. J. Nicholar and J. Herschberger. Philadelphia: W. B. Saunders Co., 1982.

Croce, P. *Stretching for Athletics*. New York: Leisure Press, 1983.

Deming, H. "A 20-Minute Stretch-Flexibility Warm-up Program." *Athletic Journal* 56 (1976): 32–33.

DeVries, H. *Physiology of Exercise for Physical Education and Athletics*. Dubuque, Iowa: Wm. C. Brown Co., 1980.

Dominiquez, R. "A Surgeon's Warning: Don't Do These Stretches." *Sportsmedicine*, 1984.

Jackson, A., and A. Baker. "The Relationship of the Sit and Reach Test to Criterion Measures of Hamstring and Back Flexibility in Young Females." *Research Quarterly* 57 (1986): 183–6.

Tyne, P., and M. Mitchell. *Total Stretching*. Chicago: Contemporary Books, 1983.

Zimmermans, H., and M. Martin. "Top Ten Potential Dangerous Exercises." *Journal of Health, Physical Education, Recreation, and Dance* 58 (1987): 29–31.

LABORATORY 5.1

The Sit-and Reach-Test

PURPOSE: To measure flexibility of the back and hamstring muscles.

SIZE OF GROUP: Two

EQUIPMENT: Testing box, and a yardstick

PROCEDURE

1. Remove your shoes, and place your feet against the box as shown in Figure 5.1, being sure to keep your knees straight throughout the test.
2. Place one hand on top of the other so the middle fingers are together and the same length.
3. While your partner keeps your knees from bending, lean forward and place your hands on top of the box.
4. Slide your hands along the measuring scale as far as possible without bouncing, and hold for at least one second.
5. Repeat the test two more times and record your highest score to the nearest centimeter. Compare your results with the norms in Table 5.3.

Figure 5.1 The Sit-and-Reach Test

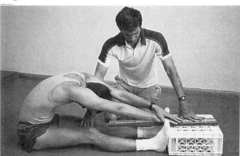

TABLE 5.3 NORMS FOR THE SIT-AND-REACH TEST		
College Females (inches)	**Performance Standards**	**College Males (inches)**
8 or above	Excellent	7 or above
5 to 7	Good	4 to 6
1 to 4	Average	1 to 3
0 or negative	Poor	0 or negative

LABORATORY 5.2

Testing Flexibility

PURPOSE: To test various aspects of flexibility.

SIZE OF GROUP: Alone, or with a partner

EQUIPMENT: A straight-back chair and a stick

PROCEDURE

The following are a few simple flexibility tests that you can administer by yourself, or with a partner. The scoring is "yes or no." Consult the pictures to help you complete this lab.

1. *Neck Flexibility.* Normal neck flexibility will allow you to use your chin to sandwich your flattened hand against your chest.
____Yes   ____No

2. *Elbow and Wrist Flexibility* (Figure 5.2). You should be able to hold your arms out straight with palms up and little fingers higher than your thumbs.
Right arm/wrist ____Yes   ____No   Left arm/wrist ____Yes   ____No

3. *Groin Flexibility* (Figure 5.3A). While standing on one leg, raise the other leg to the side, as high as possible. You should be able to achieve a 90-degree angle between the two legs.
Right leg ____Yes   ____No   Left leg ____Yes   ____No

4. *Groin Flexibility* (Figure 5.3B). While sitting, put the soles of your feet together and draw your heels as close to your body as possible. Try to touch your knees to the floor or to press your upright fists to the floor using your knees.
____Yes   ____No

5. *Trunk Flexibility* (Figure 5.4). While sitting in a straight chair with your feet wrapped around the front legs, twist your body 90 degrees without allowing your hips to move.
Right twist ____Yes   ____No   Left twist ____Yes   ____No

6. *Hip Flexibility* (Figure 5.5). While standing, hold a yardstick or broom handle with your hands shoulder width apart. Without losing your grasp, bend down and step over the stick (with both feet, one at a time) and then back again.
____Yes   ____No

7. *Shoulder Flexibility* (Figure 5.6). In a standing position, attempt to clasp your hands behind your back by reaching over the shoulder with one arm and upward from behind with the other. Repeat, reversing the arm positions.
Right arm top ____Yes   ____No   Left arm top ____Yes   ____No

Continued on next page

LABORATORY 5.2
Continued

Testing Flexibility

Figure 5.2   Elbow and Wrist Flexibility

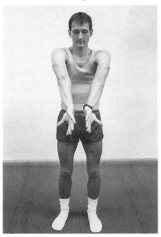

Figure 5.3A   Groin Flexibility

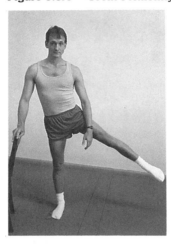

Figure 5.3B   Groin Flexibility

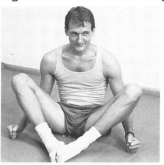

Figure 5.4   Trunk Flexibility

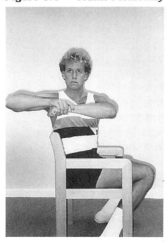

Figure 5.5   Hip Flexibility

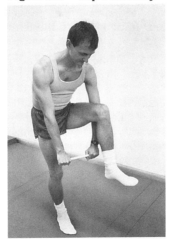

Figure 5.6   Shoulder Flexibility

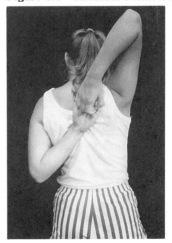

CHAPTER SIX

NUTRITION

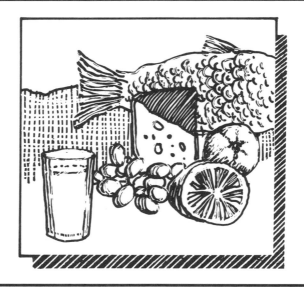

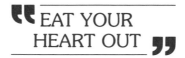EAT YOUR
HEART OUT

? HAVE YOU EVER WONDERED ABOUT:

What's wrong with the American diet?

How to make sure you are eating properly?

How to reduce your cholesterol, salt, and sugar intake?

How much iron and fiber you need?

How to read a food label?

Nutrition during pregnancy?

Nutrition and disease prevention?

The special needs of the exercising population?

How to acquire more energy through nutrition?

How to choose the best cereals?

Whether carbonated drinks are harmful?

KEY TERMS

Amino acids: essential and
nonessential

Carbohydrate loading

Complete and incomplete
proteins

Crude fiber

Dietary fiber

Electrolytes

Fat-soluble vitamins

Fetal Alcohol Syndrome

Glucose

Glycogen

Indicator nutrients

Megavitamin approach

Nutritional density

P.S. ratio

RDA

Saturated fat

U.S. RDA

Water-soluble vitamins

Evidence linking nutrition to health and well-being is mounting. The cliche "you are what you eat" is taking on new meaning as fast food outlets capture more and more of our food dollars. Some experts are of the opinion that the eating habits of the American people have never been worse. The public remains ill-informed in spite of the voluminous material available on sound nutrition. Even those "in the know" are slow to change deeply rooted eating habits and continue to practice poor nutrition.

It is not difficult to identify the problem areas. The typical American diet is too high in calories, too high in fats, too high in protein, too high in salts, too high in sugars, and too low in fresh fruits, grains, vegetables, and water. Teaching people how to correct these eating problems is easy; getting them to actually do it is not.

This chapter summarizes sound nutritional practices for individuals of all ages, dispels common myths, and discusses the special needs of the active, exercising population.

NUTRITION AND YOUR HEALTH

Sound nutritional practice has been accurately summarized by the U.S. Department of Agriculture and the U.S. Department of Health and Human Services in the brochure *Nutrition and Your Health: Dietary Guidelines for Americans* (1981). The application of these principles discussed in this report has considerable impact on health and vitality, and provides a solid nutritional base for people of all ages. Consider each of the seven dietary goals, and decide whether they can be adapted to your eating patterns.

EAT A VARIETY OF FOODS

You need about 40 different nutrients to stay healthy. These include vitamins and minerals, as well as amino acids (from proteins), essential fatty acids (from vegetable oils and animal fats), and sources of energy (calories from carbohydrates, proteins, and fats). These nutrients are in the foods you normally eat.

Most foods contain more than one nutrient. Milk, for example, provides proteins, fats, sugars, riboflavin and other B-vitamins, vitamin A, calcium, and phosphorus—as well as other nutrients.

No single food item supplies all the essential nutrients in the amounts that you need. Milk, for instance, contains very little iron or vitamin C. You should, therefore, eat a variety of foods to ensure an adequate diet.

The greater the variety, the less likely you are to develop either a deficiency or an excess of any single nutrient. Variety also reduces your likelihood of being exposed to excessive amounts of contaminants in any single food item.

One way to assure variety and a well-balanced diet is to select foods each day from each of the four basic food groups listed in Table 6.1.

Fruits and vegetables are excellent sources of vitamins, especially vitamins C and A. Whole-grain and enriched breads, cereals, and grain products provide B-vitamins, iron, and energy. Meats supply protein, fat, iron, and other minerals, as well as several vitamins including thiamine and vitamin B_{12}. Dairy products are major sources of calcium and other nutrients.

There are two major categories of minerals: those required in large amounts such as sodium, potassium, calcium, phosphorus, magnesium, sulfur, and chlorides, and those needed by the body in small amounts (trace minerals). Approximately 15 such trace minerals must be consumed daily: iron, iodine, copper, fluorine, and zinc are the most important.

TABLE 6.1 FOUR BASIC FOOD GROUPS

Basic Food Group	Sources	Daily Serving Needs
Milk	Milk, cheese, yogurt, ice cream	1 cup (8 ounces) milk; 1 to 2 ounces cheese; adults—2 servings, children—3 servings
High proteins	Meat, poultry, nuts, grain protein, dry beans, and peas.	2 to 3 ounces cooked meat, fish, or chicken; 1 cup cooked legumes; 2 servings
Fruits and vegetables	Dark green, leafy or orange vegetables 3 to 4 times weekly, fruit daily	½ cup fruit, vegetable, or juice; 4 servings
Grain	Whole grain, fortified and enriched grain products: bread, cereal, flour	1 slice bread; ½ cup cooked cereal; 1 cup ready-to-eat cereal; 4 servings

Vitamins are essential in helping chemical reactions take place in the body but are required in only small amounts. **Water-soluble vitamins** (vitamin C and the B complex vitamins) are easily eliminated from the body in the urine, and do not accumulate to toxic levels unless enormous overdoses are taken. Since storage is not possible, vitamin C and the B complex vitamins must be consumed on a daily basis. **Fat-soluble vitamins** (vitamins A, D, E, and K) cannot be eliminated if consumed in excess; instead they are stored in the liver and fat cells of the body. Because of this storage capacity, fat-soluble vitamins do not need to be consumed on a daily basis; however, excess consumptions produces toxcity. Vitamins provide no direct source of energy. Most individuals can consume them daily through a balanced diet. Tables 6.2 and 6.3 describe the role of the fourteen known vitamins.

There are no known advantages to consuming excess amounts of any nutrient. You will rarely need to take vitamin or mineral supplements if you eat a wide variety of foods. There are a few important exceptions to this general statement:

Women in their childbearing years may need to take iron supplements to replace the iron they lose with menstrual bleeding. Women who are no longer menstruating should not take iron supplements routinely.

Women who are pregnant or who are breastfeeding need more of many nutrients, especially iron, folic acid, vitamin A, calcium, and sources of energy (calories from carbohydrates, proteins, and fats). Detailed advice should come from their physicians or from dietitians.

Elderly or very inactive people may eat relatively little food. Thus, they should pay special attention to avoiding foods that are high in calories but low in other essential nutrients—for example, fats, oils, alcohol, and sugar.

Infants also have special nutritional needs. Healthy full-term infants should be breastfed unless there are special problems. The nutrients in human breast milk tend to be digested and absorbed more easily than those in cow's milk. In addition, breast milk may serve to transfer immunity to some diseases from the mother to the infant.

Normally, most babies do not need solid foods until they are three to six months old. At that time, other foods can be introduced gradually. Prolonged breast or bottlefeeding without solid foods or supplemental iron can result in iron deficiency.

TABLE 6.2 WATER-SOLUBLE VITAMINS

Vitamins	Deficiency Syndrome		Physiological Role	Food Source	Recommended Daily Allowance[1]	
	Disease	Symptoms			Men	Women
C (Ascorbic acid)	Scurvy	Rough, scaly skin; anemia; gum eruptions; pain in extremities; retarded healing	Collagen formation and maintenance; protects against infection	Citrus fruits, tomatoes, cabbage, broccoli, potatoes, peppers	60	60
B₁ (Thiamine)	Beriberi	Numbness in toes and feet, tingling of legs; muscular weakness; cardiac abnormalities	Changes glucose into energy or fat; helps prevent nervous irritability; necessary for good appetite	Whole-grain or enriched cereals, liver, yeast, nuts, legumes, wheat germ	1.4	1.0
B₂ (Riboflavin)	Ariboflavinosis	Cracking of the mouth corners; sore skin; bloodshot eyes; sensitivity to light	Transports hydrogen; is essential in the metabolism of carbohydrates, fats, and proteins; helps keep skin in healthy condition	Liver, green leafy vegetables, milk, cheese, eggs, fish, whole-grain or enriched cereals	1.6	1.2
Niacin	Pellagra	Diarrhea; skin rash; mental disorders	Hydrogen transport; important to maintenance of all body tissues; energy production	Yeast, liver, wheat germ, kidneys, eggs, fish; can be synthesized from the essential amino acid trypotophan	18	13
B₆ (Pyridoxine)	—	Greasy scaliness around eyes, nose, and mouth; mental depression	Essential to amino-acid and carbohydrate metabolism	Yeast, wheat bran and germ, liver, kidneys, meat, whole grains, fish, vegetables	2.2	2.0
Pantothenic acid	—	Enlargement of adrenal glands; personality changes; low blood sugar; nausea; headaches; muscle cramps	Functions in the breakdown and synthesis of carbohydrates, fats, and proteins; necessary for synthesis of some of the adrenal hormones	Liver, kidney, milk, yeast, wheat germ, whole grain cereals and breads, green vegetables	Not known	
Folacin (Folic acid)	—	Anemia yielding immature red blood cells; smooth, red tongue; diarrhea	Necessary for the production of RNA and DNA and normal red blood cells	Liver, nuts, green vegetables, orange juice	0.04	0.04

TABLE 6.2   WATER-SOLUBLE VITAMINS—Continued

Vitamins	Deficiency Syndrome		Physiological Role	Food Source	Recommended Daily Allowance[1]	
	Disease	Symptoms			Men	Women
B$_{12}$ (Cyano-cobalamin)	Perni-cious anemia	Drop in number of red blood cells; irrit-ability; drowsiness and depression	Necessary for pro-duction of red blood cells and nor-mal growth	Meat, liver, eggs, milk	3.0[2]	3.0[2]
Biotin	—	Scaliness of skin; pain in muscles; sensitivity to light; can possibly lead to eczema	Important in carbo-hydrate metabolism and fatty-acid syn-thesis; probably es-sential for biosyn-thesis of folic acid	Same as other B vi-tamins	Not known	
Choline	—	None observed and identified in man	Synthesis of protein and hormones of adrenal gland; im-portant in mainte-nance of normal nerve-impulse trans-mission	Brains, liver, yeast, wheat germ, egg yolk	Not known	

[1]Values are given for men and women ages 18 to 22 (in milligrams unless otherwise indicated).
[2]Micrograms.
SOURCE: Values are taken from *Recommended Dietary Allowances,* 9th ed. (Washington, D.C.: National Academy of Sciences Publication 1980).

You should not add salt or sugar to the baby's foods. Infants do not need these encourage-ments—if they are really hungry. The foods them-selves contain enough salt and sugar; extra is not necessary.

Some college students, especially those who tend to eat on the run and who have difficulty with meal planning, may also benefit from a vitamin supplement.

MAINTAIN IDEAL WEIGHT

If you are too fat, your chances of developing some chronic disorders are increased. Obesity is asso-ciated with high blood fats (triglycerides and cho-lestrol) and the most common type of diabetes. Each of these, in turn, is associated with increased risk of heart attacks and strokes. Thus, you should

try to maintain ideal weight. (See Chapter 7 for a detailed discussion of weight control through diet and exercise.)

AVOID TOO MUCH FAT, SATURATED FAT, AND CHOLESTEROL

If you have a high blood cholesterol level, you have a greater chance of having a heart attack. Other factors can also increase your risk of heart attack—high blood pressure and cigarette smok-ing, for example—but high blood cholesterol is clearly a major dietary risk indicator.

Populations like ours, with diets high in **sat-urated fats** (found in animal products, nuts, beans, grains, oils, and other substances) and cholesterol (found only in animal fats and oils), tend to have

TABLE 6.3 FAT-SOLUBLE VITAMINS

Vitamin	Deficiency	Excess	Physiological Role	Food Source	Recommended Daily Allowance	
					Men	Women
A	Night blindness; growth decrease; eye secretions cease	Swelling of feet and ankles; weight loss; lassitude; eye hemorrhages	Maintenance of epithelial tissue; strengthens tooth enamel and favors utilization of calcium and phosphorus in bone formation	Milk and other dairy products, green vegetables, carrots, animal liver; carotene in vegetables is converted to vitamin A in the body	1,000[1]	800[1]
D	Rickets; a softening of the bones causing bow legs or other bone deformities	Thirst, nausea, vomiting; loss of weight; calcium deposits in kidney or heart	Promotes absorption and utilization of calcium and phosphorus; essential for normal bone and tooth development	Fish oils, beef, butter, eggs, milk; produced in the skin upon exposure to ultraviolet rays in sunlight	5[2]	5[2]
E	Increased red cell destruction	—	May relate to oxidation and longevity, as well as a protection against red blood cell destruction	Widely distributed in foods; yellow vegetables; vegetable oils, and wheat germ	10[3]	8[3]
K	Poor blood clotting (hemorrhage)	Jaundice in infants	Shortens blood-clotting time	Spinach, eggs, liver, cabbage, tomatoes; produced by intestinal bacteria	Not known	

[1]Retinol Equivalents.
[2]Micrograms.
[3]Milligrams.
SOURCE: Values are taken from *Recommended Dietary Allowances,* 9th ed. (Washington, D.C.: National Academy of Sciences Publication 1980).

high blood cholesterol levels. Individuals within these populations usually have greater risks of having heart attacks than people eating low-fat, low-cholesterol diets.

Eating extra saturated fat and cholesterol will increase blood cholesterol levels in most people. However, there are wide variations among people, related to both heredity, and the way each person's body uses cholesterol.

Some people can consume diets high in saturated fats and cholesterol and still keep normal blood cholesterol levels. Other people have high blood cholesterol levels even if they eat low-fat, low-cholesterol diets.

There is controversy about what recommendations are appropriate for healthy Americans. But for the United States population as a whole, a reduction in the current intake of total fat, saturated fat, and cholesterol is sensible. This suggestion is especially appropriate for people who have high blood pressure or who smoke.

The recommendations are not meant to prohibit the use of any specific food item or to prevent you from eating a variety of foods. For example, eggs and organ meats (such as liver) contain cholesterol, but they also contain many essential vitamins and minerals, as well as protein. Such items can be eaten in moderation as long as your overall cholesterol intake is not excessive. If you prefer

whole milk to skim milk, you can reduce your intake of fats from foods other than milk.

To properly manage your blood cholesterol level:

1. Reduce total body fat.

2. Reduce cholesterol intake—U.S. Dietary Goals suggest an intake of 300 mg. or less daily (see Table 6.4 for the cholesterol content of common foods).

3. Adjust the ratio of polyunsaturated to satu-

TABLE 6.4   CHOLESTEROL CONTENT OF FOODS

Food	Serving Size	Cholesterol (mg)
Milk		
Skim milk	1 c	7
Whole milk	1 c	25
Ice cream	¼ c	50
Meat		
Beef, lean, cooked	3 oz	110
Chicken, flesh only, cooked	3 oz	90
Egg, whole (50 g)	1	255
Egg white (33 g)	1	0
Egg yolk (17 g)	1	255
Fish fillet, cooked	3 oz	60
Heart, cooked	3 oz	130
Kidney, cooked	3 oz	320
Lamb, lean, cooked	3 oz	110
Liver, cooked	3 oz	260
Lobster, cooked	3 oz	170
Mutton, lean, cooked	3 oz	130
Oysters, raw	3 oz (15)	165
Pork, lean, cooked	3 oz	140
Shrimp, flesh only, cooked	3 oz	105
Veal, lean, cooked	3 oz	180
Caviar	1 oz	85
Cheddar cheese	1 oz	30
Creamed cottage cheese	¼ c	9
Cream cheese	1 oz	35
Fat		
Butter	1 tsp	12
Margarine, all vegetable	1 tsp	0
Margarine, ⅔ animal fat, ⅓ vegetable fat	1 tsp	3
Lard or other animal fat	1 tsp	5

SOURCE: Eva May Hamilton and Eleanor Whitney. *Nutrition Concepts and Controversies.* St. Paul: West, 1979. Used by permission.

rated fat (**P:S ratio**) in favor of polyunsaturates (see Table 6.5).

For optimum health, total fat intake should not exceed 30 percent of total diet, with 10 percent coming from saturated fat (usually solid), 10 percent from monounsaturated fat (liquid), and 10 percent from polyunsaturated fat (liquid). Monounsaturated fat, found in olive oil, and polyunsaturated fat, found in vegetable and fish oils, are considered healthy alternatives to saturated fat and cholesterol.

EAT FOODS WITH ADEQUATE STARCH AND FIBER

The major sources of energy in the average American diet are carbohydrates and fats. (Proteins and alcohol also supply energy, but to a lesser extent). If you limit your fat intake, you should increase your carbohydrate calories to supply your body's energy needs.

Complex carbohydrates (fruits, vegetables, and grains) are our major source of vitamins, an important long-term source, and our only source of roughage or fiber. Only vitamin B_{12} is not found in carbohydrates. Complex carbohydrates burn efficiently, leave no toxic waste, and do not tax the liver or raise blood triglyceride levels. Fruits, vegetables, and grains are also foods of high **nutritional density,** providing many nutrients and few calories.

Complex carbohydrates, commonly known as starches, should comprise approximately 48 percent of the American diet. The intake of simple carbohydrates, currently 24 percent of the American diet, should be reduced to 10 percent.

In trying to reduce your weight to ideal levels, carbohydrates have an advantage over fats: carbohydrates contain less than half the number of calories per ounce than fats. Complex carbohydrate foods are better than simple carbohydrates in this regard. Simple carbohydrates, such as sugars (refined and natural) provide calories but little else in the way of nutrients. Complex carbohy-

TABLE 6.5 P:S RATIO

High (more than 2½ times as much polyunsaturated as saturated fat)	almonds corn oil cottonseed oil linseed oil margarine, soft mayonnaise (made with any of the oils in this group)	safflower oil sesame oil soybean oil sunflower oil walnuts
Medium-high (about twice as much polyunsaturated as saturated fat)	chicken breast, skin, thigh freshwater fish	peanut oil semisolid margarines
Medium (about equal amounts of polyunsaturated and saturated fat)	beef, heart and liver chicken heart hydrogenated or hardened vegetable oils	peanut butter pecans saltwater fish solid margarines
Low (about a tenth to a half as much polyunsaturated as saturated fat)	chicken liver lard olive oil	palm oil pork
Very Low (less than a tenth as much polyunsaturated as saturated fat)	beef, both lean and fat butter coconut oil	egg yolk milk and milk products mutton, both lean and fat

SORUCE: Eva May Hamilton and Eleanor Whitney. *Nutrition Concepts and Controversies.* St. Paul: West, 1979. Used by permission.

drate foods, such as beans, peas, nuts, seeds, fruits and vegetables, and whole-grain breads and cereals, contain many essential nutrients in addition to calories.

To date, there is no easy, accurate method of measuring the dietary fiber of various foods. The fiber content of food can easily be determined in a laboratory through use of acids and bases; the portion that cannot be dissolved or broken down into a liquid is referred to as **crude fiber.** When a human being consumes food, the action of the body's enzymes leaves more undigested residue than the lab tests. This is called **dietary fiber.** Dietary fiber is generally two to three times higher than crude fiber. There are no RDAs for dietary fiber but experts recommend approximately 20–30 grams daily from fruits, vegetables, and grains.

There is no reason to add fiber to foods that do not already contain it (see Table 6.6 for the fiber content in various food groups). There is a danger of going overboard and adding large daily amounts of concentrated forms of fiber. Excess fiber decreases the transmit time of food through the digestive system with some components of the fiber binding with trace minerals and rushing them through the system without a chance for absorp-

tion. A reduced absorption of needed calcium and zinc can occur. Once again, moderation is suggested with emphasis on a balanced diet.

AVOID TOO MUCH SUGAR

The major health hazard from eating too much sugar is tooth decay (dental calories). Sweet rolls for breakfast, candy bar snacks at noon, soft drinks in the afternoon, cake and ice cream at mealtime, and one last cookie before going to bed are the kinds of snacking habits that cause tooth decay, gum disease, and even the loss of your teeth. Let's take a look at exactly how it happens.

Decay begins with colonies of bacteria (called plaque) sticking to your teeth. When you eat, the bacteria break down food and change sugar to acid with this sticky bacterial plaque holding the acid to the teeth and attacking the enamel.

Plaque + Sugar = Acid
Acid + Tooth Enamel = Tooth Decay

Luckily, a few things are known about plaque. We can use these facts to help avoid problems:

1. Whether the process will destroy enamel depends upon the hardness of your tooth

Figure 6.1   Fruits, vegetables, and grains should comprise forty-eight percent of daily food intake.

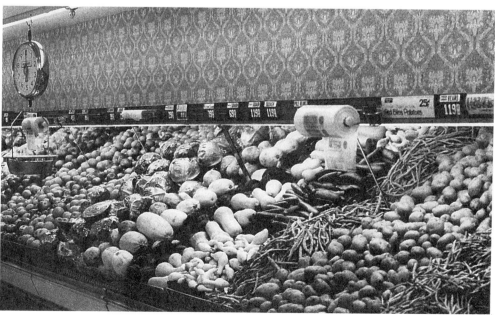

TABLE 6.6   FOODS HIGH IN DIETARY FIBER

Food Item	Approximate Fiber Content	High Fiber Food Examples
Beans	14–18 g per ½ cooked cup	Garbanzo, kidney, baked, lima
Grains	1–3 g per serving	Whole wheat bread, whole grain crackers, oat bran, popcorn
Cereals	3–12 g per serving	Shredded Wheat, oatmeal, Fiber One
Fruits	1–3 g per piece	Fresh fruit with skins (apples, apricots, peaches, peas, plums, orange, banana, dried fruits, etc.)
Nuts and Seeds	2–5 g per ounce	Peanuts, walnuts, peanut butter
Vegetables	3–5 g per ½ cup	Raw vegetables (broccoli, carrots, celery, lettuce, potato, tomato, radishes, mushrooms) and steamed vegetables

Although no RDAs exist for dietary fiber, 10–30 grams daily are recommended from the above food selections.

enamel, the strength of the acids, and the length of time the acids are on your teeth.

2. Most of the damage is done within the first 20 minutes after eating sweet foods. With repeated attacks, enamel is broken down and bacterial plaque reaches the body of the tooth, producing a cavity.

3. A cavity is a bacterial infection that can only be prevented by proper diet and oral hygiene.

4. The more often you snack on high sugar foods, the more often acids form on your teeth and the more often you get cavities. The *amount* of sugar you eat, *how often* during the day you eat it, and the *physical form of the food* (sticky caramel that remains in the mouth is the worst) determine how likely you are to get cavities. When you snack, acids remain for at least 20 minutes. With three meals, you have a 60-minute daily acid attack (3 × 20 minutes = 60 minutes). If you snack on three occasions, you add 60 more minutes for a grand total of 2 hours of acid attack per day—plenty of time to do some damage.

Here are a few things you can do to reduce your chances of plaque buildup and bacterial infection (tooth decay):

1. Reduce the amount of sugar you eat (table sugar is most readily used by bacteria to produce acid and damage teeth) to starve the bacteria. Avoid cough drops, breath mints, and candies that remain in your mouth a long time. These foods feed the bacteria and prolong the attack.

2. Reduce the number of times daily you snack on sugar foods.

3. "Swish" immediately after you drink or eat sugar foods. Rinse the mouth vigorously with water. Remember, the first 20 minutes are the most destructive, and you can remove a lot of the sugar before it starts to form acid.

4. Floss and brush daily to break up plaque before it hardens and organizes into colonies.

5. Eat a balanced diet.

6. Use flourides daily (toothpaste and drinking water).

7. Get topical flouride treatment from your dentist once a year.

The risk of cavities is not simply a matter of how much sugar you eat. The risk increases based on the frequency with which you eat sugar and sweets, especially if you eat between meals and eat foods that stick to the teeth. For example, frequent snacks of sticky candy, dates, or soft drinks may be more harmful than adding sugar to your morning cup of coffee—at least as far as your teeth are concerned.

Obviously, there is more to healthy teeth than avoiding sugars. Careful dental hygiene and exposure to adequate amounts of flouride in drinking water are especially important.

A second major health hazard from excess sugar intake is obesity. Estimates indicate that Americans use on the average more than 130 pounds of sugars and sweeteners a year. This means the risk of tooth decay is increased not only by the sugar in the sugar bowl but by the sugars and syrups in jams, jellies, candies, cookies, soft drinks, cakes, and pies as well as sugars found in products such as breakfast cereals, catsup, flavored milks, and ice cream. Frequently, the ingredient label will provide a clue to the amount of sugars in a product. Sugar intake should be carefully controlled in infancy. Children begin to show a preference for it by age 1 to 1½ years. Their desire (some experts call it addiction) increases until age 19 to 20; it slowly decreases thereafter. The empty calories of sugar are not needed. Consult Appendix C on the sugar content of selected foods as you try to reduce your daily intake.

Contrary to widespread opinion, too much sugar in your diet does not seem to cause diabetes. The most common type of diabetes is seen in obese adults, and avoiding sugar without correcting the overweight factor will not solve the problem. There is also no convincing evidence that sugar causes heart attacks or blood vessel diseases.

AVOID TOO MUCH SODIUM

Table salt contains sodium and chloride—both are essential elements. Sodium is also present in many beverages and foods that we eat, especially in certain processed foods, condiments, sauces, pickled foods, salty snacks, and sandwich meats. Baking soda, baking powder, monosodium glutamate (MSG), soft drinks, and even many medications (many antacids, for instance) contain sodium.

Approximately one-third of our salt occurs naturally in food, another third comes from processed food, and the remaining third comes from the salt shaker. High salt intake has been associated with high blood pressure and an increased risk of coronary heart disease for some individuals. In addition, salt intake must be reduced for those who already suffer from heart, liver, or kidney diseases.

Recognizing the dangers of high salt intake, the Surgeon General of the United States has set as a national health objective the reduction of average daily salt ingestion (as measured by excretion) for adults to 1.6–4 grams (½–1½ teaspoons). Recent analysis of dietary intake has shown that the average salt ingestion for adults, excluding salt added at the table, was within the Established Safe and Adequate Daily Dietary intake range of 1100 to 3300 milligrams set by the National Academy of Sciences in 1980. Salt intake for children appears to be above these guidelines.

Figure 6.2   Breakfast and luncheon meats are high in salt and should be consumed sparingly.

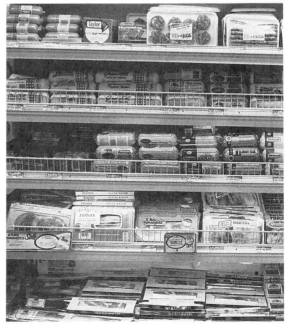

Although a decrease in salt intake has occurred in the United States in the past few years, some experts still feel the typical diet contains three to six times more salt than is necessary. If you wish to reduce your salt intake, consider using less salt in cooking and substitute other spices and flavorings such as garlic, pepper, onion, or lemon; taste food before adding table salt; reduce consumption of cured meats (bacon, ham), luncheon meats, sausages, canned fish (crab, salmon, tuna), American cheese, instant potatoes, potato chips, pretzels, salted nuts, and popcorn; remove salt from the table; and learn to count the milligrams of sodium consumed daily to stay within the recommended ranges.

IF YOU DRINK ALCOHOL, DO SO IN MODERATION

Alcoholic beverages tend to be high in calories and low in other nutrients. Even moderate drinkers may need to drink less if they wish to achieve ideal weight.

On the other hand, heavy drinkers may lose their appetites for foods containing essential nutrients. Vitamin and mineral deficiencies occur commonly in heavy drinkers—in part because of poor intake, but also because alcohol alters the absorption and use of some essential nutrients.

Heavy drinking may also cause a variety of serious conditions such as cirrhosis of the liver and some neurological disorders. Cancer of the throat and neck is much more common in people who drink and smoke than in people who don't.

One or two drinks daily appear to cause no harm in adults. If you drink, you should do so in moderation.

ASSESSING THE GOALS

As previously mentioned, there is little doubt that the application of these goals leads to better health. A good question is whether the 1981 report went far enough in its conclusions.

The Surgeon General of the United States, Dr. C. Everrett Koop, recently referred to an elaborate 712-page *Report on Nutrition and Health* by the Public Health Service (1988) as a landmark

effort that he hoped would have as strong an impact as the 1964 report on Smoking and Health. Although findings did not differ from those presented in *Dietary Guidelines for Americans,* the recommendations cited bring a stronger emphasis to the importance of nutrition and health. Of particular concern in the report is the overconsumption of certain dietary components. The association of an excessive intake of dietary fat to coronary heart disease, some forms of cancer, diabetes, high blood pressure, strokes, and obesity, is strongly stated. Indeed, a reduction in fat is cited as the number one dietary priority (see Table 6.7 for suggested percent fat of dietary intake).

Critics of the goals, while accepting the overall movement toward awareness of consumption, have pointed out several key omissions. In the discussion of obesity, the importance of exercise is not stressed. Iron intake is not listed as a major goal in spite of the fact that national surveys indicate widespread deficiency. Other health hazards such as smoking and sedentary living are also not mentioned.

Still, despite these valid criticisms, the goals do suggest a change toward a more healthful diet, and represent sound nutritional advice.

PROTEIN

Although this is not one of the seven dietary guidelines for Americans, the association of excess protein to a number of diseases in our society is evidence of the need for some people to reduce their protein intake (see Table 6.7 for the suggested percent protein of dietary intake). For others, such as strict vegetarians and the poor, adequate protein is lacking in the diet.

Protein, from the Greek word *proteios,* or "primary," is critical to all living things. In the human body it is used to repair, rebuild, and replace cells. More specifically, protein aids in growth, fluid balance, salt balance, acid/base balance, and in providing needed energy when carbohydrates and fats are insufficient or unavailable.

Protein is produced in the body through protein building blocks called **amino acids.** Some amino acids are produced in the body; others are derived from food sources. **Nonessential** amino acids can be manufactured by the body if not

TABLE 6.7 DIETARY GOALS FOR AMERICANS

		Recommended Percent of Intake
Fat	30	
Saturated		10
Monounsaturated		10
Polyunsaturated		10
Carbohydrate	58	
Simple		10
Complex		48
Protein	12	
Cholesterol		300 mg
Salt		less than 3 g

obtained from the diet. **Essential** amino acids, eight to ten of which must be present in the body in the proper amount and proportion to the non-essential amino acids for normal protein metabolism, cannot be manufactured by the body and must be acquired in our diet. All 22 amino acids must be present simultaneously in order for the body to synthesize them into body proteins that will be used for optimal maintenance of body growth and function.

Humans obtain protein from both animal and plant foods. In general, animal protein is superior to plant protein since it contains all the essential amino acids and contains them in the proper proportions. If one essential amino acid is missing or in the incorrect proportion, protein construction may be blocked. Milk, cheese, meat and eggs are excellent protein choices containing the essential amino acids. Protein exists in vegetables in smaller quantities and may be low in three essential amino acids (lysine, methionine, and tryptophan). Without careful planning it is difficult to consume adequate protein from only vegetable sources since all vegetables and grain products lack some essential amino acids in sufficient quantity. Vegetables and grains must be eaten in proper combinations to provide a balanced supply of amino acids. Rice and beans, for example, represent a complete protein in one meal from vegetables alone.

When this and other correct combinations are included in one meal, vegetarian diets provide all the essential amino acids necessary for human nutrition.

Protein containing all of the essential amino acids is termed high-quality or **complete protein**. Protein from most vegetable sources (such as wheat and corn) that are low in some amino acids and will not support growth and development when used as the only source of protein are termed low-quality or **incomplete protein**. Terms such as *low and high biological value* are also used to describe the quality of protein.

Approximately 54 grams of protein are recommended daily for males and 46 to 48 grams for females in the 15 to 65 age group. Larger individuals, pregnant and lactating women, adolescents, and those who are ill may need slightly more protein. Athletes generally do not need additional protein unless the weather is hot and profuse sweating occurs which produces additional nitrogen loss. Individuals living in extremely hot climates may also need slightly more protein. Approximately 12 percent of calories in the American diet should come from protein.

RECOMMENDED DAILY DIETARY ALLOWANCES

Every five years the Food and Nutritional Board of the National Academy of Sciences' National Research Council reviews for possible revision the **recommended dietary allowances (RDAs)** of certain essential nutrients. The RDAs are categorized for males and females. RDAs are recommendations, not minimum requirements, and represent generous levels of intake of essential nutrients considered to be adequate to meet the known nutritional needs of practically all healthy persons in the United States.

RDAs vary with age, medical conditions, and pregnancy. Individuals with medical problems may have different RDA needs. The margin of safety is substantial and it is estimated that two-thirds of the recommended amounts is adequate for most healthy people. Failing to meet Recommended Daily Allowances for one day does not mean you have a deficient diet; however, RDAs should average out over a five to eight-day period.

RDAs are based on the needs of the average adult male (154 pounds or 70 kilograms). An adult male who weighs 180 pounds will need more of the RDA; a 120-pound male will need less. Women and children also need to adjust their RDA needs accordingly. You can use Appendix D to determine whether your basic nutritional needs are being met. Table 6.1 provides a recommended daily pattern of servings form the basic food groups. Consult this table to determine whether you are eating foods from each of the basic categories.

The **U.S. RDA** is nothing more than a simplified RDA appearing on the labels of food products (see food labeling section of this chapter) showing the percentage of the RDA provided by one serving. The U.S. RDA is a useful guide in meal planning.

NUTRITION LABELING

You now have enough knowledge about RDAs for carbohydrates, fat, protein, vitamins, and minerals, salt, sugar, cholesterol, and calories to evaluate the contents of a food item from the label. In 1973 a law was passed that established a set of standards enabling Americans to base choice of food products upon sound nutritional information. This set of standards resulted in nutritional labeling—the listing on the label of major nutrients found in a food product. The law requires every food label to state:

The common name of the product

The name and address of the manufacturer, packer, or distributor

The net contents in terms of weight, measure, or count

The ingredients in descending order of predominance by weight, prominently displayed in ordinary words (a product that lists sugar as its first ingredient and whole wheat as its last, for example, has a much greater amount of sugar than whole wheat).

The nutrition labeling section of the law states that if a nutrient is added to a food, or if any claim is made on the label, an informational panel must be provided that complies fully with the nutrition labeling requirements. The panel must conform to the following format under the heading "Nutrition Information":

Serving or portion size

Servings or portions per container

Food energy in Calories per serving

Carbohydrate and fat, in grams per serving

Protein, vitamins, and minerals as percentages of the U.S. RDA (a claim may not be made that a food is a significant source of a nutrient unless it provides a minimum of 10 percent of the U.S. RDA in a single serving)

Amounts per serving of the **indicator nutrients** (major nutrients for which intake assumes coverage of all needed nutrients)

The indicator nutrients are:

Required Listings	Optional Listings
Protein	Vitamin D
Vitamin A	Vitamin E
Thiamin (B_1)	Vitamin B_6
Riboflavin (B_2)	Folacin
Niacin	Vitamin B_{12}
Vitamin C	Phosphorus
Calcium	Iodine
Iron	Magnesium
	Zinc

If you choose these eight indicator nutrients in sufficient quantities from the basic four food groups, you are likely to be obtaining 100 percent of the other nutrients also.

A number of terms have been standardized and manufacturers must conform if the terminology is used: *sodium free* (must be less than 5 mg/serving); *very low sodium* (35 mg or less per serving); *reduced sodium* (processed to reduce the regular amount by 75 percent or more); *unsalted* (processed with the normally used salt); *low in Calories* (no more than 40 Calories per serving or 0.9 Cal per gram); *reduced-Calorie food* (at least a third lower in Calories than the food it most closely resembles); *enriched* (returning the mineral iron and the B vitamins thiamin, riboflavin, and niacin to refined products); *fortified* (nutrients have been added to the food that may or may not have been in the original product).

Information on saturated and polyunsaturated fats and cholesterol may also be provided. Protein is listed twice, once in grams and also as a percentage of the U.S. RDA. The percentage is the most important listing since not all protein quality is identical. Eight grams of protein in milk—a complete protein—yield 20 percent of the U.S. RDA for protein, while an identical amount of protein in spaghetti—an incomplete protein—yields only 10 percent of the U.S. RDA.

Study the label carefully. On some items, portion sizes are purposefully large to increase the percentage of RDAs. On others, portion sizes may be small to emphasize a low-calorie food or drink. Keep in mind also that sugar (sucrose, fructose, lactose, levilose, cane sugar, corn syrup, beet sugar, etc.) is listed under a number of different names. Several of these may appear on the same label as the third, fifth, and eighth items, for example, when the cumulative total would force sugar to be listed first. You should also be able to easily identify nutritionally dense foods. Take your time for several weeks until your skill and knowledge improve. Eventually you will become an excellent consumer, needing little more than a glance at the label to tell you what you are buying.

NUTRITION AND PREGNANCY

Although eating for two does not mean doubling your food intake, it does mean that you need additional vitamins, minerals, protein, and calories for you and the growing fetus. Once again, the four food groups serve as your basis for a well-rounded diet. Your physician will counsel you on the need for dietary supplements such as iron, folacin, or vitamins. Six to eight glasses of fluid daily are also an important phase of your diet program.

Daily caloric intake should increase 300 to 350 Calories during pregnancy and 500 Cal during lactation. For most women, exercise may continue during the early stages of pregnancy and resume while they are still lactating.

Most physicians prefer a slow and steady weight gain of 22 to 27 pounds over the full term of the pregnancy. Your physician knows you best and will monitor weight gain and nutritional habits. You may need nutritional guidance for nausea, constipation, and vitamin, mineral, caloric, and fluid needs. Use the physician's services fully; you are paying for them.

FETAL ALCOHOL SYNDROME (FAS)

If you drink too much alcohol during pregnancy, you run the risk of permanently damaging your baby. Everything that affects the mother also affects the baby. Alcohol entering the bloodstream of the mother also enters the baby's bloodstream. With a much smaller liver, and baby must work overtime to sober up—time that cannot be devoted to developing. A number of things could then go wrong with the baby: the baby may be extremely small at birth, the face may not develop properly, eyes may be widely spaced and small, speech may be slurred as the child develops, physical coordination may be impaired, and the baby may be mentally retarded. You can prevent this danger by following these guidelines:

1. Avoid drinking any alcohol during pregnancy if possible.

2. If you must drink, three ounces of alcohol per day (three three-ounce glasses of wine, three cans of beer or three mixed drinks) is the maximum; drinking two one day does not mean you can drink four the next.

3. Avoid drugs unless they are prescribed by a physician.

4. Consult your friends, relatives, husband, and doctor if you cannot control your drinking.

There is no safe drinking limit. The one way to guarantee your baby will avoid **fetal alcohol syndrome** is not to drink at all.

NUTRITION AND DISEASE

Nutrition has been associated with a number of diseases. Excess protein, for example, is now suspected of contributing to osteoporosis, heart disease, and certain types of cancer. When too much protein is ingested, the kidneys excrete more calcium—50 percent more when protein intake is doubled. Such losses over an extended period of time could lead to osteoporosis. The high saturated fat content in meat protein elevates blood cholesterol and contributes to heart disease. High protein intake also increases the incidence of certain types of malignant tumors and accelerates tumor growth. One way to regulate protein intake is to plan at least two meatless meals weekly, reduce egg consumption to two or three weekly, and cut down on dairy products.

Choosing the right foods can lower your risk of heart disease and heart attacks. High intake of animal products such as egg yolks, meat, and organ meats, and saturated fat such as fatty meats, butter, cream, whole milk, chocolate, coconut, and palm oils, raises blood cholesterol. Excess calories increase body weight and fat and may also increase cholesterol and blood pressure. Increasing your consumption of complex carbohydrates contributes to a healthy heart by aiding weight and fat control and replacing harmful saturated fat in your diet. In addition, certain types of fiber such as oat bran may lower blood cholesterol levels. Research also indicates that it may be wise to reduce your consumption of caffeine, alcohol, and salt.

Elaborate research is now underway to clarify the role of diet and nutrition in the development of cancer. Although no direct cause-and-effect relationship has been established, statistical data show that eating some foods and avoiding others may increase or decrease the risks for certain types of cancer. The American Cancer Society offers the following recommendations:

(1) *Avoid obesity.* Those who are 40 percent or more overweight increase their risk of colon, breast, prostate, gallbladder, ovary, and uterine cancers.

(2) *Cut down on total fat intake.* High-fat diets may be a factor in the development of certain cancers, particularly breast, colon and prostate.

(3) *Eat more high-fiber foods* such as whole-grain cereals, fruits and vegetables. Diets high in fiber may help reduce the risk of colon cancer and provide a good substitute for foods high in fat.

(4) *Include foods rich in vitamins A and C in* your daily diet. Dark green and deep yellow fresh vegetables and fruits, such as carrots, spinach, sweet potatoes, peaches, and apricots, are sources of vitamin A. Oranges, grapefruit, strawberries, and green and red peppers—good sources for vitamin C—may help lower the risk for cancers of the larynx, esophagus and the lung. Vitamin C tablets are not recommended because of possible toxicity.

(5) *Include cruciferous vegetables* (flowers with four leaves in the pattern of a cross) in your diet. Cabbage, broccoli, brussels sprouts, kohlrabi and cauliflower may keep certain types of cancers from developing.

(6) *Eat moderately of salt-cured, smoked, and nitrate-cured foods.* A higher incidence of cancer of the esophagus and stomach has been found in areas of the world where these foods are frequently consumed. The American food industry has now developed new processes to help avoid possible cancer-causing by-products in some of these foods.

(7) *Keep alcohol consumption moderate.* Heavy use of alcohol, especially when accompanied by cigarette smoking or smokeless tobacco, increases the risk of cancers of the mouth, larynx, throat, esophagus and liver.

Additional foods and vitamins are currently being studied:

Artificial sweeteners	Saccharin in large doses has caused bladder cancer in lab animals. Aspartame has not been shown to be carcinogenic.
Caffeine	No link has been found to date although some studies suggest a higher rate of bladder and pancreas cancer among heavy coffee drinkers.
Heat-charred meats	Although the effect on the human body is unknown, browned parts of meat or meat cooked at high temperatures by frying, grilling, or broiling contains substances that may be carcinogenic.
Selenium	Preliminary findings indicate that selenium (found in meat, seafood, chicken, grains, and egg yolks) lowers the rate of liver, colon, and breast cancer in laboratory animals; cancer rates are also high in areas of the world where selenium intake is low.

Vitamin E There is no evident that vitamin E, found in wheat germ, margarine, vegetable oils, whole-grain cereals, and green-leaf vegetables, provides any protection.

SPECIAL NEEDS OF THE ACTIVE INDIVIDUAL

Active people who follow the dietary guidelines discussed previously have very few special nutritional needs. There are only four other areas of concern for the exercising individual:

1. Eating enough calories for energy and body repair in order to fully benefit from the conditioning program

2. Drinking sufficient fluid to prevent dehydration and early fatigue

3. Replacing electrolytes lost in perspiration (potassium, sodium, and chloride)

4. Using iron supplements (for females)

EATING ENOUGH CALORIES DAILY

If you are neither losing nor gaining weight, you are taking in the correct number of calories daily to maintain your present weight and fat level. Weigh yourself at exactly the same time of day and under the same conditions, preferably in the morning upon rising. If no weight gain or loss is occurring, there is no real need for complicated record keeping of caloric intake and expenditure, unless you wish to lose or gain weight.

You can estimate the number of calories you need from Table 6.8. Multiply your body weight times the calories recommended per pound for your activity level. This is only an estimate of your needs. Your body has an infallible computer that accurately registers your caloric intake daily: the printout is body weight changes.

REPLACING FLUIDS (WATER)

Water needs depend upon the individual and factors such as body weight, activity patterns, sweat loss, loss through expired air and urine, and the amount of liquid consumed through other foods and drinks. Your body contains about 10 gallons of water. Loss of only 10 percent (one gallon) is disabling, and a 15 percent loss can cause death.

The active individual needs a minimum of six to eight glasses (1½ to 2 quarts) of water daily—much more in hot, humid weather. Drinking too much water generally poses no problem; water is rarely toxic and the kidneys merely excrete it ef-

TABLE 6.8 APPROXIMATE NUMBER OF CALORIES NEEDED DAILY PER POUND OF BODY WEIGHT

Age Ranges	7–10	11–14	15–22	23–35	36–50	51–75
Males:						
Very Active	21–22	23–24	25–27	23–24	21–22	19–20
Moderately Active	16–17	18–19	20–23	18–19	16–17	11–15
Sedentary	11–12	13–14	15–18	13–14	11–12	10–11
Females:						
Very Active	21–22	22–23	20–21	20–21	18–19	17–18
Moderately Active	16–17	18–19	16–18	16–17	14–15	12–13
Sedentary	11–12	13–14	11–12	11–12	9–10	8–9

Sedentary—No physical activity beyond attending classes and desk work.
Moderately Active—Involved in a regular exercise program at least three times weekly.
Very Active—Involved in a regular aerobic exercise program 4–6 times weekly, expending more than 2,500 calories per week during physical activity.

ficiently. The kidneys are also capable of conserving water when the body is deprived by excreting more highly concentrated urine. If the color of your urine is darker than a manila folder, you need to consume additional water (not fluid from other drinks). Surveys of Virginia Commonwealth University undergraduate students suggest that college students are becoming a "waterless society" as Kool-Aid, sodas, coffee, tea, cocoa, beer, and juices dominate our palates. The average daily intake of water, as revealed in a June 1980 survey, was slightly less than two glasses. More soda, coffee, tea, and beer were consumed than water. Again, the body needs plain water for heat regulation and proper functioning of the various systems.

If you exercise in hot, humid weather, thirst sensations will underestimate your needs. By the time you are thirsty, a water deficit has been created that cannot be undone for several hours. Forced drinking, even when no thirst sensation exists, will minimize water deficit, result in more efficient performance, and delay fatigue. Attempt to force an extra 8 to 10 ounces down on each

Figure 6.3   Drink water freely before, during, and after exercise.

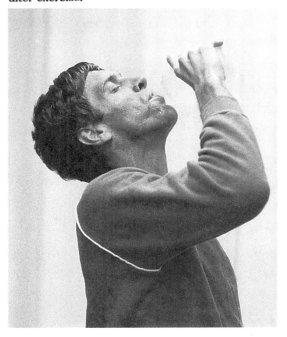

occasion less than 15 minutes before you begin to exercise. Earlier consumption (30 minutes) may fill the bladder and make you uncomfortable during activity. Water will in no way interfere with your performance; drink it freely before, during, and after activity. It is the single most important substance in preventing heat-related illnesses and in restoring the body to normal following exercise in hot, humid weather. For the quickest absorption of fluid, drink plain water (sugar slows absorption) chilled to about 40 degrees Fahrenheit. For additional discussion on water and its role in preventing heat exhaustion, muscle cramps, and heat stroke, see Chapter 8, Table 8.2, and Appendix G.

MAINTAINING ELECTROLYTE BALANCE

Electrolytes—water, sodium, potassium, and chloride lost through sweat and through water vapor from the lungs—should be replaced as rapidly as possible. It is the proper balance of each electrolyte that prevents dehydration, cramping, heat exhaustion, and heat stroke. Too much salt without adequate water, for example, actually draws fluid from the cells, precipitates nausea, and increases urination and potassium loss. A salt supplement is rarely needed in spite of the weather or intensity and duration of exercise. Salt in food and table salt will provide sufficient sodium even for active individuals.

Potassium is critical to maintaining regular heartbeat and also plays a role in carbohydrate and protein metabolism. Profuse sweating over several days can deplete potassium stores by as much as 3 milligrams per day. The average diet provides only 1.5 to 2.5 milligrams daily. If you are a profuse sweater and exercise almost daily, you may need five to eight servings of potassium-rich foods each day. Excellent sources of potassium include orange juice, skim milk, bananas, dried fruits, and potatoes (see Appendix C for additional sources). A potassium supplement is not recommended since too much potassium is just as dangerous as too little.

In the stomach, ionic chloride is part of hydrochloric acid and serves to maintain the strong acidity of the stomach. Loss of too much chloride upsets the acid/base balance of the body. The adding of chlorine to public water provides humans with this valuable element and makes water safe for human consumption.

Water alone will not restore electrolyte balance. One alternative is to use commercially prepared drinks; such as Gatorade or Quick Kick, providing you alter their contents. These drinks are much too high in sugar and should be diluted with water to twice the normal amount for two reasons: to reduce sugar intake and avoid the body's release of insulin and possible reduction in quick energy sources in the blood, and to increase absorption time when the sugar content is less than 3 percent.

While useful before exercise, the addition of electrolytes to water is of minimal value during a workout. Research findings suggest that electrolyte replacement is also secondary in importance to water replacement during rehydration after exercise. Fruit juices have the same pitfalls as commercial drinks and should be diluted with at least twice the amount of water suggested on the can.

REPLACING IRON

Iron deficiency can lead to loss of strength and endurance, early fatigue during exercise, shortening of attention span, loss of visual perception, and impaired learning. Each of these consequences can result in poor sports performance. At a time in our society when the need for iron is increasing, iron intake is reduced due to the removal of iron-containing soils from the food supply and the diminished use of iron cooking utensils. While animals can secure iron from muddy water and soil ingestion, our sanitary society cleans all food carefully and thereby restricts iron intake to selected foods and supplements.

Iron needs and uses vary according to age and sex. It is the only nutrient needed in greater quantity by the female than by the male. Table 6.9 is a summary of these variables to allow you to determine your specific needs. Approximately 85 percent of daily iron intake is used to produce new hemoglobin, with the remaining 15 percent used for new tissue growth or held in storage.

Adolescent girls are more apt to be iron deficient at an age when great concern exists for body figure and appearance. Consequently, food intake may be restricted leading to iron deficiency. During the menstrual period, female athletes of all ages should use an iron supplement.

Iron is more easily absorbed from meat, fish, and poultry than from vegetables. Twice the volume of vegetable iron is absorbed when vegetables and meats are consumed in the same meal. The iron content of 50 common foods is shown in Table 6.10. Estimate your daily intake and compare it to the recommended daily needs.

TABLE 6.9 IRON NEEDS		
Group	**Daily Needs**	**Comments**
Nongrowing adult males	10 mg	Little need for iron; absorb about 10% of iron ingested; daily loss of about 1 mg
Menstruating females	18 mg	Great need for iron; absorb about 20% of iron ingested; daily loss of 5 to 45 mg during menstrual period
Adolescent boys and girls	18 mg	Slightly greater need than that of menstruating females
Preadolescents	4 to 10 mg	

TABLE 6.10 FOOD SOURCES OF IRON SELECTED TO SHOW A RANGE OF VALUE

If You Eat This Size Serving Of:	You Will Receive This % Of Your Need[a] Of IRON:	If You Want 100% Of Your Need[a] Of IRON From This Food:	You Will Have To Eat This Size Serving:
Oysters, raw (1 c, 160 cal)	93%	Parsley, chopped fresh	5 c (100 cal)
Sirloin steak, lean (8 oz, 480 cal)	42	Spinach, cooked	2.9 c (119 cal)
Spinach, cooked (1 c, 41 cal)	35	Oysters, raw	1.1 c (176 cal)
Lima beans, cooked (1 c, 260 cal)	32	Bok choy cabbage, cooked	10 c (200 cal)
Braunschweiger sausage (2 pcs, 205 cal)	30	Beet greens, cooked	6.7 c (268 cal)
Beef liver, fried (3 oz, 185 cal)	29	Dandelion greens, cooked	10 c (350 cal)
Peach halves, dried (10, 311 cal)	29	Mushrooms, raw sliced	20 c (360 cal)
Navy beans, cooked dry (1 c, 225 cal)	28	Clams, raw meat only	21 oz (455 cal)
Soy beans, cooked dry (1 c, 235 cal)	27	Broccoli, cooked	10 c (460 cal)
Hamburger patty + bun (4 oz, 445 cal)	27	Beef liver, fried	10.3 oz (629 cal)
Kidney beans, canned (1 c, 230 cal)	25	Braunschweiger sausage	6.7 pcs (697 cal)
Parsley, chopped fresh (1 c, 20 cal)	20	Lima beans, cooked	3 c (780 cal)
Split peas, cooked (1 c, 230 cal)	19	Navy beans, cooked dry	3.6 c (810 cal)
Beet greens, cooked (1 c, 40 cal)	15	Soy beans, cooked dry	3.7 c (870 cal)
Clams, raw meat only (3 oz, 65 cal)	14	Kidney beans, canned	4 c (920 cal)
Dandelion greens, cooked (1 c, 35 cal)	10	Peach halves, dried	34 halves (1057 cal)
Broccoli, cooked (1 c, 46 cal)	10	Sirloin steak, lean	19 oz (1152 cal)
Bok choy cabbage, cooked (1 c, 20 cal)	10	Split peas, cooked	5.3 c (1219 cal)
Whole wheat bread (1 sl, 70 cal)	5	Whole wheat bread	20 sl (1400 cal)
Mushrooms, raw sliced (1 c, 18 cal)	5	Hamburger patty + bun	15 oz (1691 cal)
Sole/flounder, baked (3 oz, 120 cal)	2	Apple, fresh medium	100 apples (8000 cal)
Apple, fresh medium (1, 80 cal)	1	Cheddar cheese	100 oz (11,400 cal)
Cheddar cheese (1 oz, 114 cal)	1	Nonfat milk	too much (too many cal)
Nonfat milk (1 c, 86 cal)	<1	Sole/flounder, baked	too much (too many cal)

[a]"Your need" is defined here as the U.S. RDA, 18 mg of iron.

SOURCE: Eva May Hamilton, Eleanor N. Whitney and Frances S. Sizer, *Nutrition: Concepts and Controversies* (West, 4 ed., 1988). Used by permission.

CARBOHYDRATE LOADING

The body has an adequate supply of energy available—in the form of glucose and glycogen—for performing regular exercise, or competing in a sport. **Glucose** (sugar in the blood available for energy) and **glycogen** (the chief storage form of carbohydrate) are available in the blood, muscles, and liver, and provide sufficient energy for most workouts. Energy available in the average individual is as follows:

Blood glucose

5 grams × 4 calories per gram = 20 calories

Muscle glycogen

300 grams × 4 calories per gram = 1,200 calories

Liver glycogen

75 grams $\times$ 4 calories per gram = 300 calories

Total Energy in Calories = 1,520 calories

Individuals who compete in marathons, triathalons, and other endurance contests lasting several hours need additional energy and can benefit from a technique referred to as **carbohydrate loading**. This consists of three to four days of vigorous exercise and a high protein/fat, low carbohydrate diet (the depletion stage), followed by three days of little or no exercise and a high-carbohydrate diet (the loading stage). New evidence indicates that the depletion stage is unnecessary. By merely increasing carbohydrate intake three to four days before the contest, liver glycogen stores will double and muscle glycogen stores will more than double. Such an increase provides approximately 3,040 to 3,640 calories of energy—enough for practically any endurance event. Two large, high-carbohydrate meals (300 grams, 1,200 calories per meal) are recommended daily for three to four days.

FREQUENTLY ASKED QUESTIONS

Can nutritional changes add years to your life?

Conclusive data on the effects of different kinds of nutrition are lacking, although long-range studies are now being conducted in the United States. Evidence linking overnutrition to numerous diseases and decreased lifespan is available. There is also some evidence that the lifespan of rats can be doubled by nutritional changes such as "undernutrition;" it is theorized that undernutrition approaches, such as a two-day fast every week (supplemented with a multiple vitamin and sufficient water) or eating only every other day, would prolong life by as much as 40 to 50 years in humans. Only time will tell.

Why is there such concern over cereals?

Cereal manufacturers have long realized that children, not parents, choose the brand. Sales are more dependent upon catchy names (peanut butter smacks, strawberry balls, chocolate squares), prizes inside the packages, games on the outside, items to be purchased with box tops, colorful boxes, and taste than they are upon nutrition.

Read the contents carefully. There are some tasty and nutritious cereals on the market. Some provide nearly 100 percent of daily vitamin and mineral needs with one serving. Some, like those on the market 5 to ten years ago, provide nothing more than pleasant taste, high sugar and calories, and low roughage.

The ideal cereal is low in sodium (none or just a trace); low in fat (one gram or less); low in sugar (two grams or less); moderately low in calories (110 or less); and high in fiber (minimum of three grams) and protein (minimum of two grams). The 1987 results of tests by *Consumer Report* (based on a one-ounce serving without milk) revealed the five most nutritious, least nutritious, and most popular cold cereals:

Most Nutritious	Least Nutritious	Most Popular
Shredded Wheat Flakes in Bran (Nabisco)	Cap'N Crunch (Quaker Oats)	Corn Flakes (Kellogg)
Spoon Size Shredded Wheat (Nabisco)	Cocoa Puffs (General Mills)	Frosted Flakes (Kellogg)
Shredded Wheat (Nabisco)	Trix (General Mills)	Cheerios (General Mills)
Fiber One (General Mills)	Honey Nut Cheerios (General Mills)	Raisin Bran (Kellogg)
Frosted Mini-Wheats (Kellogg)	Golden Grahams (General Mills)	Shredded Wheat (Nabisco)

Do active individuals need more protein?

Since active people have more muscle mass and since muscles are made of protein, logic follows that protein intake should be increased. Once again, the American public pursues the simplistic view that if a little of something is good, a whole lot of it will be fantastic. Let's examine the logic more carefully.

Protein is a poor source of fuel for muscular work; only in starvation or semi-starvation conditions is it burned for energy. Athletes have been shown to perform equally well on 50 grams, 75 grams, 100 grams, or 150 grams of protein daily (approximately 100 to 150 grams are recommended daily). There is no evidence available to suggest that increasing protein intake will improve strength, or muscular or heart-lung endurance.

Acquiring muscle mass is important to individuals in contact sports (football, rugby, lacrosse, etc.) and weight events (decathalon, disc, hammer, shot put, etc.). The nutritional approach to increased muscle has been high protein consumption. Unfortunately, such a diet does not favor muscle growth. Muscles grow in response to one stimulus only: muscle work. To gain one pound of muscle mass, you need to gradually acquire an extra 3,500 calories of food from a balanced diet and engage in an exercise program. If you merely want to gain weight, a high-fat diet is the fastest approach. About one-half pound of muscle weight per week is as much as you should attempt to gain.

Protein is not stored; excess amounts are merely excreted through urination. A high-protein diet is expensive, provides no extra fuel for energy, is high in cholesterol, and is not helpful in gaining muscle mass. For weight gain, energy, and increased muscle mass, the emphasis should be on increased calories from the basic four food groups and a sound strength-training program.

Are carbonated drinks harmful?

Let's analyze the contents of a 12-ounce can of cola. From the view of a nutritionist, it is a poor choice. It contains 40 to 70 milligrams of caffeine, approximately 9 teaspoons of sugar, and 150 calories. In addition, the carbonation irritates the stomach lining. Weight problems, gas, tooth decay, and stomach irritation are some of the possible effects of drinking three to four sodas daily. In addition, caffeine produces a number of other physical changes.

Almost everything you drink, except water, contains approximately 150 calories per 12-ounce serving (juices, beer, sodas, whole milk). While some of these drinks provide necessary vitamins and minerals, most, like carbonated beverages, do not. Sodas merely provide empty calories and approximately one pound of fat for every 23 to 25 cans consumed. With per capita consumption at 493 cans in 1976, the average person is drinking nearly 1½ sodas daily and enough extra calories in non-nutritious fluid to add over 21 pounds of body fat per year.

Are liquid meals helpful before exercise?

Liquid meals, in the form of a 12½-ounce can of protein, fat, carbohydrates, and all known vitamins and minerals, come in chocolate, vanilla, cherry, and strawberry flavors and taste like a milk shake. Each container has approximately 400 calories or about ⅑ of a pound of fat. Examine different brands for taste, caloric content, balance, nutritional value, and shelf life before making a selection. Avoid those that include only predigested foods such as glucose, dextrins, peptides, and amino acids. Manufacturers will provide sample cans if requested.

Let's examine the claims for liquid meals. They are used basically to:

1. Maintain weight balance during the season by increasing caloric intake (two to six cans daily for athletes who have a tendency to lose weight), by decreasing caloric intake at mealtime for the overweight athlete (one can served after each practice to curb appetite), and by controlling and helping to hold present weight
2. Improve endurance during an athletic contest
3. Prevent nausea and cotton mouth during a contest
4. Prevent sluggishness during play
5. Provide a pregame meal that will be burned or used during play; a solid meal is not absorbed and lies in the stomach producing no energy during play, whereas a liquid meal is absorbed in about three hours.
6. Provide a beneficial meal replacement while traveling
7. Provide the necessary nutrients to wrestlers while dieting to ''make weight.''

Liquid meals are effective for weight gain, weight loss, or weight maintenance, and as a pregame meal. Research indicates that they are also reasonably effective in the other areas described above. One study even reported fewer muscle cramps and cases of game sickness with use of a liquid meal.

A liquid formula that can be made in your home vacates the stomach in about two hours (contents: ½ cup nonfat dry milk, 2 to 3 cups skim milk, 1 cup water, ¼ cup sugar, 1 teaspoon vanilla flavoring). This is a less expensive approach that is just as helpful and is very tasty when served cold.

When using liquid meals, be sure to eat a balanced diet from the four basic food groups. Otherwise, you may not receive adequate nutrition.

Are processed foods inferior?

This common untruth is advanced by many health food concerns. The FDA has good control over processing procedures and you can be assured that your food contains ample quantities of vitamins. Unlike organically grown foods, you can also be sure that processed food is free of bacterial or parasitic contamination.

Don't some people actually need vitamin supplements?

Yes. The elderly are often forced to survive on funds so limited that sound nutrition from the basic food groups is impossible. Some women and children may need an iron supplement; lactating and menstruating women have increased needs for folic acid, iron, and calcium, and vegetarians become deficient in certain nutrients. For these groups, a multiple vitamin daily may be helpful.

MYTHS AND FALLACIES

Candy or a Coke before exercise gives you extra energy.

If you eat too much sugar at one time (an entire candy bar), the body releases insulin, starting a series of complex chemical reactions. As a result, glucose is removed from the blood and stored in the fat cells and liver. This process can leave you with less glucose for energy than you would have had without the candy. Sugar also draws fluid from other body parts into the gastrointestinal tract and may contribute to dehydration, distention in the stomach, cramps, nausea, and diarrhea. To avoid these problems, dilute fruit juices with twice the recommended water, add an equal volume of water to commercial drinks, and eat only small quantities of sugar (two to three cubes, a quarter of a candy bar, or a tablespoon of honey). Sugar is absorbed faster than the muscles can use it; thus, more frequent small amounts are preferable to single doses (no more than the small quantities cited above per hour). The body's normal stores of glucose are adequate for activities of short duration; however, for football, rugby, soccer, basketball, marathon running, cycling, and so on, eating small quantities of sugar prior to competition may be helpful. Your blood glucose level will reach a peak about half an hour after consumption, and then rapidly decline.

Honey provides quick energy for exercise.

For years, honey has been used before, during, and after exercise for quick energy and rapid recovery. Since 40 percent of the sugar in honey is fructose which is rapidly converted to glycogen, it has been hypothesized that honey will quickly restore glycogen reserves. Unfortunately, there is no evidence to support this theory. There *are* no quick energy foods, and honey (which contains two sugars—glucose and fructose) has the same limitations and advantages of any sugar.

Large doses of vitamins improve fitness.

Although it is a fact that vitamin deficiency decreases performance and that a little of something (vitamins) is good, the logic that a lot of the same thing is better is not true with vitamins. Vitamins administered in excess do not improve performance or fitness. This **megavitamin approach** (10 to 100 times daily needs) is expensive and dangerous since some vitamins are toxic and can cause illness. If you eat a balanced diet, extra vitamins are totally unnecessary. For the college student who eats on the run and has poor nutritional habits, deficiencies in iron, vitamin C, and some B-complex vitamins are common, and a vitamin supplement may be advisable.

Gelatin improves performance and fitness.

Plain dry gelatin added to some water is almost pure protein. The dessert-type gelatin contains approximately 4 grams protein and 34 grams carbohydrate. Athletes consider gelatin a good source of protein and a precursor for the formation of phosphocreatine, which helps provide anaerobic energy (quick energy). The theory advanced is that gelatin may help form phosphocreatine in the muscle. Research is conflicting, with some findings suggesting beneficial effects and others reporting no effects. The findings of recent research indicate no beneficial effect upon performance.

Wheat germ oil (vitamin E) improves fitness.

While there is some favorable evidence available, most claims for wheat germ oil and vitamin E are greatly exaggerated. As you might suspect, most so-called "miracle" foods are not backed up by scientific research. The following findings by researchers have come to light:

1. Vitamin E is related to muscular function and reproduction. Its exact purpose is not fully understood, although a deficiency can cause sterility.
2. Vitamin E is widely distributed in foods—vegetable oils, wheat germ oil, and green leaves of vegetables—and it can be stored in the body.
3. Large doses of vitamin E produce no toxic effect and are apparently not harmful.
4. Vitamin E appears to be important to physical effort and may assist in delaying fatigue when combined with physical conditioning.
5. When intake is accompanied by exercise, improvements in middle-aged men are noted in blood pressure and electrocardiogram readings.

The unknown factors associated with wheat germ oil are commonly promoted. Some champion athletes do use wheat germ oil and feel it is helpful. According to heart specialists, its use is not considered helpful in repairing the heart after an attack, in preventing heart attacks, or as a treatment for any related disease. A great deal of research is now in progress, and it should be pointed out that there are users from all walks of life (physicians included) who are strong believers in the power of vitamin E. One jar of 500 tablets (a four-month supply) costs over $20, which would buy a lot of nutritious food that also has vitamin E.

Alcohol keeps you warm and improves performance.

First, alcohol is a depressant or sedative, *not* a stimulant. Although the initial one or two drinks seem to improve physical and mental functions, they are actually depressing ability in these areas one to two minutes after consumption. Typing, arithmetic problem solving, memorization, and recall are hindered. The body can oxidize and remove ⅓ of an ounce of alcohol per hour with no ill effects. This is the amount of alcohol in 1 glass of beer, 3 ounces of wine, or 1 ounce of 100-proof whiskey. For this reason, for every two drinks taken, a three-hour waiting period is suggested before driving or performing any complex task.

Second, alcohol does *not* help to warm you up on a cold day. The initial increase in warmth comes from dilation of blood vessels near the skin. Actually, heat loss is increased and you are more susceptible to chilling.

Third, alcohol is not a good source of energy, although it is rapidly absorbed. There are also many other reasons why you should not drink beer or alcohol:

1. Reaction time, strength, and skill are impaired by its use. Even alcohol taken the night before will decrease performance in a contest the following day.
2. Alcoholic drinks are high in calories and may cause a weight problem.
3. A balanced diet is rarely attained by those who overuse alcohol.
4. Numerous serious diseases are related to overuse of alcohol.
5. Alcohol consumed before a contest, a common practice in some countries, increases the likelihood of violence during play.

Milk cuts your wind and brings on early fatigue.

Some people believe that milk, especially when taken before exercise, will cut your wind, hinder performance, or curdle in the stomach and cause cotton mouth (dryness and discomfort).

Drinking milk or putting it on cereal does not result in fatigue or loss of fitness. The flow and condition of the saliva are related to perspiration, water loss, and emotions rather than to any type of food. Also, milk curdles in the stomach as a necessary part of digestion—no upset stomach occurs. In fact, milk is an alkaline and may buffer or neutralize excess acid.

More than 30 million Americans are intolerant of milk. For these individuals, other dairy products (yogurt, hard cheeses, and other products with a lower lactose content) can sometimes be substituted. A relatively new product called Lact-Aid can be added to a quart of milk to provide the deficient lactose enzyme and make milk tolerable. Skim milk, lower in calories and saturated fat, is a wise choice for most college students.

Caffeine improves heart-lung endurance.

Coffee, tea, cola, and cocoa have one common ingredient: caffeine, a member of the speed, pep pill, and amphetamine group. Coffee contains the most caffeine (100 to 150 milligrams), whereas tea (60 to 70 milligrams), cola drinks (35 to 55 milligrams), and cocoa (50 milligrams) contain somewhat less. Caffeine stimulates the nervous system, particularly the brain. A number of other bodily changes occur:

1. Resting heart rate increases.
2. Metabolism of body cells increases 10 to 25 percent, accelerating the burning of food for energy and raising oxygen requirements.
3. Appetite is decreased.
4. Blood pressure rises.
5. Arteries to the brain and head region are constricted (this aids in relieving headaches since many headaches are caused by over-dilated arteries that stretch the small nerve fibers to the artery walls; heavy coffee drinkers may develop headaches that are relieved after a cup of coffee.

The controversy continues over the value of caffeine. Many long-distance runners swear by their one to two cups of coffee an hour before the big race, convinced that fatigue will be delayed and performance will improve. Research findings are conflicting, with some studies supporting the use of caffeine and others revealing no benefits in strength and endurance activities. It is sound nutritional practice to limit coffee intake to one to two cups daily and to avoid consumption on an empty stomach (eat breakfast or lunch first).

Bread is fattening and should be avoided.

Bread is not only nutritious (carbohydrates, calcium, iron, niacin, riboflavin, thiamine, protein) but is also low in calories (approximately 70 calories per slice). A sandwich becomes fattening as butter, margarine, cheese, mayonnaise, meat, and other items are added to it—bread gets the blame.

Large doses of vitamin C prevent the common cold.

The vitamin C (ascorbic acid) controversy lingers on. There is still no solid evidence that massive doses (up to 5,000 milligrams daily) do anything but cause diarrhea, excessive urination, and kidney stones. Handshaking (after touching a mucous membrane of nose or eyes) and breathing in the droplets from a sneeze or cough are the two leading ways a cold is spread. Having extra vitamin C in the body does not seem to be the factor that determines why one individual develops a cold and the other does not. Although extra vitamin C will not improve physical performance, it is important to consume adequate amounts daily, particularly during the growth period since ascorbic acid deficiency is associated with growth impairment.

Exercise should be avoided following a meal.

People have avoided exercise after eating for years, believing that it hindered digestion and brought on stomach cramps.

Exercise does slow acid secretion and the movement of the food downward toward the stomach during the activity period and for 1 hour or so later. After this time, there is actually an increased digestive action. In the final analysis over a 12 to 18 hour period, exercise has little effect on the speed of digestion. Performance could be hindered, although it is unlikely, from discomfort due to overeating, a feeling of lethargy, or a fullness that does not permit the diaphragm to descend completely during inhalation.

It is dangerous to swim immediately after eating.

The belief that swimming after eating will cause stomach cramps and contribute to drowning has no basis. Stomach cramps are quite uncommon compared to cramps in the feet and the backs of the lower legs. It is wise to wait approximately 45 minutes after eating if you are a beginning swimmer and become tense about the water. The real killers are panic and poor judgment, although stomach cramps get the blame.

BIBLIOGRAPHY

Consumer Reports. *1987 Buying Guide Issue.* Mt. Vernon, NY: Consumer's Union of the United States, Inc.

Dintiman, George B., and Jerrold Greenberg. *Health Through Discovery,* 4th ed. New York: Random House, 1989.

Dintiman, George B., and Robert Ward. *Train America! Achieving Peak Performance and Fitness for Sports Competition.* Dubuque, Iowa: Kendal-Hunt, 1988.

Hamilton, Eva May Nunnelley, Eleanor Ness Whitney, and Frances Sienkiewicz Sizer. *Nutrition: Concepts and Controversies.* 4th ed. St. Paul: West, 1988.

Hegarty, Vincent. *Decisions in Nutrition.* St. Louis: Mosby, 1988.

Frankle, Reva T., and Mel-Urh Yang, eds. *Obesity and Weight Control: The Professional's Guide to Understanding and Treatment.* Rockville, Md.: Aspen, 1988.

Office of Disease Prevention and Health Promotion. *The 1990 Health Objectives for the Nation: A Midcourse Review.* Washington, D.C.: U.S. Department of Health and Human Sciences, 1986.

Public Health Service. *Report on Nutrition and Health.* Washington, D.C.: U.S. Government Printing Office, 1988.

Science and Education Administration/Human Nutrition. *Nutrition and Your Health: Dietary Guidelines for Americans.* Washington, D.C.: U.S. Government Printing Office, 1981.

Williams, Melvin H. *Nutrition for Fitness and Sport.* Dubuque, Iowa: Wm. C. Brown Co., 1988.

LABORATORY 6.1

Sound Meal Planning

PURPOSE: To analyze personal eating habits.

SIZE OF GROUP: Five to seven in each group

PROCEDURE

1. Each group chooses one of the following meal or snack times:
breakfast
lunch
dinner
evening snacks

2. Each group compiles a list of the foods and portions they commonly eat for the meal or snack time selected.

3. Meals are analyzed for caloric content, saturated fat, polyunsaturated fat, sugar, ingredients from the basic four food groups, and water consumption.

4. Meals are then altered to accomplish the following nutritional objectives:
Reduce saturated fat
Reduce sugar
Reduce caloric intake
Increase polyunsaturated fat intake
Consume a variety of foods from the basic four food groups each day
Consume a minimum of six glasses of water per day

RESULTS

1. Each group summarizes its findings and gives a brief presentation to the entire class.

2. Basic suggestions are given to change eating patterns at each meal time.

3. Students are asked to follow the altered meal for at least one week and report to the instructor, in writing, their findings: how they feel, difficulty in preparing, weight changes, etc.

LABORATORY 6.2

A Survey of Nutritional Myths

PURPOSE: To uncover nutritional myths in your institution.

SIZE OF GROUP: Five in each group

PROCEDURE

1. Each group chooses one of the following subject areas:
   a. Nutrition and sport
   b. Nutrition and disease prevention and cure
   c. So-called magic foods
   d. Vitamin and mineral supplements
   e. Food additives

2. Each group develops a one-page questionnaire (open-ended) to guide interviews concerning nutritional beliefs and practices in its subject area.

3. Each group devises a plan for randomly selecting subjects on the college campus. The questionnaire and random selection procedure must be approved by the instructor before proceeding.

4. Each student in every group interviews 25–50 subjects. An interview should take less than five minutes.

RESULTS

1. Summarize your data and give a brief presentation to the class.
2. Evaluate the soundness of the nutritional knowledge of those interviewed.
3. Identify the nutrition myths on your campus and their extensiveness.

CHAPTER SEVEN

WEIGHT CONTROL

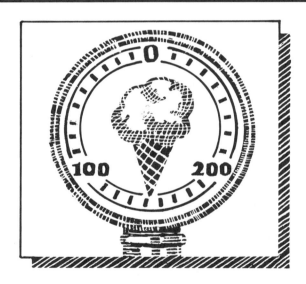

" THE BATTLE OF THE BULGE "

? HAVE YOU EVER WONDERED ABOUT:

How to measure your body fat?

How to accurately determine your frame size?

How to lose weight and body fat safely?

How exercise helps you control your weight?

The untold dangers of dieting?

Skin wrinkling and dieting?

How to determine your caloric needs?

The reason weight loss slows down after the first few days?

The importance of fat and sweets in your diet?

How to avoid getting too many fat cells?

How to get rid of stomach fat?

How to avoid weight gain when you stop smoking?

KEY TERMS

Adipose tissue
Afterburn
Anorexia nervosa
Bulimia
Cellulite

Hyperplasia
Hypertrophy
Metabolic rate
Set point theory

During the late 1800s in the United States, human muscle power provided one-third of the energy needed to run our farms, homes, and factories. Today, muscular effort contributes only one-half of 1 percent of the energy. Most Americans work in office-bound, service-oriented jobs and use business machines, pens, and pencils to accomplish their tasks. The sources of energy and the types of jobs we hold have changed over the past 100 years. However, since the human body remains the same, we are actually victims of our technology-oriented lifestyle. Approximately 50 million men and 60 million women between the ages of 18 and 79 are overweight. In addition, approximately 10 to 20 percent of the school-aged population are overweight or obese.

In the past ten years, the average weight of American adults has increased seven to ten pounds. At all ages we are growing several pounds heavier each decade. Unfortunately, this weight gain is not muscle; what we are accumulating is more body fat. This trend should be brought under control, because obesity is associated with a number of disorders including atherosclerosis, high blood pressure, diabetes, heart/lung difficulties, early heart attack, and other ailments. The death rate of obese men between the ages of 15 and 69 is 50 percent greater than that of normal-weight persons and 30 percent greater than that of persons classified as overweight. For every 10 percent above normal weight, it is estimated that lifespan is decreased by one year.

This chapter examines the critical aspects of weight control: (1) causes; (2) assessment of body weight and body composition; (3) special diets; and (4) the role of exercise in weight control to assist the student in managing his or her body weight and body fat during the critical college years.

CAUSES OF OBESITY IN THE UNITED STATES

Inactivity and overeating are the two most common causes of obesity. Activity can do much to offset weight gain and regulate tendencies to put on unwanted pounds. Weight gain of genetically obese mice, for example, is drastically reduced by treadmill exercise. In humans, a group of Harvard University students, forced to double their daily caloric intake from 3,500 to 7,000, suffered no weight gain when involved in a vigorous exercise program.

Social, genetic, and psychological factors may also result in overeating and obesity. In only a small percentage of cases are glandular and other physiological disorders related to weight problems, although many obese people blame these. Sedentary living and excessive eating are the two greatest perpetuators of obesity; both can be controlled.

SET POINT THEORY OF OVERWEIGHT AND OBESITY

The human body regulates many functions with tremendous precision. Body weight is one of these functions. Each individual appears to have an ideal biological weight (the **set point**) and will defend it against pressure to change. Those who do succeed in losing or gaining weight generally return to their set point weight in a few months or years. Within 24 hours of beginning a low-calorie diet, metabolic rate (amount of calories burned at rest) slows by 5 to 20 percent as a means of conserving energy, making it more difficult to lose weight. The body is convinced it is starving and this calorie conservation is the only way of "hanging on" for a longer period of time. In addition, once excess fat cells become depleted, they signal the central nervous system to alter feeding behavior through an increase in caloric intake so that the set point can be maintained. In other words, an internal "thermostat" regulates body fat and weight and triggers an increase in food intake when fat and weight are lowered too much. Overcoming the set point is difficult. Will power and other factors that aid in tolerating physical discomfort are poor matches for a computer-like system that never quits.

Research suggests that one of the ways to "take it off and keep it off" may be to lower the thermostat. "Seesaw" approaches to weight loss may have the opposite effect and actually result in a higher setting on the thermostat. The body now begins to defend an even higher weight. This may explain why people who complete several cycles of losing and regaining ten or more pounds find it nearly twice as hard to lose weight and twice as easy to gain weight on their next attempt. Vigorous, regular exercise combined with a sound nutritional plan appears to lower the thermostat over time and allows you to lose and maintain a lower weight.

EARLY EATING PATTERNS

Most experts agree that eating habits formed in infancy and childhood carry over to the adult years (Frankle and Yang 1988, 345–350). An experiment with rats suggests the importance of early habits. The milk of one mother was shared with four babies (plenty of milk for each), while the milk of another mother was shared with as many as twenty-two babies (enough for only small quantities for each). Rats from the smaller litter became fatter and healthier in appearance. After weaning, all rats had unlimited food available. The rats who were accustomed to eating less continued to eat less while the other rats continued to eat more. After a short period of time the thin rats overtook the fat rats in growth, showed much less heart and

vessel disease, and subsequently outlived the fat rats. In addition, the thin rats exercised daily on the treadmill while the fat rats did not.

Environmental forces influence eating patterns more than physiological forces such as hunger. Negative eating behavior may begin in infancy. Some researchers have found that bottle feeding predisposes infants to obesity. Approximately three times more bottle-fed than breast-fed babies are overweight. Bottle feeding fails to provide the solace of breast feeding and tends to produce anxiety, which provokes overeating. Breast-fed babies also learn to stop feeding after removing the richest portion of the milk (the highest fat content) which gives way to more watery milk as the session progresses. The bottle does not provide such a natural mechanism, so that bottle-fed babies require more calories to satisfy their hunger.

Perhaps a more important problem is feeding babies solid foods too early. Starting solid foods early in infancy may contribute to the production of excess fat cells. Experts recommend that parents not start their infants on solid foods before the age of six months (a month or two earlier for very large or fast-developing babies).

There is little danger that a growing child will be obese if he or she is the one who decides when to stop eating each meal. Forcing children to "clean the plate" is a mistake and is the same as forcing a child to overeat. Making sweets plentiful, using them as rewards, and placing emphasis on the "fat baby" also compounds the problem, shortens lifespan, encourages premature heart disease, forms undesirable eating habits that will be continued throughout life, and destines the child to a life of restricted eating due to a high number of fat cells formed in early life. A lean child with a great deal of energy and vitality is healthier and more likely to be healthy later in life. There is no stage in life when excess fat is desirable. It is therefore advisable to start children off right and avoid overstuffing. If their mechanism to "push up" from the table when full is destroyed, they are certain to need plenty of real push-ups in the adult years to control their weight.

FAT CELLS

Our fat cells are formed early in life and increase in both size and number until the end of adolescence. Although research is inconclusive, it appears that diet decreases only the size of fat cells, not the number. With a large number of fat cells formed, return to an overweight condition is much easier. This partially explains why adults who were heavy babies have difficulty keeping their weight down. These extra cells may affect metabolism and result in the need for fewer calories to maintain normal weight than are needed by someone who generally remains at normal weight.

The number of fat cells in the human body grows rapidly during three stages of development: (1) the last trimester of pregnancy, (2) the first year of life, and (3) the adolescent growth spurt. Fat is acquired by increasing the size of existing adipose cells (**hypertrophy**) and by new fat cell formation prior to adulthood (**hyperplasia**). It is doubtful that new fat cells are formed after age 21 or so.

There is a large difference in the number of fat cells in different people. A nonobese person has approximately 25 to 30 billion fat cells while an extremely obese person may have as many as 260 billion. A formerly obese adult is never "cured" because weight loss does not reduce the number of existing cells. Fat cell size (anytime in life) and number (before adulthood) can only be reduced by modifying nutrition and exercising regularly. Preventing excess fat cell formation centers around developing healthy eating and exercise habits early in life and during the growth spurt. Children who exercise have been found to develop fewer and smaller fat cells. In adults, the same approach will successfully reduce the size of fat cells and cause weight and fat loss.

GENETICS

It is now clear that the genes we inherit do influence our weight. Children of overweight or obese parents are much more likely to be overweight or obese. It is important to keep in mind however, that environment is still critical. How you live in terms of exercise and eating and drinking habits can overcome your genetic tendency to be thin or fat.

METABOLIC FACTORS

The number of calories burned while the body is at rest but not sleeping is referred to as **metabolic**

rate. A 10-percent decrease in metabolism would result in an annual weight gain of 26 pounds. Aerobic exercise increases metabolic rate both during and after the exercise bout. The afterburn continues for 20 minutes to several hours, depending upon the duration and intensity of the workout. Coffee, tea, cocoa, colas, amphetamines, and other drugs increase metabolic rate. In midafternoon metabolism tends to slow, making this an excellent time for tennis, walking, aerobic dance, cycling, or other activities to boost metabolic rates. As one ages, metabolism slows until, at age 50, metabolic rate may have increased significantly. This slowing is less dramatic in individuals who continue to exercise throughout their lives.

BODY COMPOSITION

Many people have an ideal image of their body that they would someday like to achieve. This image may include how they looked in high school or how they appeared during their competitive athletic years. For some individuals, such an image may be unrealistic. Regardless of your motivation to change, there are several methods derived from research or actuarial tables that may help you set realistic goals for a better-looking body.

A simple method of estimating proper body weight is to use the Metropolitan Life Insurance height-weight tables (Table 7.1). Charts of so-called ideal weight for men and women were developed by the Metropolitan Life Insurance Company based upon data associating average weights by height and age with long life. Early figures indicated that those who weighed less than average lived up to 20 percent longer. These charts, which became the national guide for determining overweight and obesity for the general public, advocated the theory that "the greater the weight, the greater the risk of death." Recent research, such as the Framingham Project, has questioned the validity of such data. Findings reveal that less-than-average weights involve health risks greater than those associated with overweight and that the American preoccupation with "thin" is not a health advantage.

Authorities do not dispute that people who are much heavier than average (more than 20

TABLE 7.1 METROPOLITAN LIFE INSURNACE HEIGHT-WEIGHT TABLES

	Men[1]					Women[2]		
Height		Small	Medium	Large	Height		Small	Medium	Large
Feet	Inches	Frame	Frame	Frame	Feet	Inches	Frame	Frame	Frame
5	2	128–134	131–141	138–150	4	10	102–111	109–121	118–131
5	3	130–136	133–143	140–153	4	11	103–113	111–123	120–134
5	4	132–138	135–145	142–156	5	0	104–115	113–126	122–137
5	5	134–140	137–148	144–160	5	1	106–118	115–129	125–140
5	6	136–142	139–151	146–164	5	2	108–121	118–132	128–143
5	7	138–145	142–154	149–168	5	3	111–124	121–135	131–147
5	8	140–148	145–157	152–172	5	4	114–127	124–138	134–151
5	9	142–151	148–160	155–176	5	5	117–130	127–141	137–155
5	10	144–154	151–163	158–180	5	6	120–133	130–144	140–159
5	11	146–157	154–166	161–184	5	7	123–136	133–147	143–163
6	0	149–160	157–170	164–188	5	8	126–139	136–150	146–167
6	1	152–164	160–174	168–192	5	9	129–142	139–153	149–170
6	2	155–168	164–178	172–197	5	10	132–145	142–156	152–173
6	3	158–172	167–182	176–202	5	11	135–148	145–159	155–176
6	4	162–176	171–187	181–207	6	0	138–151	148–162	158–179

[1]Weights at Ages 25–59 Based on Lowest Mortality. Weight in Pounds According to Frame (in indoor clothing weighing 5 lbs, shoes with 1″ heels).

[2]Weights at Ages 25–59 Based on Lowest Mortality. Weight in Pounds According to Frame (in indoor clothing weighing 3 lbs, shoes with 1″ heels).

SOURCE OF BASIC DATA: *1979 Build Study* Society of Actuaries and Association of Life Insurance Medical Directors of America, 1980. Courtesy of the Metropolitan Life Insurance Company.

percent above ideal weight) obtain health benefits from weight reduction. For those in normal health who are at average or near average weight, there is no health benefit in losing weight. In fact, one should beware the lean-and-hungry look. The key factor that determines what is too much or too little is body fat (**adipose tissue**), not total body weight.

DETERMINING IDEAL BODY WEIGHT FROM HEIGHT-WEIGHT CHARTS

Check your weight according to Table 7.1. Frame size can be estimated by wrapping the thumb and index finger around the opposite wrist. If the thumb and finger do not meet, you have a large frame. If they just meet or barely overlap, you have a

medium frame, and if they overlap, you have a small frame. For a much more accurate indicator of frame size, follow the directions in Table 7.2 to obtain the exact width of your elbow.

Use Table 7.3 to find your ideal weight range. Since height-weight charts provide only a rough guide to the determination of ideal weight, use the lowest weight to the midpoint from Table 7.1 as the range for your desirable body weight. See how your actual weight compares. If you fall 20 percent below or above the range for your height, you are roughly classified as underweight or overweight; 30 percent above classifies you as obese. Keep in mind that this table provides only a rough guide to desirable weight and it is not uncommon for an individual to be fall considerably above a weight range and still possess normal or even below-normal body fat. This is particularly common in muscular men and women.

TABLE 7.2 APPROXIMATING FRAME SIZE

Men		Women	
Height in 1″ Heels	**Elbow Breadth**	**Height in 1″ Heels**	**Elbow Breadth**
5′2″–5′3″	2½″–2⅞″	4′10″–4′11″	2¼″–2½″
5′4″–5′7″	2⅝″–2⅞″	5′0″–5′3″	2¼″–2½″
5′8″–5′11″	2¾″–3″	5′4″–5′7″	2⅜″–2⅝″
6′0″–6′3″	2¾″–3⅛″	5′8″–5′11″	2⅜″–2⅝″
6′4″	2⅞″–3¼″	6′0″	2½″–2¾″

Extend your arm and bend the forearm upward to a 90 degree angle. Keep fingers straight and turn the inside of your wrist toward your body. If you have a caliper, use it to measure the space between the two prominent bones on *either side* of your elbow. Without a caliper, place thumb and index finger of your other hand on these two bones. Measure the space between your fingers against a ruler or tape measure. Compare it with these tables that list elbow measurements for *medium-framed* men and women. Measurements lower than those listed indicate you have a small frame. Higher measurements indicate a large frame.

SOURCE: 1979 *Build Society* of Actuaries and Association of Life Insurance Medical Directors of America, 1980. Courtesy of the Metropolitan Life Insurance Company.

DETERMINING THE PERCENT OF BODY FAT

A more important consideration in goal setting for a better looking and healthier body does not involve body weight, but the amount of fat (adipose tissue) you have accumulated. It is possible to be within the range of suggested weight on a height-weight chart and still possess excessive fat. Weight control is simply another name for "fat-control," and the measurement of body fat is essential in setting goals for your body.

Current records show that the average percent of body fat is approximately 25 percent for females and 20 percent for males. Individuals are considered obese if they possess more than 30 percent (men) or 35 percent (women) body fat. Ideal percentages are 20 percent for women and 15 percent for men.

Since most body fat lies just under the skin, it is possible to pinch certain body parts, measure the thickness of two layers of skin and the connected fat, and estimate the total percent of fat on the body.

Figures 7.1A to 7.1D show how to measure skinfolds using a set of fat calipers. You may obtain these calipers from a local university's health and physical education department. Another possibil-

ity is to use any type caliper that measures the thickness of wood or metal. The procedure for measuring skinfold thickness is to grasp firmly with

TABLE 7.3 IDEAL WEIGHT RANGE: WORKSHEET AND EXAMPLE

Example

Subject (female) height	5′4″ + 1″ = 5′5″
Actual weight	150 pounds
Frame size	medium
Ideal range	127 to 134
Your height	+ 1″ =
Actual weight	
Frame size	
Ideal range (low to mid)	

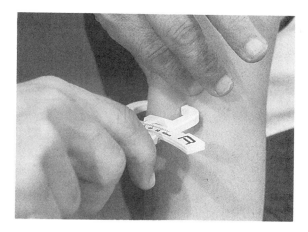

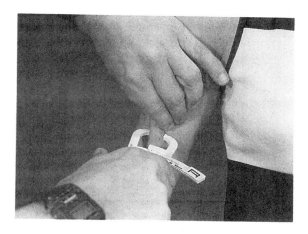

Figure 7.1C   Subscapula Skinfold

Figure 7.1D   Suprailiac Skinfold

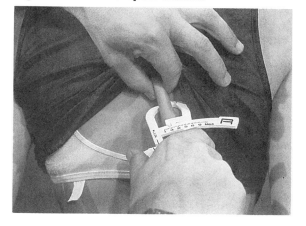

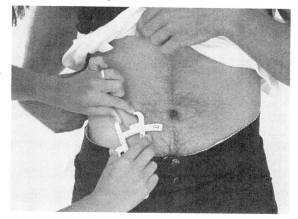

the thumb and forefinger a fold of skin and sub-cutaneous fat (fat just under the skin), pulling it away from the underlying muscle tissue. Attach the jaws of the calipers one centimeter below the thumb and forefinger. If there is ever a question as to whether the pinch encompasses muscle, the tester should ask the subject to contract the underlying muscle. Take all measurements on the right side of the body with the subject standing.

1. Using a skinfold caliper, obtain measurements at the following sites:
   Triceps. With the arm resting comfortably at your side, take a vertical fold parallel to the long axis of the arm and midway between the tip of the shoulder and the tip of the elbow.

Biceps. With the arm in the above position, take a vertical fold halfway between the elbow and top of the shoulder on the front of the upper arm.

Subscapula. Just below the scapula (shoulder blade), take a diagonal fold across the back.

Suprailiac. Just above the crest of the ilium (hip bone), take a diagonal fold following the natural line of the iliac crest.

2. Add these four measurements and find your percent of fat based upon Table 7.4.

Now that you have estimated your percent of body fat, consider the standards for body fat presented in Table 7.5.

TABLE 7.4   FAT AS A PERCENTAGE OF BODY WEIGHT BASED UPON THE SUM OF FOUR SKINFOLDS, AGE, AND SEX

Skinfolds (mm)	Percent of Fat, Males (age in years)				Percent of Fat, Females (age in years)			
	17–29	30–39	40–49	50+	16–29	30–39	40–49	50+
15	4.8	—	—	—	10.5	—	—	—
20	8.1	12.2	12.2	12.6	14.1	17.0	19.8	21.4
25	10.5	14.2	15.0	15.6	16.8	19.4	22.2	24.0
30	12.9	16.2	17.7	18.6	19.5	21.8	24.5	26.6
35	14.7	17.7	19.6	20.8	21.5	23.7	26.4	28.5
40	16.4	19.2	21.4	22.9	23.4	25.5	28.2	30.3
45	17.7	20.4	23.0	24.7	25.0	26.9	29.6	31.9
50	19.0	21.5	24.6	26.5	26.5	28.2	31.0	33.4
55	20.1	22.5	25.9	27.9	27.8	29.4	32.1	34.6
60	21.2	23.5	27.1	29.2	29.1	30.6	33.2	35.7
65	22.2	24.3	28.2	30.4	30.2	31.6	34.1	36.7
70	23.1	25.1	29.3	31.6	31.2	32.5	35.0	37.7
75	24.0	25.9	30.3	32.7	32.2	33.4	35.9	38.7
80	24.8	26.6	31.2	33.8	33.1	34.3	36.7	39.6
85	25.5	27.2	32.1	34.8	34.0	35.1	37.5	40.4
90	26.2	27.8	33.0	35.8	34.8	35.8	38.3	41.2
95	26.9	28.4	33.7	36.6	35.6	36.5	39.0	41.9
100	27.6	29.0	34.4	37.4	36.4	37.2	39.7	42.6
105	28.2	29.6	35.1	38.2	37.1	37.9	40.4	43.3
110	28.8	30.1	35.8	39.0	37.8	38.6	41.0	43.9
115	29.4	30.6	36.4	39.7	38.4	39.1	41.5	44.5
120	30.0	31.1	37.0	40.4	39.0	39.6	42.0	45.1
125	30.5	31.5	37.6	41.1	39.6	40.1	42.5	45.7
130	31.0	31.9	38.2	41.8	40.2	40.6	43.0	46.2
135	31.5	32.3	38.7	42.4	40.8	41.1	43.5	46.7
140	32.0	32.7	39.2	43.0	41.3	41.6	44.0	47.2
145	32.5	33.1	39.7	43.6	41.8	42.1	44.5	47.7
150	32.9	33.5	40.2	44.1	42.3	42.6	45.0	48.2
155	33.3	33.9	40.7	44.6	42.8	43.1	45.4	48.7
160	33.7	34.3	41.2	45.1	43.3	43.6	45.8	49.2
165	34.1	34.6	41.6	45.6	43.7	44.0	46.2	49.6
170	34.5	34.8	42.0	46.1	44.1	44.4	46.6	50.0
175	34.9	—	—	—	—	44.8	47.0	50.4
180	35.3	—	—	—	—	45.2	47.4	50.8
185	35.6	—	—	—	—	45.6	47.8	51.2
190	35.9	—	—	—	—	45.9	48.2	51.6
195	—	—	—	—	—	46.2	48.5	52.0
200	—	—	—	—	—	46.5	48.8	52.4
205	—	—	—	—	—	—	49.1	52.7
210	—	—	—	—	—	—	49.4	53.0

In two-thirds of the instances the error was within ± 3.5% of the body-weight as fat for the women and ± 5% for the men.

SOURCE: J. V. G. A. Durnin and J. Womersley. "Body Fat Assessed from Total Body Density and Its Estimation from Skinfold Thickness." *British Journal of Nutrition* (published by Cambridge University Press, Cambridge) 32 (1974): 95. Used by permission.

TABLE 7.5 FATNESS RATINGS OF COLLEGE MEN AND WOMEN BY PERCENT BODY FAT

Rating	Men	Women
Very low fat	5 to 7.9	12 to 14.9
Low fat	8 to 10.9	15 to 17.9
Ideal fat	11 to 14.9	18 to 21.9
Above ideal fat	15 to 17.9	22 to 24.9
Over fat	18 to 22.9	25 to 27.9
High fat	23+	28+

If you are overfat according to the guidelines above, you may want to consider an exercise and diet regimen to lose body fat and body weight. When setting goals for body fat loss, you can expect to lose about .5 millimeter of body fat per week with an appropriate combination of diet and exercise. For example, if you are now classified as "above average fat," it is realistic to expect to reach the "average fat" category after a 10-week program.

Now take the time to estimate how many calories you need to maintain your present body weight based on the formula described below. These figures will help you determine how much to increase your daily energy expenditure and how much to reduce your daily caloric intake. Rate your level of physical activity from the list below and honestly estimate your activity level:

Very inactive (sedentary)	13 points
Slightly inactive (occasional physical activity)	14 points
Moderately active (frequent physical activity)	15 points
Relatively active (almost always on the go, physically active)	16 points
Frequent strenuous activity (at least daily hour of running or other physical activity)	17 points

Multiply your rating times your actual weight. In our example from Table 7.3, assume the female is sedentary (13 points). To maintain a body weight of 150 pounds she would take in 1950 calories per day (150 × 13). In theory, if she is consistently eating more than 1950 calories a day, she is gaining weight. Now, multiply your physical activity rating times your ideal weight from Table 7.3 (use the low point on the range). This new figure is the number of calories you need per day to maintain that ideal weight. Our sedentary female would need 1651 calories to maintain 127 pounds. The difference between her "actual" weight maintenance intake and "ideal" weight maintenance intake is 299 calories of energy that she will need to cut back per day to arrive at and maintain her ideal weight. If our sedentary female also increases her daily energy expenditure through a more active lifestyle by 299 calories a day, it would take her only half as long to reach her ideal weight. Now complete these calculations for yourself.

With the methods given here in addition to your feelings of how much you should weigh, you can arrive at a realistic weight and body fat goal to maintain throughout your life.

SPECIAL DIETS

You may want to lose weight when you notice that you can pinch more than an inch anywhere, possess too much body fat, or have increased your weight by 5 percent or more. When you take in more calories per day than you expend, these extra calories are stored as fat. For example, with the accumulation of about 3,500 excess calories, one pound of fat is stored.

Four factors determine where body fat forms when overeating and underexercising occur:

1. *Sex.* Men have a lower percentage of fat to body weight than women. Men tend to add fat around the waist. Women deposit fat around the buttocks, upper arms, thighs, breasts, and stomach.

2. *Genetic influences.* Each individual inherits a certain body type, making some people more likely to be overfat than others.

3. *Exercise habits.* In general, the more physically active individuals are, the leaner they will be.

4. *Endocrine secretions.* In only a small percentage of cases, glandular disorders lead to excess fat deposits.

Excess calories are stored as fat, usually in areas of the body where musculature is understimulated. Fat gain often occurs over extended periods of time. As we age, we generally become less active and our metabolism slows. By age 70, we need about 15 percent fewer calories than we needed at age 20. Ideally, you should be 5 to 10 pounds lighter at age 50 than at age 25.

Weight loss that occurs slowly is more likely to be permanent. If you are a considerably overfat person, allow a minimum of three months to reach your target weight. A weight loss rule of thumb is to lose no more than two to three pounds weekly. Rapid weight loss by crash diets or fasting is dangerous and should be avoided. If you plan to lose more than 5 percent of your body weight, consult a physician before you begin. Spreading weight loss over time allows you to learn and adjust to new, sensible eating habits that you are more likely to maintain in the future.

HOW TO CHOOSE A DIET

Although there are hundreds of diets published in magazines and books, it is still difficult to choose a safe, effective plan that you can follow. *Consumer Guide Magazine* states that the best choices are balanced diets that have an adequate amount of protein, not more than 20 percent of fat (predominantly unsaturated fats), no less than 60 grams of carbohydrates daily, and a minimal amount of sugar.

Remember that calories do count, and the difference between the number of calories you consume daily and those you burn will determine the amount of weight you lose. Daily caloric intake should be at least in the 1200 to 1800 range.

Consider the following suggestions for a safe, effective diet:

1. Using Table 7.3, and the system offered to determine caloric needs (Chapter 6), decide how much you would like to weigh. Carefully count calories and do not exceed this daily target. If you reduce your caloric consumption, weight loss will occur.

2. Eat three meals each day from the four basic food groups (see Table 6.1, Chapter 6).

3. Consume a minimum of six glasses of water daily.

4. Do not skip meals, and avoid snacking between meals.

5. Eat a light meal in the evening (less than one-third of your daily caloric intake.) Evidence from research suggests that eating a heavy meal at night is not conducive to losing weight.

6. Avoid laxatives, stimulants, and diuretics, and use a multiple vitamin each day.

There are a number of reasons why the average diet lasts only five to seven days: boredom, monotony, lack of energy, fatigue, depression, complicated meal planning and purchasing, and failure to lose weight and body fat. These problems are much less likely to exist with individuals who are on a sound diet. Unfortunately, diet choices are generally a direct result of wide magazine, book, or television publicity that reveals some secret, easy method of shedding pounds and fat. The publicity and the gimmick that just might work are too much for many consumers to resist. Once again, the writer gets rich and consumers endanger their health. Table 7.6 summarizes and evaluates the special claims of many of the widely publicized diets. Study the table carefully before running the risk of illness, permanent health damage, or worse. Consult your physician for a sound, nutritionally well-balanced diet and an exercise program that are right for you before using anything found in best sellers or home magazines.

Table 7.7 lists some sound diet choices that don't include the detriments found in fad diets. Study the table to review the characteristics of a good diet. Before attempting any of these diets, however, it is best to consult a physician about your personal needs.

Combating hunger is one of the greatest hardships for the dieter. Unfortunately, poor diet choices and practices add to the problem. Eating only one or two meals a day, for example, causes hunger to become intense and may actually result in the consumption of more calories in two meals than would have been consumed in three. A sound alternative to skipping meals is to eat a good breakfast and to eat less at lunch and dinner. Eating smaller portions and having six meals per day in-

TABLE 7.6 SUMMARY AND EVALUATION OF WIDELY PUBLICIZED DIETS

Diet	Special Claims	Allowable Foods	Evaluation
Gimmick Diets Pritikin Program	Low-fat diet and exercise combine to produce weight loss.	Whole grains, vegetables, legumes, fruit; snack on raw vegetables all day and one portion from dairy, grain, and fruit groups	High fiber content causes gas and diarrhea, low protein is insufficient, diet difficult to follow. Contains one-quarter normal fat intake, fairly well-rounded, devoid of cholesterol, salt, and artificial sweeteners.
Save Your Life Diet	Fiber added to six different foods (1 cup of bran daily), claims weight loss is increased through fast transport of food through the digestive tract.	Vegetable group emphasized plus adding 1 cup of bran to six foods; meats and eggs deemphasized	Side effects may include flatulence, frequent defecation, and soft, bulky stools. Too much fiber binds to some trace minerals and may result in their passing through the system without being absorbed.
Nibbling Diet	Eating smaller portions will result in fewer calories than three meals per day and snacking.	Low carbohydrate, high protein, and nutritious snacking	With careful calorie counting, weight loss is likely to occur; difficult to get a balanced diet, and not easy to follow for long periods of time.
Cellulite Diet	Promises removal of the "fat gone wrong" (so-called fat, water, and toxic wastes).	High in fruits and vegetables; low-fat and carbohydrate intake, involves kneading the skin and massage under heat lamps to melt the fat away	No medical condition known as cellulite exists. The fat being described as cellulite cannot be eliminated by a combination of diet and massage (see the Cellulite section of this chapter).
Cooper's Fabulous Fructose Diet	"Fructose" is used as a crutch to help lose weight comfortably, to maintain constant blood sugar level, keep up energy, and satisfy the sweet tooth.	High protein intake and 1 to 1½ ounces of fructose supplement	Weight loss may occur from caloric deficit, not from use of a fructose supplement. Fructose does not help you consume fewer calories and contains the same number of calories as sucrose (4 per gram).
Lecithin, Vinegar, Kelp & B$_6$ Diet	Grapefruit and lecithin burn off excess fat by regulating metabolic rate.	One teaspoon of vinegar with each meal	No claim (grapefruit or vinegar) can be supported.

TABLE 7.6   SUMMARY AND EVALUATION OF WIDELY PUBLICIZED DIETS—Continued

Diet	Special Claims	Allowable Foods	Evaluation
The Body Clock Diet	Claim is made that when you eat is nearly twice as important as the number of calories you consume. Lose by eating breakfast like a "king," lunch like a "prince," and dinner like a "pauper."	Any type of food can be consumed or any diet can be adapted to the body clock diet.	There is no convincing evidence that eating the big meals early in the day will cause significant weight loss without very close calorie counting. The somewhat hidden implication that calories do not count is inaccurate.
High Protein Diets New You Diet Doctor's Quick Weight Loss Diet Complete Scarsdale Medical Diet Miracle Diet for Fast Weight Loss Easy No Flab Diet	"Specific Dynamic Action" (SDA) is the basis for some high protein diets: extra calories are burned through the process of digesting protein.	Lean meats and poultry, fish, seafood, eggs, and low-fat cheese; no calorie counting	SDA has no basis. Protein calories are no more or less important than carbohydrate calories. Diets are boring, hard to follow, lacking in vitamins, minerals and fiber, and can increase blood serum cholesterol levels; dangerous for pregnant women and a poor choice for everyone who wants weight loss to be permanent after a change in eating habits.
High Fat Diets Dr. Atkin's Super Energy Diet Calories Don't Count Diet	In the absence of carbohydrates, stored fat is mobilized and burned for energy. Fat mobilizing hormone (FMH) is said to be activated to fuel your body with the fat stores.	Unlimited fatty foods: bacon, meat, mayonnaise, rich cream sauces, etc.; no calorie counting and avoidance of fruits, vegetables, sugars, starches, bread, and potatoes	Carbohydrates are needed to completely oxidize fat. If in short supply, fat cannot be used completely and fatigue occurs. Ketone bodies build up in the blood and are excreted in the urine. The existence of a fat mobilizing hormone (FMH) has never been substantiated. The diet neglects the four food groups, is dangerous for pregnant women, is high in cholesterol, and is likely to produce mostly water weight loss that is temporary.

TABLE 7.6 SUMMARY AND EVALUATION OF WIDELY PUBLICIZED DIETS—Continued

Diet	Special Claims	Allowable Foods	Evaluation
Low Carbohydrate Diets			
Diet of a Desperate Housewife The Drinking Man's Diet No Breakfast Diet Dr. Yudkin's Lose Weight, Feel Great Diet The Brand New Carbohydrate Diet	Claims are similar to those stated for high protein diets—a state of ketosis[1] provides a condition more favorable for fat loss.	Protein in unlimited amounts with little or no carbohydrates permitted	Most weight loss is water and temporary, fatigue results from insufficient carbohydrate intake and is potentially dangerous over prolonged periods of time. These diets fail to provide adequate foods from the basic four food groups and are difficult to follow.
One Food Diets			
Grapefruit, egg, poultry, melon, banana, steak, beer, fruit, juice, yogurt, rice, etc.	Dieters must concentrate on the food they choose, use a multiple vitamin, and drink plenty of fluid.	Only the one food is permissible.	It is impossible to obtain the proper nourishment even with a vitamin supplement, boring, nearly impossible to follow, fails to change eating habits, and it is a short-term approach and potentially very dangerous.
Pill Diets			
Dexedrine, Dietac, Dexatrim, VitaSlim Capsules, PVM, Appedrine	Appetite is depressed and/or fluid loss occurs.	Medication is designed to restrict total caloric intake. Often used in conjunction with a variety of specific diets.	Amphetamines may curb appetite and cause exhilaration. These pills are members of the "pep" or speed group and possess the same dangers. Diuretics result in fluid loss and may cause dehydration. Nervousness, tremors, insomnia, hypertension, depression, and dependence are some of the possible side effects of heavy amphetamine use.

TABLE 7.6 SUMMARY AND EVALUATION OF WIDELY PUBLICIZED DIETS—Continued

Diet	Special Claims	Allowable Foods	Evaluation
Starvation and Fasting Diets The Zip Diet Lockjaw Zen Macrobiotic Diet Liquid Protein Diet	Diets eliminate practically everything but liquids. Jaws are sometimes wired shut (lockjaw diet) to aid will power; with no calories from chewable foods, weight loss will occur rapidly.	Liquids and some foods	These diets are extremely dangerous, lacking in vitamins, minerals, and roughage. Anemia is likely. The Liquid Protein Diet may have caused over 60 deaths. Weight loss is dramatic at first, then slows considerably even though you are practically consuming no calories. Quality of weight loss is poor; too much loss of lean-muscle mass along with fat loss keeps you flabby and unfirm.
Vegetarian Diets	People become vegetarians for numerous reasons: moral—opposition to the killing of animals; religious—eating meat is against beliefs; health—reduction in animal fats and cholesterol and less likelihood of excess body fat and heart disease.		Studies in the United States indicate that vegetarians have heart attacks 10 years later in life than meat eaters. An excellent, healthy way to lose weight and keep it off. The diet is safe, providing sufficient protein, iron, calcium and vitamin B_{12} can be consumed (an iron and B_{12} supplement may be needed). Have your physician confirm that you do not have a peptic ulcer or other inflammation of the digestive tract. On the negative side, the new habits of cooking, purchasing, and eating are not easy to follow at first.
Pure Vegetarian		Only foods of plant origin including seeds, grains, nuts, fruits, and vegetables	

TABLE 7.6   SUMMARY AND EVALUATION OF WIDELY PUBLICIZED DIETS—Continued

Diet	Special Claims	Allowable Foods	Evaluation
Lacto-vegetarian		Foods above of plant origin plus foods made of milk (yogurt, cheese, and cream)	
Lacto-ovo-vegetarian		All plant origin foods plus dairy products and eggs	
Very Low Calorie Formula Diets			
Cambridge Diet Plan	Rapid weight loss due to only 330 Calories daily from liquid, containing all necessary vitamins, minerals, carbohydrates, and proteins.	None—one-meal-per-day supplement after the first two weeks	This diet is dangerous for those with heart problems, diabetes, gout, pregnant or nursing mothers, and others. The FDA reports weakness, dizziness, dehydration, low blood pressure, and cardiac irregularities in some. It is a poor choice, since it results in no change in eating habits and causes lean muscle tissue loss. The FDA warns of danger of serious illness and death for some people.

[1]A condition brought about by a drastic reduction in carbohydrate intake that appears to make stored fat more available for energy; potentially dangerous.

SOURCE: Dintiman and Greenberg, HEALTH THROUGH DISCOVERY, © 1983, Addison-Wesley Pub. Co. Inc., Reading, Ma. pages 174, 175 & 176, Figure 8.4. Reprinted with permission.

stead of three is a useful approach for some individuals. The six-meals-a-day habit has been shown to result in more weight loss than the standard three meals a day.

Drastic reduction in daily intake to below 1,000 calories per day can be dangerous and should be avoided. Even when vitamin supplements are used and eight glasses of water are consumed, such low caloric intake daily is grossly deficient for young people. It is safer to simply reduce caloric intake by 500 calories a day or by 3,500 per week and to increase energy expenditure by 500 calories per day. Hunger can be better controlled when more realistic reductions in caloric intake are made. Other possible ways to control hunger include the following:

1. Eat at a leisurely pace to allow blood sugar levels to rise before you finish eating (20 to 30 minutes).

2. Eat bulky foods such as lettuce, celery, fruits, and carrots as your between-meal snacks.

3. Keep yourself occupied and busy. Take

TABLE 7.7 · SOUND DIET CHOICES

Diet	Special Claims	Allowable Foods	Evaluation
UCLA Diet (California Slim)	Low-fat controlled portion of 1,200 Cal/day	Variety of foods plus unlimited salads, and emphasis on fresh fruits and vegetables	Balanced diet, safe and effective
New Canadian High Energy Diet	Exchange system used to guarantee adequate nutrition intake[1]	Complex carbohydrates are emphasized	Safe and effective; provides adequate energy
Weight Watchers	Balanced diet based on exchange system and the four food groups[1]	Variety of foods from the basic four food groups	Safe and effective, emphasizes behavioral change and support groups
High Roughage Reducing Diet	2 teaspoons of bran are taken with each meal.	Low fat, low Calorie food	Too few milk products are included, diet appears safe and effective

[1]Exchange systems group foods together by nutrient similarity. Foods in such systems allow high nutrient value at a low Calorie cost.

frequent coffee breaks and drink diet and sugar-free beverages.

4. Avoid midnight snacks. Go to bed early while dieting.

5. Consume six to eight glasses of water to keep the stomach full.

HOW EXERCISE HELPS

A pleasant occurrence that often accompanies weight losses over 5 to 10 pounds is enhanced self-concept and increased energy levels. Remember, the weight you choose as a target is one that, once reached, will have to be maintained for the rest of your life. So it is not just weight loss *per se*, but the acceptance of a healthy lifestyle for yourself that is most likely to keep your "thinself" going in the future. Regular, vigorous exercise is an essential part of this healthy, holistic lifestyle.

If you expect to maintain a lower body weight, you will have to both diet and exercise. If you remain or become physically active, you will be able to eat a greater number of calories daily. The alternative is to remain mildly hungry most of your life. There are numerous other reasons why both diet and exercise should be included in a weight loss or weight management program.

EXERCISE DEPRESSES APPETITE

Weight loss through exercise is greater than would be expected through the direct expenditure of energy. This suggests that exercise acts on the body to further increase energy expenditure (through change in metabolism), or to decrease energy intake (through changes in appetite). Studies with both humans and animals suggest that physical activity decreases appetite. This was first reported in 1954, in a study that showed that female rats decreased food intake and body weight with exercise. These findings have been confirmed with other studies but the effect varies according to the sex of the animal and the nature of the activity. Evidence with humans is more sparse, but still suggests the same effect. Strong correlations have been found between physical inactivity and high body weight, and decreases in appetite have been shown to be associated with periods of regular aerobic exercise. Food intake has also been shown

Figure 7.2 The combination of sedentary living and high calorie food and drink are certain to produce weight and fat gain.

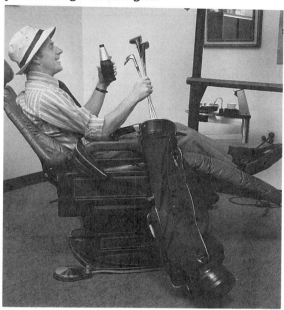

to decrease by scheduling recess in schools before rather than after lunch.

EXERCISE MAXIMIZES FAT LOSS AND MINIMIZES THE LOSS OF LEAN TISSUE

There is a difference between weight loss in terms of pounds and fatty tissue loss in terms of inches (weight loss vs. fat loss). A diet without exercise can result in about 70 percent fatty tissue loss and 30 percent lean muscle loss. With exercise and diet, fatty tissue loss can be increased to 95 percent. A greater percentage of free fatty acids are used for energy during exercise; 50 percent of the fuel for exercise bouts of from 30 to 60 minutes and as high as 70 to 85 percent for longer sessions come from free fatty acids.

EXERCISE ON A REGULAR BASIS CHANGES THE WAY YOUR BODY HANDLES FATS

For the young adult and middle-aged male and female, total serum cholesterol and tryglycerides may decrease with regular aerobic exercise, HDL

(the "good cholesterol") increases, and the ratio of HDL to total cholesterol improves. High HDL counts and a high ratio (1:4 or higher) of HDL to total cholesterol have been associated with a lower incidence of heart attacks. Ideally, at least 25% of total cholesterol should be of the HDL variety. (See Chapter 1 for more on exercise and cholesterol).

EXERCISE BRINGS NEEDED CALCIUM TO THE BONES

As a result of normal aging and weight loss, bones lose calcium and become more brittle. It takes adequate calcium intake *plus* exercise to bring the calcium to the bones.

EXERCISE BURNS A HIGH NUMBER OF CALORIES

Exercise burns calories both during the activity and for two to four hours after exercise ceases (**afterburn**). A three-mile run or walk (both burn approximately the same number of calories) will expend 250 to 400 calories depending upon the individual. For the next two to four hours following exercise, an additional 30 to 50 calories per hour (60 to 200 total) will be burned due to an increase in metabolic rate. The total caloric benefit of the three-mile walk or run then is 310 to 600 calories. Four to five such workouts weekly would produce a body weight/fat loss of approximately 3 pounds monthly and 36 pounds per year.

The best system of controlling body weight is to change your eating habits and to begin an exercise program you enjoy and are likely to continue throughout life. If you change your behavior in these two lifestyle areas, you may go through life at your ideal body weight and fat. Body weight is carefully regulated by complex forces, but the formula for weight control is simple. If you eat more calories than you burn through activity, a positive caloric balance exists and produces weight gain. If you burn up more calories than you eat, a negative caloric balance exists and weight and fat loss will occur.

Table 7.8 shows the number of days required to lose 5 to 25 pounds by exercising and lowering daily calorie intake. These charts do not reflect the additional effects of afterburn.

TABLE 7.8   DAYS REQUIRED TO LOSE 5 TO 25 POUNDS BY EXERCISE AND LOWERING DAILY CALORIE INTAKE

Walking*

Minutes Of Walking	+	Reduction Of Calories Per Day (in kcal)	Days To Lose 5 lbs.	Days To Lose 10 lbs.	Days To Lose 15 lbs.	Days To Lose 20 lbs.	Days To Lose 25 lbs.
30		400	27	54	81	108	135
30		600	20	40	60	80	100
30		800	16	32	48	64	80
30		1,000	13	26	39	52	65
45		400	23	46	69	92	115
45		600	18	36	54	72	90
45		800	14	28	42	56	70
45		1,000	12	24	36	48	60
60		400	21	42	63	84	105
60		600	16	32	48	64	80
60		800	13	26	39	52	65
60		1,000	11	22	33	44	55

*Walking briskly (3.5–4.0 mph), calculated at 5.2 Cal/minute.

Bicycling*

Minutes Of Bicycling	+	Reduction Of Calories Per Day (in kcal)	Days To Lose 5 lbs.	Days To Lose 10 lbs.	Days To Lose 15 lbs.	Days To Lose 20 lbs.	Days To Lose 25 lbs.
30		400	25	50	75	100	125
30		600	19	38	57	76	95
30		800	17	34	51	68	85
30		1,000	13	26	39	52	65
45		400	22	44	66	88	110
45		600	17	34	51	68	85
45		800	14	28	42	56	70
45		1,000	12	24	36	48	60
60		400	19	38	57	76	95
60		600	15	30	45	60	75
60		800	13	26	39	52	65
60		1,000	11	22	33	44	55

*Bicycling calculated at 6.5 Cal/minute, at approximately 7 mph.

From EXERCISE EQUIVALENTS OF FOODS by Frank Konishi, copyright © 1974 by The Southern Illinois University Press. Reprinted by permission of The Southern Illinois University Press.

TABLE 7.8 DAYS REQUIRED TO LOSE 5 TO 25 POUNDS BY EXERCISE AND LOWERING DAILY CALORIE INTAKE—Continued

Swimming*

Minutes Of + Swimming	Reduction Of Calories Per Day (in kcal)	Days To Lose 5 lbs.	Days To Lose 10 lbs.	Days To Lose 15 lbs.	Days To Lose 20 lbs.	Days To Lose 25 lbs.
30	400	23	46	69	92	115
30	600	18	36	52	72	90
30	800	14	28	42	56	70
30	1,000	12	24	36	48	60
45	400	19	38	57	76	95
45	600	15	30	45	60	75
45	800	13	26	39	52	65
45	1,000	11	22	33	44	55
60	400	16	32	48	64	80
60	600	14	28	42	56	70
60	800	11	22	33	44	55
60	1,000	10	20	30	40	50

*Swimming at about 30 yards per minute, calculated at 8.5 Cal/minute.

Jogging*

Minutes Of + Jogging	Reduction Of Calories Per Day (in kcal)	Days To Lose 5 lbs.	Days To Lose 10 lbs.	Days To Lose 15 lbs.	Days To Lose 20 lbs.	Days To Lose 25 lbs.
30	400	21	42	63	84	105
30	600	17	34	51	68	85
30	800	14	28	42	56	70
30	1,000	12	24	36	48	60
45	400	18	36	54	72	90
45	600	14	28	42	56	70
45	800	12	24	36	48	60
45	1,000	10	20	30	40	50
60	400	15	30	45	60	75
60	600	12	24	36	48	60
60	800	11	22	33	44	55
60	1,000	9	18	27	36	45

*Jogging—Alternate jogging and walking, calculated at 10.0 Cal/minute.

TABLE 7.9 ACTIVITY RATING CHART (CALORIES BURNED PER HOUR)

Activity	110 lbs. M	110 lbs. F	120 lbs. M	120 lbs. F	130 lbs. M	130 lbs. F	140 lbs. M	140 lbs. F	150 lbs. M	150 lbs. F
Sleeping, reclining		45		50		54		58	68	62
Very light: sitting, standing, driving		65		72		77		83	102	88
Light: walking on level, shopping, golf, table tennis, carpentry, light housekeeeping		130		143		153		166	197	177
Moderate: walking, weeding, cycling, skiing, tennis, dancing		205		226		242		262	292	279
Heavy: walking uphill, shoveling, basketball, swimming, climbing, football, jogging, running		400		440		472		512	571	544

Courtesy of Safeway Stores, Incorporated © 1988.

Walking, bicycling, swimming, dancing, and jogging are all effective means of exercise for weight loss. This chart also helps you decide how long you need to exercise daily to attain your weight loss goal.

Some types of physical activity and sports are relaxing and enjoyable. Other activities are superior in weight loss and aerobic benefits. Table 7.9 rates various sport and physical activities for caloric expenditure. When you choose a particular program, consider the following points:

1. Select activities that you enjoy doing.
2. Activities that expend a high number of calories per minute are best for weight loss.
3. Lifelong physical-recreational sports that provide heart/lung benefits are superior.
4. The choice you make should allow you to start at your present fitness level and progress to higher levels later.

FREQUENTLY ASKED QUESTIONS

How can I be certain that my caloric intake is not excessive?

Weigh yourself—at exactly the same time of day and under the same conditions, preferably in the morning upon rising. When the total daily caloric intake is equal to energy expenditure and calories lost in excreta, a caloric balance has been attained and no weight loss or gain will occur. When you eat more calories than you use, these excess calories are stored as fat. With the accumulation of approximately 3,500 excess calories, one pound of fat is stored. Remember, the body is extremely thrifty. Every unused calorie is stored as fat.

Often a change to an alternate food or drink will cause weight loss. An individual who drinks three glasses of whole

TABLE 7.9   ACTIVITY RATING CHART (CALORIES BURNED PER HOUR)—Continued

160 lbs.		170 lbs.		180 lbs.		190 lbs.		200 lbs.		210 lbs.		220 lbs.		230 lbs.	
M	F	M	F	M	F	M	F	M	F	M	F	M	F	M	F
72	66	77	70	81	75	86	78	90	83	95		99		104	
110	95	116	100	123	107	129	112	137	118	143		150		158	
212	190	223	200	238	213	250	224	264	237	276		290		305	
314	300	331	316	353	336	370	353	391	373	409		430		452	
613	584	647	616	689	656	722	688	764	728	798		840		882	

milk daily (165 calories per 8-ounce glass), for example, takes in nearly one pound of fat per week in milk (3,465 calories). A change to skim milk (85 calories per glass) results in a weight reduction of one-half pound weekly or two pounds monthly.

Unused calories are not only placed into a fat bank, they also cannot be withdrawn at a moment's notice. Only after weeks of proper nutrition and regular exercise can they be removed. To top it off, you have to carry the bank around with you until a withdrawal is made.

Is it helpful to have some fat on the body?

Yes. Athletes engaged in contact sports should try to keep their weight slightly higher than normal rather than becoming "one piece of lean meat." Fat deposits around the kidneys and other major organs offer needed protection from hard blows that could otherwise prove serious. Fat is not all bad; when the ratio of fat to muscle mass is normal, fat has a vital role in providing both insulation and protection.

Is it true that the major part of excess weight is water?

No. Do not restrict your water intake in any way. Water is essential to the proper function of every body system. Drinking water immediately before, during, or immediately after an exercise session will have no effect upon weight loss.

Retention of fluids is common while dieting since water remains in the spaces freed by the disappearance of fat. This fluid generally remains for two to three weeks and often obscures actual weight loss. Drink water freely at all times, particularly when you are restricting your calories.

The majority (about 80 percent) of excess weight is fat, not water. If fat individuals would replace between-meal and "binge" eating with water, there would never be any misunderstanding.

Does alcohol stimulate the appetite?

Only indirectly. Since alcohol is a depressant it encourages relaxation, and relaxation improves appetite. Alcohol contains calories (200–225 per ounce, about 150 per 12-ounce can of beer) and can cause a weight problem without stimulating the appetite. Some individuals consume four to six beers at one sitting. Such a feat adds about 750 calories; five such sittings add one pound of hard-to-remove fat. The body doesn't care whether alcohol or increased appetite gets the blame.

Are sweets important in my diet?

No. Most people get enough sugar in natural foods and do not need "empty calories" that only serve to destroy appetite and restrict intake of important foods. A common mistake of parents is to reward children with candy, immediately establishing the fallacy that sweets are better than other food. This reward procedure associates warmth and love with an undesirable food— a link that remains throughout life. Since food and emotions are associated in the child's mind, it would be far better to establish the association between good foods and reward.

Small amounts of candy elevate blood sugar level and curb appetite, a benefit to dieters who want to control hunger. But as an important source of energy and cell building, or as an aid to the function of body systems, candy rates low. It also can form an eating habit that will keep you fat in the future.

Do sugar-free drinks eliminate hunger?

Sugar-free drinks do temporarily aid in reducing hunger by filling the stomach and giving the sensation of fullness for a short time. Such drinks are valuable to a diet, and three to four 12-ounce bottles daily are likely to cause no harm. These drinks are not a substitute for water. Continue to drink 6 to 8 glasses daily.

On the negative side, it must be said that the controversy is not over. Even though saccharin has been replaced by Nutrasweet® in most products, there are concerns about the safety of this new product.

After dieting for two weeks, my weight has dropped only one pound. What am I doing wrong?

Nothing. Stay with it. You are experiencing a temporary retention of water because of the release of an anti-diuretic hormone that obscures the actual measurable weight loss occurring in the early stages of your diet (vacated fat cells fill with water). This temporary water retention can be discouraging and cause the scales to record only moderate weight loss even when strict dieting has been followed. However, actual weight loss has occurred and will be more noticeable in terms of reduced pounds following this 2 to 3-week period. Do not discontinue your diet before this phenomenon passes.

Some sound diets requiring the consumption of 6 to 10 glasses of water daily avoid this reaction since increasing water consumption results in the elimination of water and actually counteracts this tendency. A more accurate measure of weight loss during the initial stages of your diet is the reduction of fatty tissue. Avoid weighing yourself every day the first three weeks of your diet. Pinch yourself instead in the areas where you want to lose fat. You should notice a difference within a week.

How much time is needed to lose 25 pounds?

As a general rule, weight loss should not exceed 2 to 3 pounds weekly. A physician should be consulted when the desired weight loss exceeds 5 percent of your body weight. A return to an obese or overweight state tends to occur within a time period proportional to that spent losing a specific amount of weight. Reducing over an extended period of time (a minimum of three months) is preferred and generally results in the acquisition of sensible eating habits that are more likely to be continued in the future. Rapid weight loss, through fasting and other crash programs, can be dangerous and often results in a rapid return to old eating habits and an overweight condition. The extended period of time also involves the pleasant personal adjustment to clothes and new positive self-image so vital to weight control. Slow, controlled weight loss, then, has the advantages of safety, permanency, and little or no loss of strength and endurance for the athlete. Don't try to take it off any faster than you put it on.

Everyone wants fast results. What's wrong with diets that promise rapid weight loss?

In addition to being potentially dangerous to your health—possibly life threatening—there are other concerns:

1. The pounds you lose very fast will be gained back very fast since no change in eating habits takes place and you soon return to the old ones.
2. Rapid weight loss followed by weight gain makes you fatter. You may not weigh more, since losing 10 pounds and regaining 10 leave you at your original weight. You will, however, have more body fat in the 10 pounds you regained than in the 10 pounds you rapidly lost. Keep this up and your percent of total body fat will continue to increase with each cycle. It isn't weight you really want to lose, but fat.
3. After two to three cycles of rapid weight loss and regain (10 pounds or more), it becomes nearly twice as difficult to lose weight and twice as easy to gain weight the next cycle.
4. Rapid weight loss diets fail to tell you that most of the initial weight you lose is only water. If you lose 10 pounds in the first week of a diet, for example, you are a long way from having lost 10 pounds of fat. To lose 10 pounds in 7 days requires a daily caloric deficit of 5,000. If your daily needs are 2,500, you are still about 50 percent short of losing 10 pounds in one week. Your ten pounds of weight loss more likely consists of a maximum of 2 pounds of fat, 1 pound of lean muscle tissue, and 7 pounds of fluid. The 7 pounds of fluid can be reacquired so quickly it will shock you.

Rapid weight loss at a pace faster than 2 to 3 pounds weekly over several months makes little sense and is the furthest approach from the answer to your long-term weight problems.

Is fasting useful in losing weight?

Long-term fasting should be attempted only in a hospital under close supervision. This approach is used in various clinics for the extremely obese. It is best to avoid reducing caloric intake below a basic metabolic rate (approximately 800 to 1,800 calories depending upon the individual). Consuming fewer calories is unsafe: it may cause the body to begin conserving energy through a slowing of metabolic rate, and may predispose a person to binge eating (Frankle and Yang 1988).

Fast only under the supervision of a physician. It is also wise to use a multiple vitamin daily. Even wiser is an attempt to eat sensibly, thus avoiding an obese condition and the need for fasting.

Will dieting cause skin wrinkling?

Since young people have elastic skin, this is rarely a problem for the under-30 age group. For older individuals, wrinkles and folds do occur, but they will, depending upon age and the amount of weight loss, disappear over a substantial period of time. Slow weight loss over a long period of time is less apt to result in wrinkling and fat folds.

Several factors determine the extent of wrinkles and folds that may appear:

1. *Speed of weight loss.* A minimum of two to six months is recommended when attempting to remove more than 5 percent of body weight. With weight loss under 5 percent, a wise approach is to eat a balanced diet and engage in regular aerobic exercise daily.
2. *Age.* The older the individual, the more prone to wrinkles and less resilient is the skin.
3. *Amount of weight to be lost.* Fifty, 75, 100, 150 and 200-pound reductions can result in such ugly appearance in the stomach area that surgery may be needed to remove excess skin.
4. *Exercise.* Daily aerobic exercise is needed to maintain muscle tone, increase fatty tissue loss, and decrease lean tissue loss.

The basic problem is that skin is stretched and it remains stretched after weight loss, so it just does not fit the body—much the same way a baby's skin appears at birth.

Will eating only one or two meals daily help me lose weight?

No. It is nearly impossible for most people to skip a meal and lose weight. Their hunger becomes so intense by the next scheduled meal that more calories are consumed than would have been eaten in three meals. It also is difficult to get the necessary daily vitamin requirements with one or two meals daily. Breakfast is the most commonly missed meal. After approximately twelve hours without food, it is the one meal that is absolutely necessary in your diet. Research indicates that late morning fatigue is likely if breakfast is missed. The noon meal is the next most commonly missed and also represents a poor attempt at weight reduction. A ten-hour period of activity without food is too long and will result in tremendous overeating at the evening meal.

Do not skip a meal. Eat less, eat from the basic four food groups, or eat six meals per day instead of three, consuming even smaller portions at each. This approach has been shown to result in more weight loss than the three-meal-per-day method.

Should carbohydrates be eliminated from my diet?

No. The dieter should restrict carbohydrate intake, not eliminate it. Exercise will draw from available carbohydrate supply for energy; if the supply is limited, the body must resort to fat for fuel and the result is a loss of fatty tissue. In addition, the brain needs a constant supply of glucose (obtained from sugar and carbohydrates). This need is so essential that the body has a built-in mechanism to convert protein to carbohydrates when the supply is absent. Cut down on your simple carbohydrate (sugars) intake but do not completely avoid these foods.

Athletes need to include some simple carbohydrates in their diet to provide ample energy for exercise. Long-term energy should come from adequate intake of complex carbohydrates (fruits, vegetables, and grains), not simple carbohydrates. Some experts suggest that for athletes in vigorous training, about 65 percent of food calories should be carbohydrates.

Should fat be completely excluded from the diet?

No. Fat plays a vital part in digestion and in the transportation of vitamins, and is the main fuel of some muscle fibers in most muscle groups. It would be nearly impossible to eliminate fats from the diet. Meat is far from pure protein and is often tenderized with fat (marbelized) to improve taste. Unless one resorts to artificial foods, fats cannot be avoided.

Fat has the highest concentration of energy (one gram of fat = 9 cal., one gram of protein = 4 cal., one gram of carbohydrate = 4 cal., and one gram of alcohol = 7 cal.) and should be avoided in excess. One level teaspoon equals approximately 4 grams and one cup is equivalent to 100 grams. Up to 65 percent of your caloric intake should come from carbohydrates, 10 to 15 percent form protein, and the remaining percentage from fats.

In terms of performance, energy derived from fats is less economical than energy drawn from carbohydrates and protein. About 10 to 12 percent more oxygen is needed to utilize energy supplied from fats. Both your long-term health and athletic performance will improve if fat intake is reduced—only a magician could completely eliminate it.

Should college students drink whole milk?

The American male, the overweight female, and anyone who is vulnerable to atherosclerosis (that includes practically all of us) would be wise to drink skim milk. Resorting to skim milk reduces damaging saturated fats and calories.

There is some justification for placing children on fortified skim milk, since cholesterol buildup begins early in life, as do weight problems and the start of atherosclerosis. Keep in mind that although fortified skim milk has approximately 40 percent more calories than plain skim, it is probably the wiser choice for children.

You don't need the fat in whole milk; you consume enough in meats and other dairy products. After the initial acclimation period of one to two months, whole milk will taste like cream and be unpleasant.

Is it possible to avoid gaining weight when I stop smoking?

Yes. Kicking the smoking habit is no easy task; more than 75 percent who quit are puffing away one year later. A major reason for this relapse is weight gain. Those who quit put on an average of five to seven pounds, although the range is zero to thirty pounds. This nicotine/weight connection seems to be more pronounced in women. It appears from laboratory studies that nicotine intake decreases the consumption of sweet foods (this may be one reason teenage girls, a particularly weight-conscious group, are the fastest-growing group of cigarette smokers). In the absence of nicotine, the amount of sweet foods consumed increases in proportion to the rise in weight. Early research indicates that it may be important to restrict the type, not the quantity, of food around the ex-smoker if weight gain is to be prevented. Being alert to the problem of nervous eating, counting calories, and beginning a moderate exercise program are additional tips that can help prevent weight gain when you quit smoking.

What is anorexia nervosa?

Anorexia nervosa is a serious and potentially fatal eating disorder. A typical case involves a young woman from a middle-class family who becomes obsessed with the idea that she is fat and uses self-denial as a means of controlling her weight. This starvation approach is then carried to an extreme of undernourishment where total body weight may reach seventy pounds or less. Even then she may still feel fat and continue to starve herself. Early treatment by an experienced physician or clinic is essential if permanent health damage is to be avoided. Without treatment, approximately 10 percent of anorexics die of starvation (Whitney, Hamilton 1987). Forced feeding may temporarily improve their health, but the condition can reappear unless proper psychological and medical therapy is successful.

What is bulimia?

The recent disclosure by exercise and weight control enthusiast Jane Fonda that she was bulimic from age 12 to age 35 was shocking news to many readers. **Bulimia** is gorging oneself with food and then vomiting it. The typical profile is also similar to that of anorexics, although victims tend to be slightly older, otherwise healthy, and close to normal weight. Bulimics eat a tremendous volume of food secretly and follow the binge with vomiting or use of large quantities of laxatives to eliminate the food. Left untreated, the condition may lead to kidney failure, potassium depletion, urinary track infections, ulcers, and hernias. Although the number of treatment clinics and qualified physicians is growing, the disease is still poorly understood.

Do men suffer from anorexia nervosa and bulimia?

Very rarely. These two eating disorders are mainly prevalent among young girls and women, apparently the result of our overemphasis on slimness. Even in middle age women in our society are expected to remain beautiful. Not nearly so much social pressure is placed on men to remain youthful throughout life. These kinds of pressures, coupled with the nationwide trend of middle-aged men marrying women twenty years their junior, is a heavy burden for American women.

MYTHS AND FALLACIES

Overweight and obese people are always big eaters.

In both children and adults, studies show that the major cause of overweight conditions is inactivity, not excessive eating. Although proper eating and regular exercise are the two ingredients necessary for any successful weight loss or weight control program, many individuals could both lose and maintain ideal weight by merely increasing their energy expenditure through regular exercise.

Cellulite can be eliminated with special foods and exercises.

From a medical point of view, there is no such thing as **cellulite** as a particular form of fat. Fat is merely fat although the size and appearance of fat cells vary in different body parts. Weight reducing salons and some diet books define cellulite as a gel-like substance made up of fat, water, and wastes trapped in lumpy, immovable pockets beneath the skin. The Federal Trade Commission issued a statement that cellulite does not exist, so advertised treatments for cellulite are therefore fraudulent.

Regardless of the terminology, these lumpy deposits tend to occur in women, sometimes as early as the late teens. A somewhat thicker skin in the upper legs and buttocks keeps the fat deposits form showing through in men. Prevention is a lot easier than treatment and focuses on regular exercise and proper nutrition, maintaining normal weight, and avoiding "yo-yo" dieting (rapid weight loss and weight gain) that tends to reduce skin elasticity. Exercise programs such as swimming, jogging, cycling, rope jumping, aerobic dance, and aerobic exercise performed on a regular basis will help prevent these deposits. The girth control program described in Appendix J offers effective prevention and treatment. Massage, special foods, extra vitamin A and C, oils, water jets, minerals, body pressure wraps and other body therapy methods only remove the lumps in your wallet.

Weight charts accurately determine one's weight status.

Charts are grossly inadequate and should be used only as a guide. The major pitfalls are:

1. It is possible to be within the range of suggested weight and still be overweight.
2. It is possible to be classified as overweight (more than 20 percent above suggested ranges) or obese (more than 30 percent above suggested ranges) when you are at a desirable weight and possess little fatty tissue. Among thick-muscled athletes with low body fat, this is a common finding.
3. After age 25, some charts allow you to gain weight with age, suggesting that it is fine to be fat at age 30, 40, or 50. Actually weight should decrease with age. If an adult at 40 weighs the same now as 20 years ago, he or she is probably overfat. Lost muscle mass from earlier years has been replaced by an increased proportion of fatty

tissue. Ideally, you should be 5 to 10 pounds lighter at age 50 than your ideal weight at age 25.

4. The three categories of small, medium, and large frames encourage cheating. We have yet to meet anyone who took the recommended weight from the small frame range, yet everyone in this world cannot possibly have a medium or large frame. A woman's frame is generally small until she checks a weight chart. Men rarely consider themselves anything but large framed.

5. The key to obesity is not total body weight, but total body fat. Weight charts do not reveal the presence of fat.

Sit-up exercises will remove the fat from the stomach area.

The only way to eliminate stomach fat is through reduction of calories and through calisthenics—a frightful word to many people, since this type of exercise has been grossly misused. The purpose of a calisthenic program directed at the abdominal area is to create what is termed "definition"—to bring out the lines of musculature in the stomach area. Keep in mind, however, that it requires both reduced calories and regular calisthenic-type exercise to produce a flat stomach. An individual with a flabby stomach, for example, could do 5,000 sit-ups daily, but unless a calorie deficit occurs to produce fat loss, the flab will remain even though underneath lies a strong group of abdominal muscles. You cannot change fatty tissue to muscle tissue—they are two different types of tissue. You need to shrink the fat cells through reduced caloric intake and firm the muscles with calisthenics.

Laxatives help you lose weight.

Laxatives are no more effective than the early Roman practice of forced vomiting after a gluttonous meal to allow continuous eating and socializing. Laxatives have a similar effect; however, they are a more dangerous approach and can cause gastrointestinal trouble. You need adequate fluid intake and nutrients while dieting. A laxative, taken on a regular basis, can prevent you from obtaining either, and can cause dehydration and undernourishment. Be sensible. It is better to be fat than to be sick. It is impossible to defecate away unwanted pounds safely.

Weight-reducing pills are a safe approach to depressing the appetite.

Without careful supervision by a physician, the use of numerous drugs and drug combinations has been shown to be extremely harmful and sometimes fatal. The various drugs (prescription and patent medicine) employed to lose weight generally attempt to cause loss through (1) increasing metabolic rate or the rate at which the body burns calories while at rest, (2) curbing the appetite, or (3) causing fluid loss. Amphetamines and diuretics are the two most commonly used diet pills. Amphetamines toy with the thyroid gland, cause nervousness, speed up metabolism, and require increasingly strong doses as the body builds up a tolerance; diuretics result in rapid fluid loss. Both are a dangerous attempt at weight control.

Consult your physician before starting any type of diet, and certainly before ever using any drug for weight loss. Crash dieting with pills can destroy your health.

Reducing aids such as vibrators, body wraps, rubber suits, steam baths, and massage effectively remove fat from the body.

Gimmick approaches to weight loss promising rapid loss of body fat remain popular. Although each approach appears to provide an easy solution, each also has its limitations.

Most special apparatus used for spot reducing are of little value. Vibrators result in little caloric expenditure and do not cause weight loss. Steam baths and saunas remove body fluids and merely cause a temporary drop in body weight. Drinking water immediately after a "sweat" session results in an immediate return to normal weight.

Since exercising in a rubber suit also causes sweating, people mistakenly assume that weight loss occurs. This practice is potentially dangerous. The suit retains body heat and core temperature can rise during exercise to a dangerous level. Since the air does not contact the sweat, the most effective means of cooling the body (evaporation) is eliminated. In addition, the rubber suit does not increase the number of calories burned; therefore, no extra weight loss occurs.

Rapid weight loss due to loss of body fluid exceeding 5 percent of body weight is dangerous; it causes changes in water metabolism and in kidney and circulatory functions.

Wearing a weighted belt during exercise may burn a few extra calories. The size of the waistline and the muscle tone, however, remain unchanged after prolonged use. The effect on weight loss is negligible.

Massage also burns very few calories. It is relaxing and may slightly improve circulation.

There is no fast, easy method or device to lose weight and body fat. Save your money, and start a sound program of diet and exercise based on your individual interests.

BIBLIOGRAPHY

Dintiman, George B., and Jerrold Greenberg. *Health Through Discovery.* 4th ed. New York: Random House, 1989.

Dintiman, George B., and Robert Ward. *Train America! Achieving Peak Performance and Fitness.* Dubuque, Iowa: Kendal-Hunt, 1988.

Frankle, Reva T., and Mel-Urh Yang eds. *Obesity and Weight Control: The Professional's Guide to Understanding and Treatment.* Rockville, Md.: Aspen, 1988.

Hegarty, Vincent. *Decisions in Nutrition.* St. Louis: Mosby College, 1988.

Office of Disease Prevention and Health Promotion. *The 1990 Health Objectives for the Nation: A Midcourse Review.* Washington, D.C.: U.S. Department of Health and Human Sciences, 1986.

Whitney, Eleanor and Eva May Hamilton, *Understanding Nutrition.* 4th ed. St. Paul: West, 1987.

Williams, Melvin H. *Nutrition for Fitness and Sport.* Dubuque, Iowa: Wm. C. Brown Co., 1988.

LABORATORY 7.1

Evaluating Your Body Fat and Body Weight

PURPOSE: To determine if you are overweight or overfat

PROCEDURE

Determine your frame size accurately using the elbow breadth test. With your shoes on, determine your correct height. Now locate your weight range in Table 7.1.

For a quick estimate of your body fat, administer these two tests:

1. *The pinch test:* Using the thumb and forefinger, take a fold of skin and subcutaneous (beneath the skin) fat in these sites: back of arm, back below the shoulder blade, thigh, back of the calf, and abdomen. A fold greater than one inch indicates excessive fat.

2. *The ruler test:* For an individual who is not fat, the slope of the abdomen (when lying on the back) between the flare of the ribs and front of the pelvis is flat or slightly concave. A ruler placed on the abdomen along the midline should touch both ribs and the pelvic area.

RESULTS

1. Did you fall within the recommended weight range for your height?

2. Do you have excess fat in any body parts?

3. Did you find you fell within an acceptable weight range on the charts and still pinched more than an inch?

LABORATORY 7.2

Caloric Balance and Daily Weight Fluctuation

PURPOSE: To determine whether a "caloric balance" is in effect and to demonstrate weight changes over a 24-hour period.

PROCEDURE

1. Weigh yourself three times daily: a) in the morning after rising, without clothes, b) at noon, and c) at 11:00 P.M. or just prior to bed time.

2. Complete the three weigh-ins on both Saturday and Sunday one weekend and repeat the following weekend.

RESULTS

1. Did you weigh the same on Saturday and Sunday of the first weekend?
2. How much does your weight fluctuate in a 24-hour period?
3. How much did your weight change from one week to the next?
4. Are you in a caloric balance as indicated by less than one pound of weight fluctuation from one weekend to the next?
5. Are you gaining weight?

	Morning				**Noon**				**Evening**	

Weekend 1:

Saturday	Sunday	Change		Saturday	Sunday	Change		Saturday	Sunday	Change

Weekend 2:

Saturday	Sunday	Change		Saturday	Sunday	Change		Saturday	Sunday	Change

CHAPTER EIGHT

Injury
Prevention
and
Emergency
Treatment

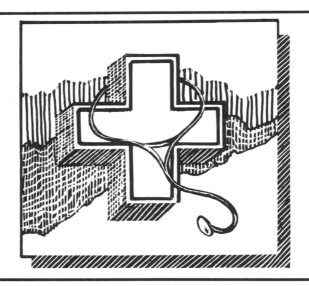

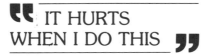 IT HURTS
WHEN I DO THIS 🙶

? HAVE YOU EVER WONDERED ABOUT:

How to protect yourself from injury and illness?
How your body tells you to stop?
The proper home treatment for common injuries?
How much the wind lowers outside temperature?
Muscle soreness?
How to prevent heat-related illnesses?
The effects of drugs on the human body?

KEY TERMS

Amphetamines
Barbiturates
Bone jolt
Cyrotherapy

Orthotics
Morton's foot
R-I-C-E
Steroids

Entering into a fitness program involves only a small risk of injury or illness. In fact, a key benefit of improved conditioning is the reduction in the incidence and severity of serious injuries during sports participation. The danger of injury increases considerably, however, when individuals fail to follow simple rules of training. For such individuals, like the "weekend athlete," exercise can be dangerous or even fatal. This chapter is designed to help you avoid common hazards and to make exercise a safe, fun experience. It includes 10 steps for injury proofing your body, provides basic treatment procedures for common injuries and illnesses, and discusses the special injury-proofing problems of women.

PROTECTING YOUR BODY FROM INJURY AND ILLNESS

Common sense and the application of some basic conditioning concepts can eliminate the majority of risk in fitness programs. The 10-point program that follows is designed to help you plan a safe fitness program.

IMPROVING YOUR GENERAL CONDITIONING LEVEL

The first step in injury proofing your body is to slowly attain a satisfactory level of general conditioning. It is important to be extra careful the first several months of a newly started exercise program as you are particularly vulnerable to muscle, ligament, and joint injuries. Injuries of all types are also more likely to occur when you are in a state of general fatigue. Fatigue causes a reduced blood supply to muscles. In addition, when you are fatigued, fibers are devitalized and easily torn, and joint stability and muscle groups are weakened. This state of general fatigue is common during the early stages of an exercise program. Strengthening the injury-prone areas such as the ankle, wrist, knee, shoulders, lower back and neck (see Chapter 4, Muscular Strength and Endurance Training) before beginning a new sport helps prevent injuries caused by fatigue.

ANALYZING YOUR MEDICAL HISTORY

If you are over 40 years of age, have been inactive for more than two or three years regardless of age, or are in the high-risk group (obese, high blood pressure, diabetic, high blood lipids), a thorough physical examination is recommended (see Chapter 3). Resting heart rate and blood pressure, and exercise heart rate and blood pressure will provide some clues to your body's response to the new fitness program. Although the chances of a serious problem are slight for college students, it's better to be safe than sorry.

WARMING UP

At the beginning of an exercise session, it is important to raise body temperature one to two degrees to prepare muscles, ligaments and tendons for vigorous movement. A few extra minutes of warm-up can prevent common muscle pulls, strains, sprains, lower back discomfort, and reduce muscle soreness occurring 8 to 24 hours later (see Chapter 3 for additional information).

COOLING DOWN

The cool-down is an important phase of the fitness workout that should be enjoyed rather than avoided. Experienced joggers or runners complete the final one-half to two miles at a slow, easy pace rather than with a "kick" or sprint. The final 5 to 15 minutes of any workout can also be used to slowly taper off and cool the body to a near resting state (see Chapter 3 for additional information).

PROGRESSING SLOWLY

Add small increments to your workout each day. Too much, too soon is a common cause of muscular injuries. Plan your program (see Chapter 9, Tailor-Made Programs for You) over a period of three to six months to maximize enjoyment and minimize pain and risk.

Your workout should not increase heart rate to more than 70 percent of your maximum (approximately 135 to 140 beats per minute at age 25) the first two to four weeks. After this acclimation period you can train at higher heart rates safely.

The popular 1.5 mile test which helps you find your aerobic fitness level can also be dangerous for the high-risk population mentioned in the previous section on medical history. For this group, it is much safer to engage in a light conditioning program for several weeks before completing a field test of this nature.

ALTERNATING LIGHT AND HEAVY DAYS

Many people make the mistake of trying to train hard every day. The body does not have adequate time to repair or rebuild, and the full benefit of your workout may not be realized. In addition, injuries, boredom, and "peaking out" are much more likely with overtraining.

Overuse injuries are more common in exercisers who have recently begun a program or who are progressing from one level to another. Brody classified runners according to mileage and pace and identifies the injuries common to each group in Table 8.1.

Within each category; injuries are often a result of excessive mileage, intensive workouts, and a rapid increase in distance. Compounding the problem is running surface (a soft level surface is preferred); running up and down curbs which increases shock to the legs, feet, and back; sloping or banked roads which force the foot on the higher part of the slope to pronate excessively, overstressing tendons and ligaments; or uphill (strains the Achilles tendon and low-back muscles) and downhill running (force to the heel strike is increased).

If you are using the sports approach to fitness, alter the length of your workout and the caliber of opponent to utilize the light-heavy concept. High-level competition on a daily basis violates the concept, hinders conditioning improvement, and makes injury more likely.

TABLE 8.1   CLASSIFICATION OF RUNNERS AND POTENTIAL INJURIES

Classification	Mileage	Potential Injuries
Jogger or Novice Runner	3–20 miles per week at 9–12 minutes per mile	Shin splints, chondromalacia (runner's knee), soreness, hamstring strains, and low back pain
Sports Runner	20–40 miles per week, participant in fun runs and races of 3–6 miles	Achilles tendonitis, stress fractures
Long Distance Runner	40–70 miles per week at 7–8 minutes per mile; may compete in 10,000 meters (6.2 miles) or marathons (26.2 miles)	More serious injuries to thigh, calf, and back; sciatica and tendon pulls
Elite Marathoner	70–200 miles per week at 5–7 minutes per mile.	Stress fractures, acute muscle strain in the back, sciatica

© Copyright 1980, CIBA-GEIGY Corporation. Reprinted with permission from CLINICAL SYMPOSIA by David M. Brody, M.D., illustrated by Frank H. Netter, M.D.

AVOIDING THE "WEEKEND ATHLETE" APPROACH TO FITNESS

One sure way to guarantee numerous injuries and illnesses is to exercise vigorously only on weekends. The older weekend athlete is particularly susceptible to heart attack, while individuals of all ages increase their chances of muscle, tendon, and ligament injuries.

Considerable publicity has been given to athletes who have died during exercise. Chuck Hughes, receiver for the Detroit Lions, and William Hill, marathon runner, died of heart attacks caused by fatty plaques in the arteries that supply blood to the heart. Karen Krantzcke, professional tennis player, died from heart arrhythmia following a victory in the Lionel Cup Tennis Tournament in Florida. Two former University of Maryland basketball players died during pick-up games in 1976. And more recently, Jim Fixx, the guru of the running boom, and "Pistol" Pete Maravich, former NBA great, died victims of heart problems while exercising. These deaths and many others like them may be attributable to congenital heart defects unrelated to fitness. There are few, if any, cases of healthy individuals dying from exercise.

Cooper (1982) describes a cardiac condition in which death occurs following unaccustomed exertion in cold weather although an autopsy reveals no signs of a heart attack. While this condition is rare, it is a possibility when men and women try to "do it all" in one weekend workout. Cold air constricts the blood vessels of the skin and increases blood pressure slightly. Vigorous exercise then also increases blood pressure, heart rate, and oxygen needs of the heart dramatically. Without proper warm-up and with the presence of hidden signs of heart disease, a heart attack may occur.

If the weekend is the only time you can exercise, avoid long bouts in hot or cold weather and strenuous exercise (jogging, running, racketball, handball, tennis, basketball, soccer, rugby, and so on) unless you take frequent breaks. Consider supplementing your weekend routine with one other workout during the week. After one month, try increasing to two workouts during the week in addition to one on weekends. If you choose an aerobic activity and progress slowly for several months, you can minimize the risk of serious illness or injury. With a total of three workouts weekly, you have the foundation for a good conditioning program.

PAYING CLOSE ATTENTION TO YOUR BODY SIGNALS

Pain and other distress signals should not be ignored. Although some breathing discomfort and breathlessness are common and minor pain may be present in an ankle, foot, knee, hip, back, or other body part, severe, persistent, and particularly sharp pain is a warning sign to stop exercising.

It is sound advice to stop exercising immediately if you notice any abnormal heart action (pulse irregularity, fluttering, palpitations in the chest or throat, rapid heart beats); pain or pressure in the middle of the chest, teeth, jaw, neck, or arm; dizziness; lightheadedness; cold sweat; or confusion. Study Appendix G on chest pains to help determine whether any pain that occurs is associated with a heart attack or, as is more common, with other muscular, skeletal, tendonous, or illness problems.

After each workout, let your body analyze the severity of your exercise. The workout was too light if sweating did not occur, and it was too heavy if breathlessness persisted 10 minutes after, your pulse rate is above 120 beats per minute 2 minutes after stopping, prolonged fatigue remains for more than 24 hours, nausea or vomiting occur, or sleep is interrupted. To remedy these symptoms in the future, exercise less vigorously and lengthen your cool-down period. When you are obviously ill or not "up to par," rest a few days and return to a lower level or easier workout.

MASTERING THE PROPER FORM IN YOUR ACTIVITY

Proper running form is important to most fitness programs. Joggers should avoid running on the toes, which produces soreness in the calf muscles. The heel should strike the ground first before rolling the weight along the bottom of the foot to the toes for the push-off. A number of other running form problems often produce mild muscle and joint strain.

Participants in racket sports are also susceptible to numerous form-related injuries (tennis elbow, shoulder and wrist inflammation, lower-back problems) from faulty stroke mechanics such as elbow-lead ground strokes, bent-elbow hits, muscles not firming at impact, and so on. A few professional lessons in your sport can help to reduce the risk of these injuries.

DRESSING PROPERLY FOR THE WEATHER

Weather extremes can cause health problems during exercise (see Appendix G on heat exhaustion, heat stroke, hypothermia, and frostbite). Consider the suggestions in Table 9.2 to reduce the risk of overheating on hot, humid days or overexposure on cold days.

If you are a runner, it is also helpful to plan your jogging course to avoid being too far out on either a hot or cold day should symptoms of heat exhaustion or overexposure occur. In cold weather, you should run against the wind on the way out; however, on the way back, when you are likely to be sweating much more, a head wind and wet clothes would draw away your body heat, so you should run with the wind.

Both weather extremes can kill. Heat stroke (core temperature may rise to 105° or 106°) symptoms are difficult to reverse unless immediate, rapid

TABLE 8.2   PREVENTIVE TECHNIQUES ON HOT AND COLD DAYS

Hot, Humid Weather	Cold Weather
1. Listen to weather reports and avoid vigorous exercise if the temperature is above 90° and the humidity is above 70 percent. Make hot days your light workout.	1. Listen to weather reports noting temperature and wind-chill factor. Study Table 8.3 carefully, and unless the equivalent temperature is in the "little danger" area, avoid outside exercise.
2. Avoid adding to normal salt intake. Do not use salt tablets. Increase consumption of fruits and vegetables.	2. Eat well during cold months; the body needs more calories in cold weather.
3. Avoid lengthy warm-up periods.	3. Warm-up carefully until sweating is evident.
4. Wear light-colored, porous, loose clothing to promote evaporation. Remove special equipment, such as football gear, every hour for 15 minutes.	4. Use two or three layers of clothing rather than one heavy warm-up suit.
5. Avoid wearing a hat (except for an open visor with brim) since considerable heat loss occurs through the head.	5. Protect the head (warm hat), ears, fingers, toes, nose, and genitals. A hat should cover the ears and face. Fur-lined supporters for men can also prevent frostbite to sensitive parts.
6. Never use rubberized suits that hold the sweat in. Increase fluid and salt/potassium loss.	6. Never use rubberized, air-tight suits that keep the sweat in. When the body cools, the sweat starts to freeze.
7. Wet clothing increases salt and sweat loss. Replace whenever possible.	7. Keep clothing dry, changing wet items as soon as possible.
8. Slowly increase the length of your workout by 5 to 10 minutes daily for nine days to acclimate to the heat.	8. Slowly increase the length of your workout by 5 to 10 minutes daily for nine days to acclimate to the cold.
9. Drink cold water (40°F) before (10 ounces 15 minutes prior to exercise), during, and after exercise. Hydrate before the workout with two or three glasses of water.	9. Drink cold water freely before, during, and after exercise. Let thirst be your guide.

cooling takes place. On the other hand, a one-degree drop in core temperature will produce pain. Should the body temperature drop to 94°, behavior becomes irrational; at 90° shivering ceases and rigidity sets in; at 75° death usually occurs from heart failure.

Properly fitting shoes, the appropriate racket, avoidance of gimmick exercise devices, and acceptable equipment for contact sports are also important to injury prevention and need special attention. A good quality shoe (jogging, tennis, team sports) is your best protection against injury to the feet, ankles, knees, hips, and lower back.

BASIC EMERGENCY AND HOME TREATMENT METHODS

The majority of exercise injuries can be managed through emergency and home treatment methods. It is also important to know what injuries and symptoms suggest physician care. Appendix G provides you with some cues for 45 common exercise injuries, illnesses and problems. Emergency treatment and initial home treatment for most muscle, ligament, and tendon strains, sprains, suspected fractures, bruises, and joint inflammation involve four simple actions known as the **R-I-C-E** approach (see Figure 8.1):

Rest—to prevent additional damage to injured tissue, stop exercising immediately; if the lower extremities are affected, use crutches to move about.

Ice—to decrease blood flow to the injured part and prevent swelling, apply ice immediately for 15 to 30 minutes (avoid direct ice contact with the skin).

Compression—to limit swelling, wrap a towel or bandage firmly around the ice.

Elevation—to help drain excess fluid through gravity, raise the injured limb above heart level.

Home treatment should begin as soon as possible. Continue to use R-I-C-E for at least 48 hours.

TABLE 8.3 OUTSIDE TEMPERATURE AND EQUIVALENT WIND-CHILL FACTOR

Wind (mph)	Temperature °F								
Calm	40	35	30	25	20	15	10	5	0
	Equivalent Chill Temperature								
5	35	30	25	20	15	10	5	0	−5
10	30	20	15	10	5	0	−10	−15	−20
15	25	15	10	0	−5	−10	−20	−25	−30
20	20	10	5	0	−10	−15	−25	−30	−35
25	15	10	0	−5	−15	−20	−30	−35	−45
30	10	5	0	−10	−20	−25	−30	−40	−50
35	10	5	−5	−10	−20	−25	−35	−40	−50
40	10	0	−5	−15	−20	−30	−35	−45	−55
Little Danger								**Increasing Danger**	

Figure 8.1   Using the R-I-C-E Approach on an Injured Ankle

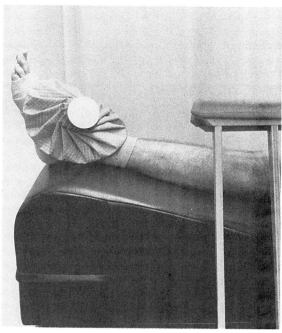

On the fourth day, discontinue cold treatments and begin to apply moist heat, dry heat, or whirl-pool twice daily for 15 to 30 minutes. Depending upon the severity of the injury, mild exercise can resume four or five days after it occurs.

SHOCK

Many injuries such as fractures, concussions, profuse bleeding, heart attack, back and neck damage, and severe joint trauma can produce shock. Shock is one of the body's strongest natural reactions to disease and injury. It slows blood flow acting as a natural tourniquet, reduces pain, and eases the body's agony in serious injury. All three types of shock can kill: *traumatic* (injury or loss of blood), *septic* (infection-induced), and *cardiogenic* (from a heart attack). Shock is much easier to prevent than to cure. Assume shock is present with the above injuries and illnesses, splint broken bones, handle the victim with care, stop bleeding, and keep the victim warm at all times.

The more common injuries, illnesses, and problems associated with exercise are discussed in

TABLE 8.3 OUTSIDE TEMPERATURE AND EQUIVALENT WIND-CHILL FACTOR—Continued							

Wind (mph)	Temperature °F						
Calm	−5	−10	−15	−20	−25	−30	−35	−40
	Equivalent Chill Temperature						
5	−10	−15	−20	−25	−30	−35	−40	−45
10	−25	−35	−40	−45	−50	−60	−65	−70
15	−40	−45	−50	−60	−65	−70	−80	−85
20	−45	−50	−60	−65	−75	−80	−85	−95
25	−50	−60	−65	−75	−80	−90	−95	−105
30	−55	−65	−70	−80	−85	−95	−100	−105
35	−60	−65	−75	−80	−90	−100	−105	−115
40	−60	−70	−75	−85	−95	−100	−110	−115

Increasing Danger
(Flesh may freeze within one minute)

Great Danger
(Flesh may freeze within 30 seconds)

SOURCE: George Sheehan. *Dr. George Sheehan's Medical Advice for Runners.* Mountain View, Cal.: Anderson World, 1978, p. 263. Reprinted by Permission from Runner's World Magazine, 1400 Stierlin Rd., Mountain View, CA 94043.

Appendix G. This chart serves as a guide for diagnosis, prevention, emergency treatment, and determining the need for a physician. If in doubt, consult your physician. Proper early care is important in preventing further damage.

FREQUENTLY ASKED QUESTIONS

Can anything be done to help prevent arthritis in later life?

For football players, those in other contact sports, and anyone who has had cartilage removed, arthritis may be one of the unavoidable hazards of the game. Mild arthritic pain is common among former footballers over the age of 30.

Arthritis has numerous causes: rheumatic fever, infection, faulty metabolism, degenerative joint disease, circulatory and nervous disorders, glandular disturbances, allergy, and trauma, to name a few. Symptoms include joint pain, swelling, tenderness, and loss of movement in the hands, wrists, fingers, knees, ankles, feet, or any other joint. A permanent cure is unknown. Arthritis patients are among the most victimized by quack cures (to the tune of $250 million annually). Medication to relieve pain and prevent further joint damage must be provided immediately by a physician. Special gadgets, apparatus, and quick cures do not work on anything but your pocketbook.

These suggestions, if followed, can help keep you from becoming an arthritis victim:

1. Maintain a high level of general health.
2. Exercise on a regular basis with a program designed to elevate heart-lung efficiency.
3. Protect the joints from injury, strain, and cold.
4. Avoid competing while injured, since repeated trauma is a causative factor.
5. Correct diseased tissues such as toenails, teeth, eyes, and infected sinuses immediately.
6. Avoid stress to weight-bearing joints (knees, ankles) later in life.
7. Dress warmly when exercising in cold weather.

Is it dangerous to use contact lenses when exercising?

It can be dangerous to participate in some sports unless you take preventive measures. Swimmers and wrestlers should not use contact lenses during practice or competition. If you are a user, be sure to keep a spare pair handy, maintain close supervision with your practitioner during the initial adjustment period, and use sanitary measures in handling lenses to avoid infection.

Is a "popping" sound in the knee a sign of serious injury?

Not necessarily. The sound results when a tendon flips over bony fulcrums. Warm-up may reduce or eliminate the sound. Bone or cartilage damage is not indicated unless other symptoms such as inflammation, swelling, fluid, and locking are present. "Joint mice," or pieces of loose cartilage, may be causing some grating at times.

Does ankle taping prevent injuries?

There is some indication that taping is helpful in preventing inversion sprains. Some experts feel that a tightly taped ankle places more stress on the knee when leg contact occurs and the foot is firmly planted. Firm taping that greatly limits ankle flexibility is not recommended.

What is the proper way to use ice therapy in the treatment of injuries?

Ice therapy (**cryotherapy**) is used immediately following an injury (for 2 to 4 days) and during the rehabilitation phase of treatment (after 4 days). Immediately following an injury, ice relieves pain by encouraging the production of endorphins, and by preventing pain messages from reaching the brain. Cold also reduces swelling, blood clot formation, and tissue damage in the first 9 to 16 minutes of application. Less blood flows through constricted arteries and temperature is decreased to reduce the metabolic requirements of the injured part. Ice should be applied immediately after any injury that causes swelling. The procedures described for R-I-C-E therapy should be used with ice applied for no longer than 19 minutes at one time and reapplied for 19 minutes every hour on the hour for four hours. It is advisable to avoid applying ice directly to the tissue.

Do walking and running create bone jolt or G-force that leads to injury?

Yes. A simple step, when the heel strikes the surface, will bow the leg bones, compress the discs between the vertebrae of your back, and bounce the base of your brain half a millimeter. Each walking step is a collision with the ground involving the body falling about two inches with 150 or more pounds of impact to create a force of approximately 30 Gs or more.

One G is equal to the force of the earth's gravity. Walking creates negative Gs from rapid deceleration when the heel strikes the ground. Hard surface walking may produce 30 Gs in the heel of a hard leather shoe. The shock wave dissipates as it passes from the shoe through the bones of the foot, through the skeleton, and on to the head (**bone jolt**). Bone, muscle, and connective tissue receive the shock as it passes at over 200 miles per hour. If the body failed to absorb the shock, you would be punch drunk in less than one block. Fortunately, the shock-absorbing system begins at the heel where nearly 80 percent of the energy is dissipated. By the time the shock wave hits the knee, it is down to 5 Gs, and down to only ½ G when it reaches the head. The repeated shock occurring in walking and running probably contributes to osteoarthritis, tendonitis, stress fractures, and low back pain.

Does an innersole help reduce the shock waves?

Yes. Certain types of protective pads appear to reduce the shock, prevent damage to the shock-absorbing system, and even permit activity while recovering from an injury. Visco-elastic polymers, made from synthetic compounds, closely resemble the body's cushioning system. The polymer has the properties of both fluids and elastic solids—the damping properties of fluids and the resilience of sponge rubber. Sorbothane is the best known polymer on the market. A Sorbothane wedge in the heel of a hard-soled walking shoe reduces the shock at the tibia by 50 percent. A full Sorbothane innersole may be more appropriate for running, tennis, and team sports. Shock waves through the body may be reduced by 50 to 80 percent with use of a polymer. This reduced shock wave may prevent some solid tissue and bone injuries.

What is orthotics?

Among individuals participating in sports involving a lot of running, knee, hip and back problems are common. In most cases, these injuries are a result of improper foot/ground contact due to excessive foot pronation (when the foot rolls inward). Miles of hard pounding on uneven road surfaces add to the problem.

A podiatrist, who may also be an orthotics specialist analyzes your problem and makes a shoe insert (orthotic) using a cast of your foot. This **orthotic** is designed to correct faulty ground contact and to eliminate injuries. Let's examine some of the common problems that orthotics can help:

1. *Excessive foot pronation and flat feet.* In the correct mechanics of running (not sprinting) you land on the heel first. Weight then transfers to the outside part of the foot as the foot moves forward. At this point, the foot rolls inward to shift body weight to the inside bottom of the foot and distribute the shock throughout the foot and leg. Runners who tend to be flat-footed over pronate and roll the foot inward too far. The most common injury from excessive pronation is pain behind the kneecap caused by the kneecap rubbing against the femur (long bone of upper leg). Check your old shoes for excessive wear on the outside back of the shoe heel.

2. *High arched feet.* These individuals have the opposite problem and fail to pronate enough to distribute body weight properly. Stress fractures and pain on the outside of the knee is common in athletes with this structural problem.

3. *Unequal leg lengths.* Even slight differences of $\frac{1}{3}$ or $\frac{1}{4}$ inch can lead to hip, back, or leg pain. You can measure overall leg length by standing erect with ankles together and having a helper measure the distance from the floor to spots marked on either side of the top of your pelvis. If the two bony protrusions of the ankle do not meet at the same point, your length difference is below the ankle. If, while sitting on a chair with feet on the floor, heels together, and toes pointed, a carpenter's level placed on both knees is uneven, your problem is above the ankle.

4. **Morton's foot.** Approximately one person in three has a short first metatarsal (big toe) and long second metatarsal (second toe). Because the second toe is longer than the big one, it must take more force of the initial foot stride (particularly in stopping and changing direction), and is more susceptible to stress fractures and irritation. Orthotics and padding to even the alignment of the first and second toes can help prevent injury.

Is an individual who has his or her wind knocked out in danger?

No. The temporary inability to breathe following a blow to a relaxed midsection will slowly subside until breathing is restored. Meanwhile the victim will gasp for breath, possibly suffer from dizziness, nausea, all-around weakness, and may even collapse. Technically, a hard blow to the solar plexus increases intra-abdominal pressure, causes pain, and interferes with the diaphragmatic cycle reflex due to nerve paralysis or muscle spasm. Obviously, breathing is temporarily affected by such a blow.

A physician or trainer should be called and emergency treatment begun immediately by instructing the victim to breathe slowly through the nose. Clothing should be lossened at the neck and waist and ice applied to the abdomen. The practice of lifting the victim up by the belt and dropping him or her to the ground is of no value and could be harmful should stomach injury be present.

It may be helpful to know that it is nearly impossible for death to occur from such an injury, which merely paralyzes the nerve control of the diaphragm. This may be little consolation to a gasping victim who is convinced that death is only seconds away. One of the most severe cases observed occurred during a rugby game in which the victim's gasping was heard throughout the playing area, suggesting a rather severe injury. Approximately 20 seconds later, normal breathing returned and not a trace of pain was evident on the victim's extremely pale face.

Are women more susceptible to injuries than men?

Physiological differences between the sexes make women somewhat more susceptible to injury and less responsive to training: (1) women have a lower ratio of strength to body weight, (2) women have more body fat, and (3) the chemical makeup of muscle tissue is different in women. These factors make women slightly more vulnerable to soft tissue injuries from contusions and strain. The female athlete can reduce the likelihood of injuries through proper conditioning and strength training.

Can swimming pools be used to rehabilitate an injury?

A swimming pool allows free movement of the injured part without the full body weight producing pain. Waist-deep water is excellent for contracting injured legs and arms and even jogging, when such movements would be painful on land.

How does aging affect injury and healing?

Unfortunately, older individuals are more easily injured and slower to heal than younger individuals. Age results in numerous physical changes that bring this about: the quality of distensibility disappears from connective tissue, limiting flexibility and increasing the possibility of injury; localized areas of cartilage soften from injury, disease, or wear, particularly in weight-bearing areas of the legs, leaving one more injury prone; muscles, ligaments, and tendons lose their elasticity and are more susceptible to injury; and broken bones heal more slowly.

Contact sports should be avoided after age 45 to 50 and substituted with vigorous activity of another nature. Again, for those who have excercised continually throughout life, injury is less likely to occur. Pushing oneself too far beyond the maximum at later ages can lead to strain.

Is it safe to use various types of Novocain derivatives to deaden pain so I can continue to exercise or compete for my team?

No. It is also against league rules at most levels of competition. Strict enforcement of this regulation is encouraged since Novocain produces a number of physiological changes: blood pressure is raised, peripheral vessels are dilated, and the warning signs of pain are masked to permit activity that may result in serious permanent danger to a body part. Repeated trauma or blows to an area are also a leading cause of bursitis, which in severe cases demands complete rest.

Although most athletes want to compete even while injured, such action should be allowed only if there is little danger of more serious injury and if pain and discomfort are mild enough to permit it. Local anesthetic in the ankle, shoulder, knee or thigh, to name a few common spots, should not be allowed by coaches, trainers, or team physicians at the high school and university levels.

Is the use of drugs dangerous for those who exercise?

Yes. Keep in mind that people react differently to drugs of all kinds. Factors that contribute to diminished performance and increase the danger include: (1) *Individual differences to medication.* Identical doses affect people differently; they may be toxic to one person and not to another, helpful to one and harmful to another. There is no such thing as a normal dose that produces predictable physical, emotional, or intellectual behavior. (2) *Sensitivity to a drug.* This unknown factor can manifest itself through skin rashes, functional disturbances, and even death. (3) *Quantity consumed.* Excessive use has a toxic effect that can interrupt the function of the body systems and lead to death.

The time of day, humidity, temperature, air movement, amount of food in the stomach, fatigue, conditioning level, other medication in the system, mental outlook, and state of health are additional factors that determine the effect of any medication on the body. Too many tranquilizers will cause sluggish performance. Overuse of stimulants will cause overexcitability and loss of fine muscular movements as well as removal of the warning signs of fatigue and pain. Use of any of the three common types (stimulants, depressants, hormone steroids) over an extended period of time can lead to liver and kidney damage, sexual atrophy and dependence.

You can be highly fit without drugs—and for a longer period of time. Don't take the chance—you may be the unlucky one whose first dose is fatal.

Is the use of amphetamines dangerous?

Yes. **Amphetamines,** the most common drug in sports, are used in medicine to stimulate the central nervous system. Their use in athletics is unethical, a breach of sportsmanship, and extremely dangerous. Use of amphetamines is hazardous because (1) doses are difficult to control, since different physiological states alter one's reaction to the drug; (2) tolerance occurs and forces you to increase the dosage for the same effect; (3) danger of addiction is present; (4) warning signs of fatigue and overstrain are unnoticed during exercise, increasing the possibility of bodily harm from overexertion; (5) vasopressor effects (elevated blood pressure) are undesirable; (6) complete circulatory collapse may occur from over use; (7) heat stroke is more common to users on hot, humid days.

You may feel pepped up after using an amphetamine, but this feeling is not likely to improve your performance. The long-term effects on the internal organs can be fatal with continuous use. Leave the illegal use of amphetamines to the horses unless you want to bet your life.

How does cocaine affect the body?

Cocaine is highly toxic, habit forming, and extremely hazardous to health. It is also very expensive. Its derivatives, procaine and Novocain, are widely used in medicine. Cocaine stimulates the central nervous system and steps up both breathing and circulation. It has been used in the sports world as a recreational drug and as a means of postponing fatigue by masking its symptoms in an attempt to increase muscular work and endurance and to speed up recovery.

Cocaine stimulation is usually followed by acute depression. Evidence revealing the use of "coke" by a number of professional athletes has prompted numerous investigations and routine drug testing. The unpredictability of the effects of cocaine on an individual, even one who has been a regular user, makes it an extremely dangerous drug capable of causing death with just one experimental attempt to see what it's like.

Is the use of barbiturates dangerous?

Yes. Overuse of **barbiturates** can lead to dependence, intoxication, and sluggishness. It is much safer to relax by eliminating caffeine-containing stimulants such as coffee, tea, cocoa, and cola, and to improve relaxation techniques, than to rely on barbiturates.

Millions of tranquilizers are used by the American public. Millions of people also chase away the drowsiness of last night's tranquilizer with wake-up pills (stimulants). Such a practice places them on a treadmill with all exits leading to the hospital. Slang terms for barbiturates include barbs, blue devils, dolls, goofers, phenies, red devils, and yellow jackets. The "sting" lasts up to four hours, except with an overdose, in which case it's very, very permanent.

Is the use of anabolic steroids and other hormones dangerous?

Steroids are drugs of great potency with many side effects. Testosterone (male sex hormone) is commonly used in athletics, particularly by weight lifters, decathlon competitors, and football players, as a means to gain weight and increase strength. Testosterone has androgenic (producing masculine characteristics) and anabolic (increasing nitrogen retention, protein building, and muscle weight) qualities. A synthetic steroid is now in use that produces an anabolic effect without much change in masculine characteristics.

Some studies have shown that steroids increase body weight and strength; others have not. Some individuals who use steroids are convinced that the drug increases muscle mass and strength. One thing is certain: steroids are dangerous and have been known to lead to serious liver damage, growth stunt in adolescents that prematurely fuses the long bones of the body, acne, sterility, stomach bleeding, and cancer.

Actual skill in any sport is not affected by use of steroids; increased strength and weight, however, do provide considerable help in sports where muscle bulk and explosive power are critical. The general feeling is that steroids retard fatigue during training and allow more work to be done.

What about LSD and PCP?

LSD (lysergic acid diethylamide) is taken orally in small quantities. It is nearly one thousand times more potent than most other drugs and affects the brain within 30 to 60 minutes for 10 to 12 hours. Body temperature, heart rate, and blood pressure increase and sweating and chills occur. Headache and nausea rarely affect the psychedelic experience. LSD is an extremely dangerous drug and has produced many "bad trips" resulting in individuals jumping in front of cars or out windows, or swimming out to sea. Heavy users may experience "flashbacks" weeks or months after taking the drug. LSD is rarely used by athletes for the purpose of improving performance or delaying fatigue. Not only would both be adversely affected, but behavior would be unpredictable and dangerous.

PCP (phencyclidine) is also a psychedelic and hallucinogenic drug that is taken orally in a capsule, smoked with tobacco, parsley, or marijuana, or injected intravenously. The drug causes symptoms similar to other psychoactive drugs. Heavy doses may produce a stupor lasting several days; overdose can result in a coma lasting several days and followed by weeks of confusion. PCP is an extremely dangerous drug.

MYTHS AND FALLACIES

When an injury occurs to most body parts, heat should be applied.

Injuries to soft tissue (muscle, ligaments, tendons), such as bumps and bruises, should be immediately treated with R-I-C-E therapy, which requires ice, not heat. To be safe, heat should be avoided for two to three days until swelling begins to subside. The practice of applying heat pads, hot towels, hot baths, whirlpool, and other forms of heat increases swelling, delays healing, and can result in serious problems that may require surgery.

Sports and exercise can damage the female breast.

Injuries to the female breast are rare. It is advisable, however, to wear a protective brassiere in sports such as fencing, racketball, squash, field hockey, team handball, basketball, and wrestling.

Exercise is harmful to the female reproductive organs.

A blow to the body or violent jarring does not cause a similar jolt to the uterus. There is at present no evidence to suggest that a healthy female of any age can be harmed by vigorous exercise.

Individuals who have a heart murmur should not exercise.

A heart murmur is an abnormal sound caused by turbulent blood flow. The difficulty may be an impaired value that fails to close completely or valve orifices that are narrowed and slow the flow of blood. A greater-than-normal load is placed on the heart, heart walls may increase in size, and tension increases inside the walls. The heart is less efficient and, in a sense, has to regurgitate blood twice. In what is termed a "functional" murmur, no structural defect is evident to account for the abnormal sounds. Although individuals with functional murmurs can generally exercise safely, it is important to consult your physician before starting a new program.

Is the use of aspirin harmful?

Not if used properly. Aspirin remains the most popular household medication for all types of aches and pains. It can be purchased plain, buffered, effervescent, candied, combined with other drugs, and in different colors.

It is effective in reducing fever, cold or flu symptoms, and pain and discomfort, and possibly in reducing the chances of recurrent heart attacks in some patients.

There is no over-the-counter (nonprescription) drug in existence that surpasses aspirin as an analgesic (pain controlling), antipyretic (fever diminishing), or anti-inflammatory (inflammation reducing) agent. Acetaminophen is available for those who cannot tolerate any form of aspirin; however, it costs more and is not an effective anti-inflammatory agent.

Aspirin can irritate the stomach and cause reactions such as hives, asthma, and mucous membrane swelling. Taking aspirin with food, milk, or even a full glass of water reduces chances of stomach upset. Most types no longer contain phenacetin, which may cause permanent, serious kidney damage. Others have caffeine added.

Numerous studies have been conducted to determine which type of aspirin is more effective in terms of speed of absorption, pain-killing ability, stomach irritation, and safety. All appear to be equally effective in the areas of concern. The main difference is price. Buy the cheapest aspirin available. Also, avoid overuse. It is much more sound to have a physician analyze what may be causing the symptom of pain than to mask it with aspirin.

Aren't the health risks of smoking reduced in those who exercise?

The risks may be slightly less for those who engage in regular aerobic exercise; however, they are certainly not eliminated. Research has shown that cigarette smoking (1) reduces the oxygen-carrying capacity of the blood due to carbon monoxide absorption; (2) reduces the ability of the lungs to take in and use oxygen by as much as 50 percent; (3) produces an increase in heart rate with only one cigarette from 2 to 52 beats per minute which remains for 30 to 45 minutes; (4) elevates blood pressure for 30 to 45 minutes; (5) constricts blood vessels; (6) drops skin temperature of the hands and feet form 1 to 9 degrees Fahrenheit; (7) damages small arteries that carry blood to the lung surface for oxygenation; (8) adversely affects performance in complex motor skills; (9) decreases altitude tolerance, making you less efficient at higher altitudes—smoking one pack per day is equivalent to living at an altitude of 8,000 feet; (10) irritates the nervous system; and (11) irritates the membranes of the throat and lungs, causing a cigarette cough and greater chance of infection.

What does all this mean? In simple terms, it means that performance in endurance-type activities is decreased by smoking. Even speed is hindered in some individuals. Why? Because oxygen must be taken into the lungs and distributed to the working muscles, and carbon dioxide eliminated, as efficiently as possible during exercise. If you smoke, you are operating like an untuned car; you cannot use fuel efficiently. Also, a rapid heart is less efficient since it does not have enough time to fill between beats, higher blood pressure forces the heart to pump against greater resistance, and constriction of blood vessels reduces the supply of blood to all body parts.

Use of tobacco in any form is an unwise health choice. Without cigarettes, you can perform at a high pace for a longer period of time. You will feel better and live a longer, healthier life. Stop smoking for a season and see for yourself—you may never light up again.

What about smokeless tobacco?

The use of chewing tobacco and snuff is under tremendous fire. Early research strongly suggests that smokeless tobacco causes cancer of the mouth, lip, gums, stomach, and other organs. In addition, evidence also indicates that a number of the undesirable physiological changes described previously for cigarette smokers also occur with the use of smokeless tobacco. As a result of recent legislation, all smokeless tobacco products carry health warning statements similar to those on cigarette packs. Don't be influenced by professional athletes who use smokeless tobacco. It is an extremely dangerous practice that can decrease fitness and destroy your health.

Is marijuana smoking harmful?

Yes. Although effects vary from one person to another, a reaction similar to that produced by alcohol occurs. The behavior of users is difficult to predict because one experiences elation as well as time, distance, and sound distortion for about four hours. Drowsiness and sleep may occur, and there is generally no hangover or physical discomfort upon waking.

Marijuana (grass, hash, hemp, joint, Mary Jane, muggles, pot, reefers, stuff, tea, weed) releases inhibitions and can make you irresponsible, unpredictable, and dangerous. Though it produces no withdrawal symptoms or physical dependency, a psychological or emotional dependency is common. Also, its use may expose you to the drug scene and probable use of more dangerous drugs. Evidence suggests that for some, marijuana is a dangerous, habituating, intoxicating drug. It is a sedative that depresses body functions and impairs physical performance. It is not a sexual stimulant and is more likely to impair sexual performance than enhance it. While some people feel it enhances creativity, it is now clear that so-called creative thoughts are not considered very creative when analyzed by users after the "high" disappears.

Fine, imprisonment, poor health, exposure to the drug scene, emotional dependence, hallucination, impaired performance and judgment, and panic reactions are some of the by-products of use. Marijuana smoking can only hinder performance and fitness. it is a much more powerful drug than early studies first indicated. No wise individual would consider even one "joint."

BIBLIOGRAPHY

American College of Sports Medicine. *Guidelines for Grade Exercise Testing and Exercise Prescription.* Philadelphia: Lea and Febiger, 1986.

Brody, David M. "Running Injuries." *Clinical Symposia.* CIBA Pharmaceutical Co. 32:4 (1980).

Brooks, G. A., and T. D. Fahey. "Fundamentals of Human Performance." New York: Macmillan, 1987.

Cohen, Sidney. *The Substance Abuse Problems.* Vol. 2, New Issues for the 80's. New York: Haworth Press, 1985.

Cooper, Kenneth H. *The Aerobics Program for Total Well-Being.* New York: M. Evans, 1982.

Dintiman, George B., and Robert Ward. *Train America! Achieving Peak Performance and Fitness for Sports Competition.* Dubuque, Iowa: Kendal Hunt, 1988.

Dintiman, George B., and Robert Ward. *Sportspeed: Speed Improvement for Football, Basketball and Baseball.* Champaign, Ill.: Human Kinetics, 1988.

Dintiman, George B., et al. *Doctor Tennis: A Complete Guide to Conditioning and Injury Prevention for all Ages.* Richmond, Va.: National Association of Speed and Explosion, 1980.

Fahey, T. D., ed. *Athletic Training: Principles and Practice.* Mountain View, Cal.: Mayfield, 1986.

Fisher, Seymour, Allen Raskin, and E. H. Uhlenhuth, eds. *Cocaine: Clinical and Biobehavioral Aspects.* New York: Oxford University Press, 1987.

O'Brien, R., and S. Cohen. *The Encyclopedia of Drug Abuse.* New York: Facts on File, 1984.

LABORATORY 8.1

Evaluating Your Potential for Foot and Leg Injuries

PURPOSE: To identify aspects in the make-up of the lower extremities that may require some adjustment to prevent injury.

PROCEDURE

Examine yourself carefully in the following areas:

1. *Length of both legs below the ankle:* Stand erect, ankles together, and ask a helper to measure the distance from the floor to a spot marked with a magic marker at the bony protrusion of the ankle.

2. *Length of both legs above the ankle:* Sit in a chair with your feet on the floor, heels together and toes pointed. If a carpenter's level placed on both knees is uneven, your problem is above the ankle.

3. *Morton's foot:* Stand erect without shoes or socks and determine whether your second toe is larger than your great toe.

4. *Excessive pronation:* Examine your running or athletic shoes for excessive wear on the outside back of the shoe heel.

RESULTS

1. Are your leg lengths identical or do they differ by less than $1/16''$?

2. Is the problem below the ankle or from the ankle to the knee?

3. Are your shoes wearing unevenly?

4. Is your second metatarsal longer than your great toe?

5. Are you experiencing pain in the lower back, hip, knee, ankle, or feet during or following exercise? If so, consult your orthopedic physician for advice on how you should change your form or athletic shoes to correct the problem.

LABORATORY 8.2

Cigarette Smoking and Heart Rate

PURPOSE: To determine the effects of smoking upon resting heart rate. To compare the resting heart rate of smokers and nonsmokers.

PROCEDURE

1. Smokers and nonsmokers are seated in separate halves of the room, as far apart as possible. Both groups remain in their seats for a minimum of 15 minutes without rising. During this period, students practice self-administering the carotid pulse check: using the tips of the three middle fingers, press up under the rear portion of the jaw bone until a pulse is felt.

2. After the rest period, each student determines his or her pulse rate for 30 seconds before doubling that count. A recorder lists the resting pulse rates separately for each group.

3. During the next 15 minutes, members of the smoking groups (regular and low tar) may light up and smoke at their normal rates until the time limit expires. No one is permitted to stand or to walk around the room. Nonsmokers should be as far away as possible and windows should be opened to reduce the effects of secondhand smoke.

4. After the 15-minute smoking period, both smokers and nonsmokers again take and record their carotid pulse.

RESULTS

1. Compare the carotid pulse rates of smokers (regardless of the type of cigarette) and nonsmokers, using only the initial count (prior to the smoking period). What is the average pulse rate of:

Smoking men ———   Nonsmoking men ———   Difference ———

Smoking women ———   Nonsmoking women ———   Difference ———

2. Compare the initial pulse rate with the second pulse rate for the smoking group:

Average pulse rate (initial pulse) for all smokers   ———

Average pulse rate (second test) for all smokers   ———

Difference   ———

Average pulse rate (initial test), regular cigarettes   ———

Average pulse rate (initial test), low tar   ———

Average pulse rate (second test), regular cigarettes   ———

Average pulse rate (second test), low tar   ———

Continued on next page

LABORATORY 8.2
Continued

Cigarette Smoking and Heart Rate

3. What effect did smoking have on heart rate?

4. Using 70 cc of blood per beat (approximate volume pumped per beat), calculate how much extra blood the smokers' hearts must pump to maintain sitting posture.

5. How effective were the low-tar cigarettes in reducing the effect of cigarettes on heart rate?

6. Compare the initial pulse rate with the second pulse rate for the nonsmoking group:

   Average pulse rate (initial test)   ——

   Average pulse rate (second test)   ——

   Difference   ——

   Did changes occur for the nonsmoking group?   ——

7. Could secondhand smoke have affected the nonsmoking group?

8. What conclusions can be drawn from this study?

CHAPTER NINE

Tailor-Made
Programs
FOR YOU

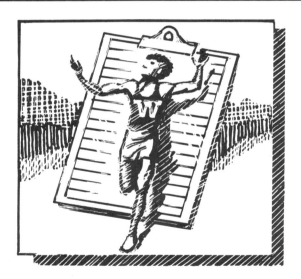

❝LOOKING OUT FOR
NUMBER ONE **❞**

? HAVE YOU EVER WONDERED ABOUT:

How to begin the exercise activity of your choice?
How to progress safely and surely?
How to reach a high fitness level?
How to keep up regular training?
How to breathe correctly while you exercise?

KEY TERMS

Exercise allergy
Exercise breathing
LSD training
Normal breathing rates

Oxygen debt
Second wind
Staleness

From the information provided in Chapters 3 through 8, you are now ready to begin an aerobic regime that will form the foundation of your fitness program. Choose an aerobic activity that you enjoy and are likely to continue for four months or more. Tables 9.1 to 9.5 are designed to allow you to enter the program of your choice at your present conditioning level and to progress systematically to as high an aerobic fitness level as you desire. Each program applies the concepts of conditioning presented in Chapter 3 to slowly, systematically, and safely improve your cardiovascular or aerobic conditioning level, help you lose body fat through high caloric expenditure, and assist you in the prevention of early heart disease.

After choosing your aerobic activity, it is necessary to determine your aerobic fitness level. If you have been inactive for six months or more or have never been involved in aerobic exercise, enter your program at the Very Beginning level and progress slowly. If you have been exercising regularly (minimum of two times weekly), turn to Chapter 3, p. 70, and plan to take the 1.5-mile test on a quarter-mile track or a measured golf course or road. Find your fitness category and begin your aerobic program.

FREQUENTLY ASKED QUESTIONS

Can you offer suggestions to assist in training regularly?

Although thousands of people initiate daily exercise programs, the majority eventually disband their efforts long before actual weight loss or physiological value is attained. For the athlete, this may become a problem in the off-season period.

Even the most ideal exercise program demands three to four weeks of systematic involvement if observable results are to accrue. A strong effort must be made in both diet and exercise habits to avoid termination before a program becomes an important part of the daily routine. The following tips will help you maintain a regular exercise program:

1. Establish an exercise goal in terms of desired objectives, and choose the program most conducive to the attainment of these objectives.
2. Set realistic starting levels well within your physical and psychological limits.
3. Fight off early desires to miss a training session.
4. Set aside a daily time for your program and prevent any type of conflict.
5. Incorporate some method of periodic self-evaluation.
6. Vary your program through alternate activities of a vigorous nature.
7. Maintain both weight and exercise progress records to ensure a systematic approach and to uncover any unusual weight changes.

TABLE 9.1 CYCLING

Week	Aerobic Training Program	Comments

I. Very Beginning

1st week	Ride for a distance of 2 miles, three times per week.	Do not be concerned with time during first weeks of your program. Cycle at a pace that allows you to finish 2 miles without undue fatigue.
3rd week	Ride for a distance of 2 miles, three times per week. Try to finish the distance in 12 minutes or less.	Time your ride and attempt to reach the target time.
6th week	Test yourself in the 1.5-mile test. If your category has changed, move on to the program for rating II. If there is no change, add one workout and cycle four times each week.	

II. Beginning

1st week	Ride for a distance of 3 miles, three times per week.	Time your ride and aim for a time of 17 minutes or less.
3rd week	Continue riding for 3 miles, but work out four times per week.	Try to lower the time for your ride to 14 minutes or less.
6th week	Test yourself in the 1.5-mile test. If your category has changed, move on to the program for rating III. If there is no change, add one workout and cycle five times each week.	

III. Intermediate

1st week	Ride for a distance of 5 miles, three times per week.	Time your ride and aim for a time of 25 minutes or less.
3rd week	Continue riding for 5 miles, but work out four times per week.	
6th week	Test yourself in the 1.5-mile test. If your category has changed, move on to the program for rating IV. If there is no change, add one workout and cycle five times each week.	

IV. Advanced

1st week	Ride for a distance of 8 miles, four times per week.	Aim for a time of 35 minutes or less.
3rd week	Add one workout and cycle five times per week.	

V. Excellent/Superior

	Continue with this workout and try to lower your time to 24 minutes or less. Take the 1.5-mile test once a month to judge the success of your program.	

TABLE 9.2 JOGGING AND RUNNING

Week	Aerobic Training Program	Comments
	I. Very Beginning	
1st week	On a track, begin running at a comfortable pace until you sense the onset of mild fatigue. Stop immediately and note the distance covered. Walk at an average pace until fatigue symptoms subside. Note the distance. Return to running until fatigue symptoms reappear. Stop. Record the total distance covered during the two running phases and one walking phase. This is your first target. Until you can run this distance nonstop, do not add any mileage to your workout.	This is a run/walk workout. Do not overdo it on the first day. After several weeks, you should be able to run the target distance nonstop. Work out at least three times weekly.
3rd week	Begin **LSD** (long/slow/distance) training. Use a pace that permits a pleasant conversation and causes only mild distress. Continue running nonstop for as long as possible. Rather than walk, slow the pace and attempt to finish the workout pleasantly tired but not exhausted. Do not be concerned about time.	Continue LSD training, add ½ to 1 minute to each workout until you can run nonstop for at least 20 minutes. Work out at least three times weekly.
6th week	Test yourself in the 1.5-mile test. If your category has changed, move on to the program for rating II. If there is no change, continue LSD training until you can run 30 minutes nonstop.	
	II. Beginning	
1st week	Use LSD training as described above, covering a minimum of 1 mile each workout (nonstop) for several weeks before walking/ running 1 or 2 additional miles at the end of each workout.	Increase the number of weekly workouts to four.
3rd week	Begin to time each mile, running at a 9:00 minutes per mile pace for as long a distance as possible. Attempt to achieve 2 miles in 18:00 or less.	Run a minimum of 6 miles weekly.
6th week	Test yourself in the 1.5-mile test. If your category has changed, move on to the program for rating III. If there is no change, continue LSD training until you can run 1 mile in 8:45 and 2 miles in 17:30.	
	III. Intermediate	
1st week	Continue LSD training at a 9:00 pace.	Increase to 10 to 12 miles weekly.
3rd week	Increase your nonstop run to 3 miles.	
6th week	Test yourself in the 1.5-mile test. If your category has changed, move on to the program for rating IV. If there is no change, continue to increase weekly mileage volume by 2 to 3 miles.	

TABLE 9.2 JOGGING AND RUNNING—Continued		
Week	**Aerobic Training Program**	**Comments**

IV. Advanced

1st week	Increase your nonstop run to 6 miles. Continue LSD training at an 8:45 to 8:30 pace.	
3rd week	Continue LSD training, picking up the pace by 5 to 10 seconds per mile.	
6th week	Test yourself in the 1.5-mile test. If your category has changed, move on to the program for rating V. If there is no change, continue the above training for two additional weeks, then retest.	

V. Excellent/Superior

If this is your test category, continue with whatever program you have been using.

Take the 1.5 mile test once a month to judge the success of your maintenance program.

Each workout at all levels begins with a slow, 1-mile, warm-up run/walk, and ends with a ¾ to 1-mile slow, cool-down jog.

8. Maintain a balanced diet, get proper rest, and avoid use of drugs to curb appetite.
9. Do not expect instant results.
10. Alternate hard and easy days. If you seem tired while exercising, slack off and make it an easy day.
11. Keep daily or weekly records of resting heart rate, distance covered, and time spent exercising.

What is the proper way to breathe during vigorous exercise?

Through your mouth. This allows air to enter and exit much faster since there is less resistance to overcome. At rest, the most efficient breathing is through the nose. Air is warmed, moistened, and cleansed of foreign particles. On hot days, however, air does not need to be warmed and so mouth breathing actually helps to cool the body. With **exercise breathing,** nose breathing cannot keep up with the increased demand for oxygen. To demonstrate this fact, you need only run a distance of a quarter mile or more with your mouth shut.

Breathing is a very simple process that involves three steps: gas exchange in the lungs, gas transport through the bloodstream to the tissues, and gas exchange between the blood and tissues. The rate of breathing is controlled by the amount of carbon dioxide in the blood rather than by the lack of oxygen. **Normal breathing rates** vary from 12 to 20 breaths per minute during rest to as high as 50 to 60 during exercise. As conditioning levels improve, breathing rate is lowered.

In general, you will be more efficient if you leave breathing to nature. At rest, each person has a rate and depth of breathing

TABLE 9.3 ROPE JUMPING

Week	Aerobic Training Program[1]	Comments[2]
I. Very Beginning		
1st week	Practice the basic jumps (described below) for 15 minutes. Then try to use the two-foot single-beat jump for a 30 second set; repeat three times. Sets are 3 seconds longer each workout.	Master the technique of each type of jump. Stop and check your heart rate after 30 seconds. If continuously jumping, rest 2 minutes between sets.
3rd week	Practice the basic jumps for 15 minutes. Then use the two-foot single-beat jump for 45 seconds; repeat three times. Sets are 3 seconds longer each workout.	Rests 2 minutes between sets.
6th week	Test yourself in the 1.5-mile test. If your category has changed, move on to the program for rating II. If there is no change, remain at this point for two more weeks.	Rest 1½ minutes between sets.
II. Beginning		
1st week	Practice the basic jumps for 15 minutes. Then use the two-foot single-beat jump for 75 seconds; repeat four times. Sets are 3 seconds longer each workout.	Rest 1½ minutes between sets.
3rd week	Same as above for 90 seconds.	
6th week	Test yourself in the 1.5-mile test. If your category has changed, move on to the program for rating III. If there is no change, remain at this point for two more weeks.	Rest 1½ minutes between sets.
III. Intermediate		
1st week	Practice the basic jumps for 15 minutes. Then use the two-foot single-beat jump, and any two basic jumps for 4 minutes; repeat twice more. Sets are 10 seconds longer each workout.	Rest 1 minute between sets.
3rd week	Same as above for 6 minutes. Sets are 10 seconds longer each workout.	Rest 1 minute between sets.
6th week	Same as above for 8 to 9 minutes. Test yourself in the 1.5-mile test. If your category has changed, move on to the program for rating IV. If there is no change, remain at this point for two more weeks.	
IV. Advanced		
1st week	Use the two-foot single-beat jump for 10 to 12 minutes; repeat twice more using two of the basic jumps. Sets are 10 seconds longer each workout.	Rest 1 minute between sets.
3rd week	Same as above for 13 to 15 minues. Add 25 seconds per workout.	Rest 1 minute between sets.

TABLE 9.3   ROPE JUMPING—Continued

Week	Aerobic Training Program[1]	Comments[2]

IV. Advanced

| 6th week | Same as above for 17 to 20 minutes, completing two sets. Sets are 30 seconds longer each workout. Test yourself in the 1.5-mile test. If your category has changed, move on to the program for rating V. If there is no change, remain at this point for two more weeks, then retest. | Rest 1 minute between sets. |

V. Excellent/Superior

If this is your test category, continue with whatever program you have been using.

Take the 1.5-mile test once a month to judge the success of your maintenance program.

[1]Each workout at all levels begins with 5 minutes of warm-up jumps and ends with a cool-down consisting of 3 to 5 minutes of slow double jumps.

[2]Workouts should be followed four times weekly.

Warm-up Jumps:

Two-foot double-beat jump After the rope passes under the feet, a small hop is taken before jumping again to clear the rope.

Two-foot single-beat jump No intermediate jump is taken.

Single-foot hop The left food is used for a specified number of jumps, following by the right foot.

Basic Jumps:

Boxer's shuffle Use alternate right-foot and left-foot jumps.

Running forward Jump while running forward.

Single-foot hops Same as warm-up jump; progress from slow to fast or pepper (very fast).

Double Jump The rope must pass under the feet twice while in the air; do one double jump, one single, one double, and so on.

Cross-overs Fully cross the arms as the rope clears the head.

most efficient for him or her; nature will find it. Since atmospheric oxygen is needed, exercise is one of the few times that it does not pay to keep your mouth shut.

What is second wind?

In some individuals, signs of fatigue such as breathlessness, rapid pulse, and sore muscles are suddenly relieved. The load that appeared strenuous and may have caused breathlessness is lightened. When this occurs, an individual is capable of additional effort. This so-called **second wind** may not take place for you, or it may happen following some types of exercise and not others. In fact, some complain that they never experience this sudden freedom from fatigue.

It is not fully understood why second wind occurs or what brings it about. The following observations may shed some light on the subject and assist you in the future:

1. Second wind occurs earlier during vigoruous exercise than during moderate exercise.

TABLE 9.4   SWIMMING

Week	Aerobic Training Program	Comments
I. Very Beginning		
1st week	Begin by using any stroke and swim for 12 to 20 minutes per session at least three times per week.	Swim until out of breath. Continue until swimming is nonstop for the allotted time.
3rd week	Swim three to five times per week. Try to use the freestyle stroke as much as possible.	Swim continuously for 20 minutes.
6th week	Test yourself in the 1.5-mile test. If your category has changed, move on to the program for rating II. If there is no change, remain at this point for two more weeks, then retest.	
II. Beginning		
1st week	Begin by using any stroke and swim for 15 to 22 minutes per session at least three times per week.	Swim until out of breath. Continue until swimming is nonstop for allotted time.
3rd week	Swim daily. Use the free-style stroke as much as possible.	Swim continuously for 22 minutes.
6th week	Swim daily for 30 minutes. Test yourself in the 1.5-mile test. If your category has changed, move onto the program for rating III. If there is no change, remain at this point for two more weeks.	
III. Intermediate		
1st week	Swim freestyle for 500 yards per workout, three times per week.	Begin to time your workouts. Aim for a time of 12 minutes. If you reach 12 minutes, then aim for 10½ minutes.
3rd week	Continue 500 yards per workout. Add one additional workout each week.	Try to reach the above target times.
6th week	Test yourself in 1.5-mile test. If your category has changed, move on to the program for rating IV. If there is no change, remain at this point for 2 more weeks, then retest.	
IV. Advanced		
1st week	Swim freestyle for 650 yards per workout, four times each week.	Aim for a time of 15½ minutes.
3rd week	Add one workout for the next two weeks for a total of six workouts per week.	
6th week	Test yourself in 1.5-mile test. If your category has changed, move on to the program for rating V. If there is no change, remain at this point for two more weeks and add 50 yards per workout, then retest.	

TABLE 9.4 SWIMMING—Continued

Week	Aerobic Training Program	Comments
	V. Excellent/Superior	
	Aim to swim freestyle for 1,000 yards per workout. Begin with 700 yards per workout and add 50 yards every two workouts.	Aim for a 1,000-yard time of under 16½ minutes.
	Take the 1.5-mile test once monthly to judge the success of your maintenance program.	If you want to improve rather than maintain present level, add 50 yards every three workouts until you reach 2,000 yards. Aim for a time of 34 minutes.

TABLE 9.5 WALKING

Week	Aerobic Training Program	Comments
	I. Very Beginning	
1st week	Walk at a slow-to-average pace for the first 5 minutes of your workout, then walk at a brisk pace for 1 mile. Do three workouts per week.	Avoid doing too much the first few weeks by walking slowly when fatigued and walking briskly when fresh. After several weeks you should be able to keep walking at a brisk pace for the entire distance.
3rd week	Increase the distance covered to 1.5 miles. Do not be concerned about time. Be sure to cover the proper distance each workout.	
6th week	Test yourself in the 1.5-mile test. If your category has changed, move on to the program for rating II. If there was no change, continue adding 0.1 mile per workout until the distance covered is 2 miles.	
	II. Beginning	
1st week	Walk at a brisk pace for 2 miles. Do three workouts per week.	Instead of one 2-mile session, you may do two workout sessions of 1 mile—that is, 1 mile in the morning and 1 mile in the evening.
3rd week	Increase your distance to 2.5 miles three times per week.	
6th week	Test yourself in the 1.5-mile test. If your category has changed, move on to the program for rating III. If there is no change, continue adding 0.1 mile per workout until the distance covered is 3 miles.	

TABLE 9.5   WALKING—Continued

Week	Aerobic Training Program	Comments
III. Intermediate		
1st week	Walk at a brisk pace for 3 miles. Do three workouts per week.	Time your walk and aim at a time of 45 minutes or 1 hour.
3rd week	Add one workout for a total of four per week. Keep your distance the same.	
6th week	Test yourself in the 1.5-mile test. If your category has changed, move on to the program for rating IV. If there is no change, continue adding 0.1 mile per workout until the distance covered is 4 miles.	
IV. Advanced		
1st week	Walk at a brisk pace for 4.5 miles. Do four workouts per week.	Time your walk and aim at a time of 1 hour and 30 minutes.
3rd week	Walk 4.5 miles five times each week.	
6th week	Test yourself in the 1.5-mile test. If your category has changed, move on to the program for rating V. If there is no change, add 0.1 mile per workout until the distance covered is 5 miles.	
V. Excellent/Superior		
1st week	Begin walking for 10 minutes, then jog for as long as possible. Do not be concerned about distance, but try to jog nonstop for 20 minutes. Do three of these workouts per week.	
3rd week	Continue jogging three times per week and add 1 minute to each workout until you can jog for 30 minutes.	
6th week	Test yourself in the 1.5-mile test and then enter the appropriate category in the jogging and running program (Table 9.2)	

2. Second wind is more likely to take place when the weather is hot, and the individual is free from chilling winds.
3. Second wind may come about sooner when a long, vigorous warm-up was used.

When second wind occurs, body temperature rises, arterioles relax and open, and energy is saved in supplying working muscles with oxygen. Stress is relieved and you are capable of continued exercise. It may be that it happens in the following manner: fatigue products accumulate in the muscles because, until the respiratory system has time to adjust, the activity is anaerobic; it is performed without enough oxygen for efficient body functioning (**oxygen debt**). In simpler terms, there is a lag in the chemical regulation of breathing. Eventually, respiration increases and catches up. This may be second wind. Actually, it is really the "first wind," as atmospheric air is finally being used efficiently.

Experiment in your training through use of a long warm-up. When you find the technique that brings about this sudden relief from physical stress, stay with it. Also, warm up properly. Most people's "second wind" is really their first: they quit much too soon even to have a second.

Is it true that some people are allergic to exercise?

Yes. In a few cases rashes occur on the skin of the neck and upper thighs, behind the earlobes, and occasionally on other parts of the body. This **"exercise allergy"** reaction may come about at the beginning of exercise and then disappear if exercise is continued, or it may be present after exercise. Generally, the rash does not last long and presents little health danger.

Why this happens is not completely understood. It is felt that the histamines produced by exercise are not as readily destroyed in the body of an allergic person. Gradually increased doses of histamine regulated by a physician do build some tolerance in allergic individuals and help to improve this condition. They are not, however, a cure.

Very few people experience an allergic reaction to exercise. The possibility could provide a good crutch for opponents of exercise, however, much the same way endocrine difficulty is blamed for obesity. If signs of allergy are present, wear clean, soft, and loose clothing for maximum ventilation, and consult your physician immediately. Some people break out in a rash just thinking about exercise; most of these people will quickly sit down until either the rash or the thought disappears.

Does weight training improve the cardiovascular system?

Although recent surveys have indicated that most individuals are aware of the positive effects of exercise on health, there remains a continual effort on the part of the American people to get the most exercise benefit with the least effort in the shortest time. Many individuals seek a "fitness pill" that produces all the physiological benefits of a sound exercise program while they watch cable TV. In the past, isometric training involving single 10-second contractions was popular for strength development. A number of 3-minute exercise programs and 30-minutes-per-week regimes were proposed in articles and books—one even hit the bestseller list. Rope jumping and yoga were once proclaimed as the ideal exercises for achieving maximum results in a short time period. Special machines and gadgets have always promised instant fitness and weight loss with little effort. More recently there has been a renewed interest in weight training. Long recognized as an effective means of improving muscular strength and endurance, weight training is now being promoted as an adequate form of aerobic exercise.

By limiting the rest period between each set and performing exercises rapidly, proponents of this system suggest that muscular strength, muscular endurance, and cardiovascular endurance can all be improved at the same time. In fact, it is even suggested that the aerobic benefits are equivalent to those produced by sound programs of jogging, swimming, and cycling. According to a number of manufacturers of strength training equipment, cardiovascular conditioning is possible with any type of activity, providing the work is intense enough to elicit an individual's target heart rate. In addition, it is argued that the one-workout concept saves considerable time and eliminates the need for several different types of training programs. In our society, it is difficult enough to convince people to exercise at all; involving the masses in several different workout routines would be next to impossible.

Opponents of weight training as an aerobic exercise program cite a number of criticisms of this approach. Although there is some research support indicating that target heart rates can be reached, it is extremely difficult to maintain that level throughout the weight training workout. It is unlikely that the average individual could sustain this intense effort for the 20 to 30 minutes necessary to bring about the desired changes of a sound aerobic program. Crowded conditions in health clubs also make it difficult to move rapidly from one exercise station to another. Additional research is needed to determine the exact number of repetitions, speed of contraction, and length of the rest interval between sets necessary to elicit and maintain target heart rates. It is doubtful that aerobic benefits such as weight and fat loss from high-caloric expenditure, reduced resting heart and respiratory rate, increased stroke volume and cardiac output, a change in the way the body handles fats, increased HDL and an improved ratio of HDL to total serum cholesterol, and assistance in preventing early heart disease will occur from a vigorous weight training program.

More research is needed before widespread aerobic claims can be made for strength training programs. Until then, you are faced with making your own decision based on the available evidence.

MYTHS AND FALLACIES

A high level of conditioning for one activity carries over to all other physical actions.

A high level of conditioning acquired in one sport does not necessarily carry over to another. Football or soccer players who have just completed their seasons will find that they are not capable of meeting the physical demands of basketball or track. A transitional period is needed before physical efficiency is reached in the new sport. Exercise programs must simulate movements used in the activity for which training is designed. You cannot improve running speed by doing push-ups, nor will sit-ups help you jump higher.

The scientific basis for this principle lies, in part, within the muscles themselves; training is specific in terms of lactic acid production during heavy muscular work. Thus, complete training transfer, regardless of the closeness of the activities, is not possible.

If you use any type of exercise program (weight training, isometrics, calisthenics, and so on) to enable you to play another sport, make sure that your conditioning program is designed to work the same muscles that are used in the game itself, and with similar intensity. Even so, you should expect a period of transition before maximum efficiency is reached in the new sport.

Staleness, or chronic fatigue, results from too much exercise.

The symptoms of staleness include:

1. Complaints of undue fatigue
2. Difficulty falling asleep, and waking up and not being able to get back to sleep
3. Irritability and bad temper
4. Loss of appetite
5. Loss of enthusiasm and drive
6. Listlessness
7. Lack of concentration
8. Constant complaints of trivial aches and pains in joints and muscles

Sometimes after you have been training on a regular basis and improvement has been steady, your ability to perform up to self-imposed standards begins to deteriorate. You keep working out, but you feel bad and you seem to be going downhill.

The usual cause of these problems (once you are sure you are not ill or injured) is not physical, but the result of emotional and situational factors. Maladjustment, lack of sleep, and worry are the most common causes of staleness and should be the focus of change when planning alterations in training to correct the situation.

Attempts to alleviate staleness may involve:

1. Change in training routine
2. Being certain never to train hard on two consecutive days (alternative hard and light days to ensure full recovery from one workout to the next)
3. An analysis of lifestyle for stress points and underlying emotional conflicts, followed by attempts to minimize or eliminate them
4. Temporary suspension of training

If you experience staleness symptoms, remember they are generally not a result of strenuous training, and they do not always require a lightening or suspension of exercise loads. Look instead at your emotional balance and any lifestyle factors that may be interfering with your physical improvement and pleasure.

No pain, no gain.

Almost everyone has heard this claim regarding exercise; it appears on Tee shirts in gyms and fitness clubs around the country. The problem with this idea is that it does not apply to most people.

For an athlete in top physical condition, further increases in fitness and strength require overload training—training at maximum strength and endurance capacity. This requires extreme intensity and this causes pain.

Overload pain is sometimes called "the burn." People who believe the no pain, no gain theory of training think an athlete must conquer the burn by pushing the muscles or the respiratory system to the limit. This kind of training can be dangerous even for the highly trained athlete, causing dizziness and a rubbery feeling in working muscles as PH drops and the acid/base balance is altered in the body. Pain is meant as a signal to protect the body.

The no pain, no gain theory is never true for the beginner or occasional exerciser. Research shows that for the novice, aerobic and muscular fitness will improve as long as the intensity of training exceeds a minimum threshold (60% maximum heart rate or 50 to 60% repetition maximum). This training to minimum threshold will provide sufficient overload to maintain steady fitness improvement.

One sure way to defeat fitness efforts in those beginning a new program is to apply the no pain, no gain theory. Injuries and dropout are the sure results.

BIBLIOGRAPHY

Astrand, P., and K. Rodahl. *Textbook of Work Physiology: Physiological Bases of Exercise.* 3d ed. New York: McGraw-Hill, 1986.

Cooper, Kenneth H. *The Aerobics Program for Total Well-Being.* New York: M. Evans and Co., 1982.

Dishman, R. K. "Exercise Adherence." In *Exercise and Mental Health,* ed. W. P. Morgan and S. E. Goldston. Washington, D.C.: Hemisphere, 1987.

Morgan, W. P., and S. E. Goldston, eds. *Exercise and Mental Health.* Washington, D.C.: Hemisphere, 1987.

Morgan, W. P., et al. "Monitoring of Overtraining and Staleness." *British Journal of Sports Medicine* 21 (1987): 319–28.

Pollock, M. L., et al. "Effects of Frequency and Duration of Training on Attrition and Incidence of Injury." *Medical Science of Sports* 9: (1987): 31–36.

Stephens, T., D. R. Jacobs, and C. C. White. "A Descriptive Epidemiology of Leisure-Time Physical Activity." *Public Health Reports* 100 (1985): 147–58.

LABORATORY 9.1

Discussing Your Aerobic Activity Program Selection

PURPOSE: To consider the types of tailor-made programs that might be best

SIZE OF GROUP: Six

PROCEDURE

1. Each group member should write the answers to the following questions:
   What exercise or sport do I enjoy the most?
   Why don't I engage in that activity now?
   What can I do about that
   What other kinds of activities might be as much fun for me?
2. Let each person report his or her answers to the rest of the group.
3. Each group summarizes its answers and makes a presentation to the class. Class data are summarized.

RESULTS

Class members will be stimulated to think about activities that are fun for them and will hear what other class members feel about their activity choices.

LABORATORY 9.2

Selecting Your Favorite Aerobic Activity

PURPOSE: To determine a tailor-made program for you to begin.

SIZE OF GROUP: Six

PROCEDURE

1. Let one group member write the names of each type of aerobic program listed in this chapter (cycling, jogging and running, rope jumping, swimming, walking) on a folded sheet of paper. Place these folded sheets in a hat.

2. Let each group member select a sheet and identify the aerobic activity to the rest of the group.

3. Each group member looks up his or her selected program in the tables contained in the chapter and records the appropriate fitness level.

4. The group members participate in the aerobic activity program for one week. (If someone in the group selects an activity he or she cannot perform, a second selection should be made.)

5. The group meets again after one week's activity, and each member describes his or her exercise activity using the following format:

Cycling
How much?
Benefits:
Problems:

Jogging and Running
How much?
Benefits:
Problems:

Swimming
How much?
Benefits:
Problems:

Rope jumping
How much?
Benefits:
Problems:

Walking
How much?
Benefits:
Problems:

6. Each group summarizes its experience with each aerobic activity and makes a presentation to the class. Class data are summarized.

RESULTS

As class members try new programs of aerobic activity and report benefits and problems to others, individuals may be encouraged to experiment with a variety of new aerobic activities.

CHAPTER TEN

SPORTS AND FITNESS

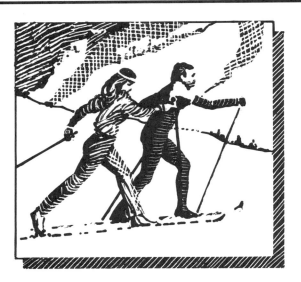

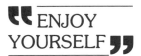

**ENJOY
YOURSELF**

? HAVE YOU EVER WONDERED ABOUT:

How to improve fitness through sports?
How to improve sports skill through fitness?
The fitness value of different sports?
The best sports for weight control/loss?
Which sports develop which body parts?
Whether there is one all-around sport for fitness?

KEY TERMS

Aerobic activities

Anaerobic activities

Skill learning, or elevation of skill level, can be an excellent method of attaining and maintaining physical fitness. A skilled person tends to seek activity throughout life, since inner motivation is present once a certain level of skill is attained. Unfortunately, mere participation in a recreational sport often adds little to one's conditioning level. It does represent a valuable and needed diversion from a regular program, but it requires careful activity selection and attention to the length and intensity of the workout. Progress, through gradually increasing work loads, is not easy since it is difficult to determine whether you performed more work one day than another or reached your target heart rate and kept it there for 20 minutes or more. As you can see, it is nearly impossible to regulate some key training variables, such as intensity or work per unit of time, to ensure improvement from day to day.

A brief discussion of sports that improve aerobic fitness and offer some potential for participation throughout life follows. Keep in mind that the *one* best method for improving fitness has not been developed. It is accurate to say, however, that your sports preference should place primary emphasis on the development of the cardiovascular system (aerobic fitness).

CHOOSING YOUR SPORT FOR FITNESS

Your best guarantee of success from the sports approach to fitness is to select an aerobic sport you enjoy and that you are likely to play a minimum of three times weekly (every other day). Start slowly the first three to six weeks, and work into more competitive, vigorous competition by choosing more advanced opponents. You may also want to supplement your sports routine with some strength and endurance activity (see Chapter 4) one time during the week, preferably in the middle of the week. Study Table 10.1 carefully to evaluate your sports choice. Notice that each sport is labeled aerobic, anaerobic, or a combination of the two (approximate percentages are given for the potential cardiovascular development, caloric expenditure, and development of the legs, abdomen, and arm and shoulders). Keep in mind that only **aerobic activities** develop the heart and lungs, expend a high number of calories, and potentially offer some protection from early heart disease. **Anaerobic activities** involve more explosive movements, and don't allow adequate oxygen uptake. Therefore, these activities can't be sustained long, and don't provide good aerobic fitness. The recommended age range for participation is offered only as a guideline; individuals in superior condition can safely continue with any sport at practically any age.

AEROBIC DANCE

Aerobic dance classes provide continuous movement in dance, calisthenic, and running and jumping activities. Target heart rates can be easily reached and maintained for 20 minutes or more. In addition, opportunities are provided to stop and take the exercise heart rate to make certain the exercise is of sufficient intensity. Instructors must pay close attention to the principles of conditioning discussed in Chapter 3 if aerobic fitness is to steadily improve. Careful planning must occur to be certain that individuals are doing more work each day by increasing either the length of continuous exercise or its intensity.

Unfortunately we are seeing a rise in such injuries as shin splints, knee problems, and back problems among aerobic dance participants. Low impact aerobics (where one foot remains constantly in contact with the floor) is now being advocated to avoid and reduce the severity of these

TABLE 10.1 RATINGS OF SPORTS

Sport	Type	Cardiovascular	Caloric Expenditure	Legs	Abdomen	Arms/ Shoulders	Age Range Recommended
Archery	Anaerobic	L	L	L	L	L	Ages 10 and up
Backpacking	50% Aerobic	M-H	H	H	M	L	All ages
Badminton	Anaerobic	L-M	H	H	L	M	Ages 7 and up
Baseball/Softball	Anaerobic	L	L	M	L	L	All ages
Basketball	15% Aerobic	M	H	H	L	L	Ages 7 to 40
Bicycling (competitive)	Aerobic	H	H	H	L	M	All ages
Bowling	Anaerobic	L	L	L	L	L	All ages
Dance (aerobic)	Aerobic	M-H	M-H	M	M	M	All ages
Canoeing/Rowing							
Recreational	Anaerobic	L	M	L	L	M	Ages 12 and up
Competitive	Aerobic	H	H	M	M	H	Ages 12 to 40
Fencing	Anaerobic	L-M	M	M	L	M	Ages 12 and up
Field Hockey	20% Aerobic	M	M-H	H	L	M	Ages 7 and up
Golf (motor cart)	Anaerobic	L	L	L	L	L	All ages
Walking	Anaerobic	L	M	M	L	L	All ages
Handball/Racketball/ Squash	Anaerobic	M	H	H	L	H	Under 45 (singles)
Hiking	Anaerobic	L-M	M	H	L	L	All ages
Ice/Roller Skating							
Speed	Anaerobic	L-M	M	H	L	L	Under 45
Figure	Anaerobic	L-M	H	H	M	M	All ages
Lacrosse	20% Aerobic	M-H	H	H	M	M	Under 45
Orienteering	50% Aerobic	M-H	H	H	M	L	All ages
Rugby	60% Aerobic	H	H	H	L	H	Under 40
Skiing (cross-country)	Aerobic	H	H	H	H	H	Under 45
Skin Diving	Anaerobic	M	M	M	M	L	All ages
Soccer	50% Aerobic	H	H	H	L	H	Under 45
Surfing	Anaerobic	L	M	H	M	M	Ages 7 and up
Tennis	Anaerobic	L-M	M	H	L	L	All ages
Touch Football	Anaerobic	L	L-M	H	L	L	Under 45
Volleyball	Anaerobic	L	L	M-H	L	M	All ages
Water Skiing	Anaerobic	L-M	M	H	L	M	All ages
Weight Training	Anaerobic	L	L	H	H	H	All ages
Wrestling	30% Aerobic	M	H	H	H	H	Under 45
Jogging	Aerobic	M-H	H	H	L	L	Ages 7 and up
Swimming	Aerobic	M	H	M	L	H	Ages 7 and up
Walking	Aerobic	L-M	M	H	L	L	All ages

H = high; M = medium; L = low

injuries. The emphasis is upon correct posture and mechanical efficiency.

BACKPACKING/HIKING

Backpacking is a pleasurable type of activity generally requiring above average muscular and aerobic endurance. How much energy you expend and the heart rate reached are dependent on the terrain and elevation, your body size and walking speed, and the weight of your backpack. Hiking or backpacking must be performed at approximately 4 miles per hour or more (15 minutes per mile) to improve aerobic fitness. Individuals who have been inactive should follow the walking starter program in Chapter 9 for at least four to six weeks before beginning the sport of backpacking.

BASKETBALL

Full-court basketball is a good sport for developing muscular and cardiovascular endurance. Half-court basketball, on the other hand, is primarily an anaerobic activity and contributes little to cardiovascular development. One limitation of full-court basketball is that it is unlikely to be continued throughout life. When you are in reasonably good condition, three 30-minute workouts weekly are sufficient to maintain your present aerobic fitness level.

BICYCLING

Cycling can be an excellent activity for improving your aerobic condition. Cycling allows you to easily check your heart rate during exercise to be certain you are working at your target for a minimum of 20 minutes each workout three times weekly. In general, you need to cycle about twice as fast as you would normally jog to produce an equivalent heart rate.

Stationary exercise bicycles are also excellent for developing aerobic fitness. In the comfort of your home, you can reach your target heart rate while reading books, listening to music, or watching TV.

CANOEING/BOAT ROWING

Canoeing and boat rowing are generally used for the pleasure of sightseeing, fishing, and camping.

Strength and endurance in the arms and shoulders make both activities easier. Regular paddling or rowing tend to develop the muscles of the arms, shoulders, and back. Whether cardiovascular improvement occurs depends upon the intensity of the paddling or rowing. Individuals who row competitively reach heart rates much higher than their target heart rates and develop a high level of aerobic fitness. It is unlikely that recreational boating will produce similar results.

FIELD HOCKEY, LACROSSE, RUGBY, SOCCER

Team sports such as field hockey, lacrosse, rugby and soccer have some common denominators: play is continuous with few time-outs or interruptions, and a field in excess of 100 yards is used. Each of these sports is predominately an aerobic activity and a wise fitness choice. Age group programs also provide opportunities for participation throughout life.

ICE/ROLLER SKATING

In general, any type of skating taxes the major muscle groups of the legs, abdomen, back, and arms to a lesser degree. Therefore, it should be supplemented with upper-body exercises. Recreational skating purely for the enjoyment of gliding over the ice on a rink or pond generally produces little change in aerobic fitness. If skating is rigorous enough, such as in speed skating or ice hockey, cardiovascular efficiency is improved.

ORIENTEERING

Orienteering is a form of cross-country racing in which participants use a map and compass to guide themselves over unfamiliar territory. It is a combination of hiking, climbing, running, jogging, and walking. The object is to complete the course as quickly as possible, hitting the various control stations in the prescribed sequence outlined on the map. A detailed topographical plan indicates the type of terrain to be encountered by the participants. A compass is used to help the orienteers establish location and stay on course as they trek through the fields and forest. When they arrive at each station, contestants punch their card with a special puncher. Each station must be completed in a designated order. The contestant who completes the prescribed course in the quickest time is declared the winner. Because you sprint on open terrain, run up hills, and scamper through thickets, you must be in superb physical condition to perform well. Orienteering improves the cardiovascular system. Only individuals who score in the good, excellent, or superior categories on the 1.5-mile test can safely engage in this activity.

RACQUET SPORTS (BADMINTON, RACQUETBALL, SQUASH, TENNIS)

Although racquet sports are primarily anaerobic activities (including singles), they are an excellent sports fitness choice. It is wise, however, to supplement play with one to two aerobic workouts weekly that will produce and maintain your target rate for 20 minutes or more. Of the four racquet sports, badminton and racquetball tend to expend the greatest amount of calories due to the length of the point. Again, much depends on whether you and your partner are of near equal ability and skilled enough to keep the ball in play. The style of play also alters the aerobic value of a sport. In a recent professional tennis tournament, both the length of each point and the rest interval between points were timed. Serve and volley players ended each point in an average of 7.1 seconds and took 22 seconds of rest between each point. Baseline players ended each point in slightly over 23 seconds before using approximately the same amount of rest time between points. Highly intense activity for 7 to 23 seconds, interspersed with 23 seconds of rest prior to the next point, is clearly an anaerobic activity. Heart rates may occasionally reach the target level; however, they never remain there for more than a few seconds.

Although not a racquet sport, handball has some of the same limitations. It is, however, more strenuous than any of the four racquet sports mentioned above, develops both sides of the upper body, and requires more skill in the early stages of the game to keep the ball in play.

CROSS-COUNTRY SKIING (NORDIC STYLE)

This sport involves rigorous pumping action of the arms and legs as the skier moves rapidly through the snow on level ground. Cross-country skiers have been purported to possess some of the highest maximal oxygen uptake values found in any sport. Caloric expenditure per minute is also perhaps the highest of any sport. Cross-country skiing obviously improves aerobic fitness. It also requires a high level of cardiovascular fitness before you can safely engage in the sport.

SKIN DIVING

Skin diving involves underwater swimming using fins, face mask, and an outside breathing apparatus called a snorkel. You either swim or float on the surface of the water and, when ready, take a deep breath, submerge and swim under water until your lungs need oxygen. After you catch your breath you repeat the dive all over again. The fitness value of skin diving depends upon the intensity of the workout: how vigorous you swim, how much you rest, and how long you stay under water.

SOFTBALL

Softball is great for maintaining agility, getting outdoors to have fun, breathing fresh air, and maybe picking up a tan, but it does not improve any measurable level of fitness because neither aerobic nor anaerobic training transpires. The incidence of softball injuries is on the rise, and poor conditioning has been cited as one of the major reasons for the increase.

SURFING AND WATER SKIING

Surfing requires excellent balance and considerable leg strength. The feat is accomplished in a standing position while the board skims along the underside of a breaking wave at an angle that varies according to the height of the wave. The surfboard is continuously manipulated by the surfer as he or she strives spontaneously to shift body weight according to the dictates of the wave. Muscular strength and endurance are especially crucial. Also, propelling the board seaward through and beyond the breaking waves is strenuous. The task of paddling back for another run works the muscles of the shoulders, back, chest, and arms immensely, as well as the cardiorespiratory systems. Surfing's aerobic value depends upon the length of the wave and the intensity of the surfer in paddling back out. It is doubtful that much improvement in the cardiovascular system occurs for most surfers.

Water skiing taxes similar muscle groups and has the same limitations as surfing.

TOUCH FOOTBALL

Like softball, touch football is another exciting and popular activity played by many. It is good for agility development but does little to improve physical fitness because too much pacing and intermittent play are involved, and no continuous exercise occurs. The number of injuries that occur during the game and the delayed soreness felt the day after leave considerable doubt as to its fitness values.

WEIGHT TRAINING

Weight training can be done by everyone, not just those interested in becoming weight lifters or body builders. Weight training increases your strength and muscle endurance as well as your overall feeling of fitness in ways that no other activity can. Specific weight training routines can be helpful in developing particular muscle groups that will improve performance in your chosen sport. Unfortunately, weight training by itself does very little for cardiovascular fitness because too many pauses occur between sets and there is no continuous effort over a long period of time. If weight training is your choice of sport, you should add some type of aerobic exercise to balance out the cardiovascular component of your fitness program.

FREQUENTLY ASKED QUESTIONS

Can golf help me lose weight?

Golf has a caloric cost of approximately 290 calories per hour for the average 150-pound person. While this expenditure is above that of carpentry, a 2.6-mile-per-hour walk, shoemaking, driving a car, sweeping, dishwashing, ironing, typing, dressing, sewing, and sitting, it is much inferior to most other sports. On the other hand, it must be said that three to four hours on the golf course and a caloric expenditure of 870 to 1160 calories (over a quarter of a pound of fat) is a significant amount. Insist on walking briskly and carrying your own bag.

Can I still participate in sports even though I'm pregnant?

There is no physiological reason why healthy pregnant women cannot safely engage in sports. A recent study in the *Journal of the American Medical Association* revealed findings that higher exercise levels than currently recommended are safe for pregnant women. The American College of Obstetricians and Gynecologists recommends that an expectant mother not exercise beyond a level that raises her heart rate to 140 beats per minute. However, the extra weight, altered equilibrium, effects of water retention, and relaxation of joints may make participation difficult. Physicians do suggest that pregnant athletes, even though they are accustomed to heavy training, curtail its intensity by their sixth month. Dr. Robert Jones, a researcher from Hershey Medical Center, says that the most important consideration is tailoring the exercise to the comfort zone of the individual.

Are cycling and jogging better for weight control than swimming?

No. Exercise physiologists report that the energy expenditure demands of swimming can be as much as four times greater than that of cycling or jogging for the same distance. A swimmer needs energy for maintaining buoyancy, for propulsion, and to overcome water resistance. The fact that you use both arms and legs for most strokes makes swimming an excellent activity to burn up calories.

Each year a number of cases of collapse and death occur during sports participation. What causes this?

Although such cases are rare, they do occur occasionally, and exercise receives the blame. Numerous causes may have contributed:

1. Use of drugs such as amphetamines that remove the warning signs of fatigue
2. Heat stroke due to hot, humid weather, heavy perspiration, limited fluids, loss of salt and potassium, and poor cooling of the body
3. Sudden vigorous exertion in a previously inactive individual
4. Presence of undiagnosed heart difficulty or other ailments
5. Aneurism (weakness in a vessel wall, which suddenly gives out)

Many of these conditions are not easily detected, and with vigorous exercise result in serious illness, injury, or death.

How does aging affect injury and healing?

Unfortunately, older people are more easily injured and slower to heal than younger individuals. Age results in numerous physical changes that bring this about:

1. The elastic properties of connective tissue are diminished, thus limiting flexibility and increasing the probability of injury. Return to complete normalcy following injury is unlikely.
2. Cartilage softens from injury, disease, or wear, particularly in weight-bearing areas of the legs, leaving one more injury prone.
3. In the healing of broken bones, age is an important factor. Bones of growing children unite more quickly and heal faster. The more rapidly a bone is growing (the younger the patient), the more quickly it unites.

Explosive movements and contact sports should be avoided after age 50 and substituted with vigorous activity of another nature. Again, for those who have exercised continually throughout life, injury is less likely to occur.

Is there one all-around sport for fitness?

Swimming (the continuous forward crawl stroke) is regarded by many exercise experts as one of the best all-around fitness activities for any age. The potential for cardiovascular development is high and a high number of calories are expended in a short time. Water temperatures between 70 and 73 degrees Fahrenheit are best for training. Although you need not be an accomplished swimmer, it is advisable that you be capable of swimming at least one pool length (25 yards) without experiencing extreme exhaustion. In early workouts, it is advisable to swim one length, get out of the pool, and return to the other end by walking. This swim-walk-swim approach will give you time to recuperate and assess your energy level before attempting another length. This practice is an excellent safety measure, especially if you classify yourself as a so-so swimmer. In time you will gradually add laps and decrease rest intervals. Eventually you will want to swim continuously for 30 to 40 minutes at least three days a week. Dr. Kenneth Cooper (1982) rates cross-country skiing as the most demanding fitness activity, followed by swimming, jogging, bicycling, and walking.

MYTHS AND FALLACIES

You can play yourself into good physical condition.

Many weekend athletes feel that participation in any sport is sufficient for developing or maintaining fitness. Unfortunately, much depends upon their definition of fitness. Health-related fitness, which has guided the development of this text, is not easily attained or maintained through the sports approach. Developing minimum levels of cardiovascular efficiency, muscular strength and endurance, flexibility, and an appropriate percentage of body fat requires a somewhat systematic approach that applies the fitness concepts described in Chapter 3. It is difficult to be certain that participation in a sport will elevate heart rate to the target heart rate and keep it there for 20 minutes or more or be more strenuous (more work per unit of time, longer workout) each workout. These two basic principles govern both development and maintenance of health-related fitness.

Fitness benefits from sports participation also depend upon your personality. Intense competitors tend to exert more energy (calories) and elevate heart rates to a higher level than do participants who emphasize the fun aspect of sport.

Golf, bowling, and archery are examples of sports contributing little to health-related fitness. Aerobic sports (soccer, rugby, lacrosse, full-court basketball, field hockey, and so on) have the potential for the improvement of health-related fitness, providing you play three to four times a week for 45 minutes or longer. Even then, there is no guarantee the two fitness principles will be met.

It is difficult to play yourself into good physical condition even by choosing one of the aerobic sports described in this chapter. The sports approach may be better suited for fitness maintenance than development. The ideal use of sports is to allow such participation to supplement a sound aerobic conditioning program (jogging/running, cycling, swimming, rope jumping, fast walking) that is used two to three times weekly.

Sports such as cycling, cross-country skiing, racket sports, soccer, and rugby are also presented as ideal lifetime activities, but each sport has its limitations. Certainly if a pool is not available, swimming is highly impractical. If you detest jogging or cannot play tennis, these also are unwise choices. Perhaps there is no single best sport for everyone. The best choice for you is an aerobic sport you enjoy and are likely to continue throughout life. Regular participation in aerobic sports will help you maintain normal weight, control body fat, and provide some protection from early heart disease.

Women are more prone to injuries than men.

Women exercise and participate in sports for the same reasons that men do—for improved appearance, conditioning, weight control, recognition, competition, and achievement. Young girls and women also face the same problems for the prevention of injuries as do males. Physiological differences between the sexes make women somewhat more susceptible to injury and less responsive to training:

1. Women are more susceptible to bruises.
2. They have a lower ratio of strength to body weight.
3. They have more body fat.
4. The oxygen-carrying capacity of the blood is lower.
5. The chemical makeup of muscle tissue is different.
6. Anaerobic (ability to sprint for extended distances) and aerobic capacity is less in women.
7. The ratio of heart weight to body weight in women is approximately 85 percent that of men.

On the other hand, some common fallacies can be overturned. For example, injuries to the breast are rare, although special protective cups are recommended for female participants in all sports. Fencing, paddleball, squash, field hockey, team handball, basketball, and wrestling are a few sports that demand the use of a protective brassiere. Large breasts are more susceptible to injury. When an injury occurs from a contusion, a hard nodule of fibrous tissue generally forms in the fatty tissue and remains for years. This nodule can be distinguished from cancer only by biopsy.

Reproductive organs, as well, are not as feeble as myth contends. The uterus is suspended by ligaments and well protected by the pelvis. A blow to the body or violent jarring does not cause a similar jolt to the uterus. There is, in effect, no evidence to suggest that a healthy female of any age can be harmed by vigorous exercise.

BIBLIOGRAPHY

Anderson, J. and M. Cohen. *The Competitive Edge.* New York: William Morrow, 1981.

Benjamin, B. E. *Sports Without Pain.* New York: Summit Books, 1979.

Carnes, R., and V. Carnes. *Sportspower.* New York: St. Martin's Press, 1983.

Cooper, K. H. The Aerobics Program for Total Well Being. New York: M. Evans, 1982.

Cooper, K. H. *Physical Fitness and Sportsmedicine.* White House Symposium newsletter, December 1980.

Darden, Ellington. *Especially for Women.* West Point, N.Y.: Leisure Press, 1977.

Dintiman, George B., and Loyd M. Barrow. *A Comprehensive Manual of Foundations and Physical Education Activities for Men and Women.* Minneapolis: Burgess, 1979.

Fisher, Garth A., and Robert K. Conlee. *The Complete Book of Physical Fitness.* Provo, Utah: Brigham Young University Press, 1979.

Getchell, B. *Physical Fitness: A Way of Life.* New York: Wiley & Sons, 1979.

Murray, J., and P. V. Karpovich. *Weight Training in Athletics.* Englewood Cliffs, N.J.: Prentice-Hall, 1956.

Rosenzweig, S. *Sports Fitness for Women.* New York: Harper & Row, 1982.

Rowes, B. "How NASA Research for Space Can Help You Be Healthier on Earth." *Family Circle* (March 1983): 58.

Siegener, R. *Shape Up For Sports.* New York: Berkley, 1978.

What Sport Is Best for the Bod? *Esquire* (October 1974): 238–39.

LABORATORY 10.1

Selecting Sports for Your Physical Fitness

PURPOSE: To identify sports you enjoy and have sufficient skill level to participate in fully.

SIZE OF GROUP: Alone

PROCEDURE

1. Decide which fitness components you wish to improve upon:
   _____ Cardiovascular _____ Muscular strength _____ Muscular endurance _____ Flexibility

2. Review the chapter and list any sports you are already skilled in. Use Table 10.1 to determine the possible benefits of each.

Sport	Type	Calories Expended	Body Area	Activity Length

RESULTS

1. Do the sports you selected target the fitness components you most want to improve?

2. In what ways could they be modified to better suit your fitness needs?

LABORATORY 10.2

Measuring Heart Rate During Sports Activity

PURPOSE: To determine play intensity while engaging in tennis or other sports.

PROCEDURE

1. Midway into the first set of your next singles tennis match, raquetball, or squash game, take your carotid pulse for 15 seconds immediately after a long rally. Multiply the number of beats counted by 4 to determine beats per minute (BPM).

2. Since your heart rate already began to slow down or recover during the 15 seconds you were inactive while taking your pulse, add 5% to your BPM to obtain a more accurate estimate of your exercise heart rate (BPM during the tennis rally).

3. Determine an estimate of your maximum heart rate by subtracting your age from 220.

    Example: Immediately after a long tennis rally, Brenda, a 20 year old student at the University of New Mexico, stood quietly, found her carotid pulse, and counted 32 beats for 15 seconds. She estimated her actual heart rate during the rally as 134 BPM (32 × 4 = 128 × 5% or 134). Brenda's estimated maximum heart rate is 220 minus 20, or 200.

    60% of maximum heart rate = 120 BPM (light intensity)
    70% of maximum heart rate = 140 BPM (medium intensity)
    80% of maximum heart rate = 160 BPM (high intensity)

RESULTS

1. Was your rally vigorous enough to be classified as light, medium, or heavy?
    a. Light (60% of maximum heart rate): Brenda's rally was classified as light intensity which is the minimum level at which some aerobic conditioning is taking place.
    b. Medium (70% of maximum heart rate): Excellent level for the development of aerobic fitness.
    c. Heavy (80% of maximum heart rate): High level suggested for those who already possess good or excellent aerobic fitness.

2. This analysis of heart rate can be conducted during any activity.

CHAPTER 11

BEYOND FITNESS

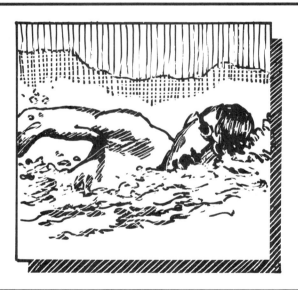

❝ THE THRILL
OF VICTORY **❞**

? HAVE YOU EVER WONDERED ABOUT:

Road race training?
Marathon training?
Triathlon training?
Advanced strength training?
Body building?
Specificity of training?
Maximum effort training?
How to improve your speed?
Long-slow distance training?

KEY TERMS

Body building
DMSO
Intervals
Long-slow distance (LSD)
Marathon

Maximum effort training
Road racing
Sprinting
Strength training
Triathlon

This chapter includes information for those desiring to go to fitness levels not necessary for health but required for competition. The previous chapters provided the information to help you progress from your current fitness level to an excellent one. When reaching the excellent level, many people want to test their limits as human beings. This is definitely not for everyone; advanced training is demanding and has a higher injury rate. By following the advanced techniques described, you will not only make significant gains but you will minimize injuries. The programs should be used only by those who have already reached a high level of aerobic or anaerobic fitness, strength, and flexibility.

COMPETITIVE AEROBICS

Although the majority of people who enter fitness programs have no desire to compete, many eventually become interested in comparing themselves to others. Such comparisons are possible in a competitive race situation. By reading this section, you have indicated a desire to make such a comparison. The information presented here is therefore designed to help you train to race the most popular **road racing** distances of 5,000 meters (approximately 3.1 miles) and 10,000 meters (approximately 6.2 miles).

The distance you select is best determined by your fitness level. For those who fall in the good to superior category on the 1.5-mile test and who are training 20 to 40 miles per week, either distance is appropriate. Those who score below the good category and who train less than 20 miles per week should consider increasing training prior to racing or limiting their effort to a slow 5K race. No matter which race is selected, your performances will be determined by your training.

5,000 METER (5K) TO 10,000 METER (10K) RACING

Training for 5K to 10K races requires that you put in sufficient mileage weekly to merely finish the race safely. If speed is desired, training also requires speed work. The amount of mileage and speed work is dependent upon your goal. Practically anyone who scores good or excellent on the 1.5-mile test can finish a 10K race and nearly anyone can finish a 5K (even slow walkers). Com-

petition infers constantly striving to improve your performance, and improvement comes with increased mileage and speed work. Minimum mileage for a strong performance is 40 miles per week but need not exceed 60 miles per week. This weekly mileage should include two days of speed work and one day for racing.

The training schedule described in Table 11.1 should not be attempted until you have reached

TABLE 11.1 TYPICAL TRAINING WEEK	
Day	**Workout**
Sunday	Long slow distance of 10 to 12 miles at a pace approximately 1 minute per mile slower than your racing pace
Monday	7 to 8 miles at a pace about 30 to 45 seconds slower than race pace
Tuesday	Speed work day: 3 to 5 miles of intervals at a pace about 20 seconds faster than your *desired* race pace (be realistic here); total workout mileage including warm-up and cool-down is 6 to 9 miles
Wednesday	6 to 9 easy miles
Thursday	Speed work day: 3 to 6 miles of intervals
Friday	4 to 6 miles of easy running if a race is planned for Saturday; 8 miles if no race is scheduled
Saturday	Race 5K to 10K distance

a good rating on the 1.5-mile test and are doing at least 35 miles per week. It would also be helpful to be timed at the 5K distance to determine your training pace.

INTERVALS

Intervals are a type of speed workout with four parts:

1. The distance to be run between each rest interval
2. The total distance to be run in the workout
3. The speed at which you run
4. The rest interval between each run

The distance to be run is determined by both your conditioning level and your desired race distance. Since this section deals with the 5K and 10K, the distance should not be less than 220 yards or 200 meters. The total distance of the workout should be 2 to 3 miles for the 5K and 4 to 6 miles for the

Figure 11.1   Road racing requires extreme dedication to training.

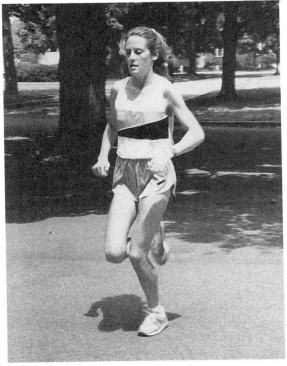

10K. The speed should be about 20 seconds faster than your desired race pace. If you want to run a 6-minute-per-mile pace, for example, you should run your quarter miles at 80 seconds, half miles at 2 minutes and 40 seconds, and miles at 5 minutes and 40 seconds. The rest interval varies according to the distance and conditions. For quarters, a set rest interval of 90 seconds is recommended. Some people, however, run a quarter and jog a quarter for rest. For longer distances, you should allow your heart rate to return below 120 beats per minute prior to running the next bout. Table 11.2 describes sample interval workouts for 5K and 10K races. These workouts will improve your conditioning to the level needed to complete the 5K and 10K race. To improve your speed (pace), follow the interval workout schedule shown in Table 11.3.

MARATHONS AND ULTRAMARATHONS

"What the mind of man can conceive and believe can be achieved." Men and women recently seem to be putting this saying to ultimate physical tests. No longer are persons satisfied with the marathon. There are 100-mile races, across-the-country races, races that involve parachuting into death valley and running out, and 24-hour races; the human mind seems to be in an endless race with the body to see which will crack first. These long-distance (endurance) contests are not new; races across the United States were waged for thousands of dollars during the 1920s and 1930s. Participants in these early races, as well as the modern-day ultra races, were few.

Although the number of races has declined in recent years, the **marathon** (26.2 miles) is still popular. The mystique of the marathon continues to draw runners of all ages and levels of conditioning. Much national attention through TV coverage has been generated by the Boston and New York marathons. Marathon participants come in all sizes and shapes; some are prepared and some, like many first time participants, are not.

Three months of training is required to run a marathon. Training requires 60 miles per week including at least one long run of 18 miles or more. If you plan to *race* the marathon, you should be running 40 miles per week prior to the final three training months. You then gradually increase your mileage (approximately 10 percent per week) to 60 miles a week during the month before the race.

TABLE 11.2   5K AND 10K INTERVAL WORKOUTS

5K Workouts	10K Workouts
1. 8 × ¼ mile	1. 12 × ¼ mile
2. 1 × ½ mile 4 × ¼ mile 6 × 220 yards	2. 16 × ¼ mile
3. 2 × ½ mile 4 × ¼ mile	3. 2 × ½ mile 8 × ¼ mile 6 × 220 yards
4. 8 × ¼ mile 4 × 220 yards	4. 4 × ½ mile 6 × ¼ mile 6 × 220 yards
5. 12 × ¼ mile	5. 1 × 1 mile 2 × ½ mile 4 × ¼ mile 6 × 220 yards
6. 2 × ½ mile 6 × ¼ mile 6 × 220 yards	6. 2 × 1 mile 2 × ½ mile 4 × ¼ mile
7. 16 × ¼ mile	7. 2 × 1 mile 2 × ½ mile 4 × ¼ mile 8 × 220 yards
8. 4 × ½ mile 6 × ¼ mile 6 × 220 yards	8. 6 × ½ mile 8 × ¼ mile 8 × 220 yards
9. 1 × 1 mile 2 × ½ mile 3 × ¼ mile 4 × 220 yards	9. 3 × 1 mile 2 × ½ mile 5 × ¼ mile 6 × 220 yards
10. 2 × 1 mile 2 × ½ mile 4 × ¼ mile	10. 1 × 2 miles 2 × 1 mile 3 × ½ mile 4 × ¼ mile
11. 1 × 2 miles 1 × 1 mile 2 × ¼ mile	11. 1 × 3 miles 2 × 1 mile 3 × ½ mile 4 × ¼ mile

There is a gradual decline during the week just before the race. If you wish to just complete the race, training using time rather than mileage is recommended. Table 11.4 provides a suggested training schedule for the marathon.

TRIATHLON

Three-event races (swimming, biking, and running), or **triathlons,** began in Hawaii and are now held throughout the United States and attract thousands of participants. To be successful, you must train in all three areas and develop what participants call "all-around fitness." Keep in mind that the triathlon is not for everyone. It is an event that requires specialized training and a tremendously high level of fitness.

For those wishing to participate, the distances vary greatly. One is as short as a 400-yard swim, a 4-mile cycle, and a 1-mile run on the beach. The Hawaii event consists of a 2.4-mile swim, a 112-mile cycle, and a 26.2-mile run.

ANAEROBIC TRAINING (INTENSE EXERCISE FOR A SHORT TIME)

Sports such as tennis, racquetball, handball, squash, football, sprinting, and baseball require all-out efforts in the form of short sprints for several seconds. To make these repetitive short sprints over a period of 30 seconds or more, you must improve your anaerobic conditioning level.

Sprinting forms the foundation of an anaerobic training program. Your first step is to apply the principle of specificity (see Chapter 3) by designing your sprints over distances similar to those occurring in your sport. Tennis players, for example, rarely must sprint all-out for more than 15 yards. A sound program for tennis, then, is a series of 15- to 50-yard sprints interrupted by short rest intervals such as those described below:

Pick-up Sprints. This type of anaerobic program involves a gradual increase from a jog to a three-quarter stride to a sprint. In early workouts, jog 10 yards, stride 10, sprint 10, and finish that repetition with a 10-yard walk. As your conditioning level

TABLE 11.3 SAMPLE INTERVAL WORKOUT FOR DEVELOPING SPEED

	Conditioned Beginner (Around 8:00 pace)	Average Runner (Around 7:00 pace)	Advanced Runner (Around 6:30 pace)
Repetitions	6	6	10
Distance	220 yards	¼ mile	¼ mile
Pace	45 to 50 seconds	100 seconds	90 seconds
Rest Interval	90 seconds	90 seconds	90 seconds
Repetitions	4	8	6
Distance	¼ mile	¼ mile	½ mile
Pace	110 seconds	100 seconds	3:00 minutes
Rest Interval	90 seconds	90 seconds	3:00 minutes

All speed workouts begin with a minimum of a mile warm-up of easy running followed by gentle stretching and some short (40 yards) running in which the pace is gradually increased to workout pace in the last 15 to 20 yards.

Most distances beyond ½ mile are done as repeats in which sufficient rest is taken to allow the heart rate to drop to 120 beats per minute. Distances for repeats can range from ½ mile to any distance at which an individual can run faster than a desired race pace, that is, 10-mile repeats could be run in preparation for a marathon. Most repeats, however, are in the ½ mile to 3 mile range.

improves, increase the number of repetitions and decrease the rest interval between each. Once weekly, use longer distances of 25, 50, and 75 yards.

Hollow Sprints. Two sprints interrupted by a hollow period of recovery such as walking or jogging are used. A sample repetition includes a 15-yard sprint, 15-yard jog, 15-yard sprint, and a 15-yard walk for recovery. Similar segments of 50, 75, and 110 yards can be used.

Sample workouts using pick-up and hollow sprints are shown in Table 11.5.

ANAEROBIC FITNESS TEST

To determine your anaerobic fitness level, complete one of the three tests below. You should score high enough to receive a rating of good if you participate in anaerobic sports such as tennis, racquetball, handball, squash, football, baseball, and so on.

Drop-off Index With all three methods below, a 15-yard running start is used to eliminate reaction time and starting ability. Attempt to reach full running stride before reaching the starting point. The best of two trials is recorded. A 15-minute formal warm-up period is used before the test, and a 10- to 30-minute rest period should be taken between the first and second trials:

Method One. Determine your 50-yard and 100-yard time (running start as described above). Double your 50-yard time. This figure should be no more than 0.1 second less than the 100-yard time. RATING: 0.1 second = excellent; 0.2 second = good; 0.3 second = fair; 0.4 second or more = poor.

Method Two. Determine your 100- and 300-yard times using the method described above. Triple your 100-yard time. This time should be no more than 3 to 5 seconds less than your 300-yard time. RATING: 3 to 5 seconds = excellent; 6 to 8 seconds = good; 9 to 11 seconds = fair; 12 seconds or more = poor.

Method Three. An individual in excellent anaerobic condition should be capable of performing a 440-yard dash (one lap around a standard track) at a pace approximately five times their best 100-yard dash effort.

TABLE 11.4   TRAINING FOR THE MARATHON

Day	Week 1	Week 2	Week 3	Week 4	Week 5	Week 6
1	10 miles	11 miles	12 miles	13 miles	14 miles	15 miles
2	0 miles	0 miles	0 miles	0 miles	0 miles	3 miles
3	6 miles	6 miles	6 miles	6 miles	7 miles	7 miles
4	7 miles	7 miles	8 miles	8 miles	8 miles	8 miles
5	6 miles	6 miles	6 miles	6 miles	7 miles	7 miles
6	7 miles	7 miles	8 miles	10 miles	10 miles	10 miles
7	4 miles	4 miles	4 miles	4 miles	4 miles	5 miles
Total	40 miles	41 miles	44 miles	47 miles	50 miles	55 miles

Basic Assumptions:

1. You are a serious runner and have been running between 25 and 40 miles a week for at least a year.

2. You have had some race experience at distances of 10K or above.

3. You have at least three months to train before the marathon you wish to run.

100-yard time	440-yard time
9.0	45.0
9.5	47.5
10.0	50.0
10.5	52.5
11.0	55.0
11.5	57.5
12.0	60.0
12.5	62.5
13.0	65.0
13.5	67.5
14.0	70.0
14.5	72.5
15.0	75.0
15.5	77.5
16.0	80.0

RATING: Within 2 seconds of 440-yard time = excellent; 3 to 5 seconds = good; 6 to 8 seconds = fair; 9 seconds or more = poor.

SPECIAL STRENGTH TRAINING PROGRAMS

A number of unique **strength training** programs have been used by athletes in various sports. Most of these approaches are extremely demanding and involve handling heavy weights. For this reason, it is highly recommended that lifting ses-

sions be done with a partner to spot (protect) you. A brief description of these programs follows.

Rest—Pause   A single repetition is performed at near maximal weight (1 RM) before resting 1 to 2 minutes, completing a second repetition, resting again, and so on until the muscle is fatigued and cannot perform even one repetition.

Set System   The use of multiple sets is one of the most popular advanced training methods. Several repetitions are performed before repeating the exercise, resting, and repeating it again. Three to four sets of approximately 5 to 6 repetitions are generally used for each exercise.

Burnout   For each exercise, 75 percent of the maximal weight is used to complete as many consecutive repetitions as possible. Without any rest interval, 10 pounds are removed from the starting weight and another infinite set is performed. Again, without any rest period another 10 pounds are removed and a third set is undertaken. This procedure is repeated over and over until the muscle is nonresponding (burned out). Each designated muscle group is put through the same demanding process. It is highly recommended that a partner be close at hand to help remove weights and assist should premature fatigue occur.

TABLE 11.4   TRAINING FOR THE MARATHON—Continued

Day	Week 7	Week 8	Week 9	Week 10	Week 11	Race Week
1	15 miles	15 miles	20 miles	15 miles	15 miles	15 miles
2	4 miles	4 miles	0 miles	5 miles	5 miles	5 miles
3	7 miles	7 miles	6 miles	6 miles	6 miles	6 miles
4	9 miles	10 miles	10 miles	10 miles	10 miles	5 miles
5	7 miles	7 miles	7 miles	7 miles	7 miles	4 miles
6	10 miles	10 miles	10 miles	10 miles	10 miles	3 miles
7	6 miles	7 miles	7 miles	7 miles	7 miles	RACE DAY
Total	58 miles	60 miles	60 miles	60 miles	60 miles	

Basic Assumptions Continued:

4. If you plan to race the marathon, you will do one speed workout a week (middle of the week) and will race (no longer than 13.1 miles) every other week.

5. If you miss a workout, you will not double up the next day to make up for it. You will, however, get one long run (15 miles) in a week beginning in the second month and will try to have two double-digit runs (10 or more miles) per week.

Wipeout   For each exercise, 50 percent of the maximal weight is used to complete as many consecutive repetitions as possible. There is no rest interval or weights to remove with this method. The number of repetitions is infinite until the designated muscle group fails. An assistant should be close at hand in the event there is premature fatigue. As a variation, a one-minute rest is taken before attempting a second or third set. Your ultimate goal is to completely exhaust the muscle group.

Supersets   A set of exercises for one group of muscles is followed immediately by a set for their antagonist. A variation of this method is known as

TABLE 11.5   SAMPLE PICK-UP AND HOLLOW SPRINTS

Early Season (Initial 3 to 5 Workouts):	Second and Third Weeks:	Fourth to Eighth Weeks:	In-Season Workout:
Walk/jog 2 miles; jog 15 yards, stride 15, walk 15—repeat 5 times; end workout with a 1 mile jog/walk.	Jog 1 mile nonstop; jog 15 yards, stride 15, sprint 15, walk 15—repeat 6 to 12 times; repeat above with 10-yard sprints 6 to 12 times; end workout with a 1 mile jog/walk.	Jog 1 mile; jog 15 yards, stride 15, sprint 15, walk 15—repeat 6 to 12 times; sprint 50 yards; jog for 10 to 12 seconds—repeat 4 times to complete a 440-yard run on the track in less than 90 seconds—repeat 6 to 8 times (in later workouts try to reduce the total 440-yard time to 75–80 seconds using the sprint/jog cycle); cool down with a 1 to 2 mile slow jog.	Jog 1 mile; jog 15 yards, stride 15, sprint 15, walk 15—repeat 3 to 5 times; jog 25, sprint 15, jog 25, sprint 15, jog 25, sprint 15, jog 25, sprint 15— repeat 6 times; 300-yard all-out run—repeat 2 to 6 times; cool down with a 1 mile slow jog.

super multiple sets and consists of performing three sets of an exercise for one group of muscles followed by the same number of sets for their antagonists. A short rest is taken between sets. For example, one set of arm curls (bicep muscle-antagonist) is followed by a set of bench presses (tricep-antagonist).

Groves' Super Overload Method

This procedure has the potential for superior strength gains and is highly applicable to the bench press, leg press, and ankle exercises. The following steps must be taken:

1. Establish your 1 RM.
2. Add 25 percent more weight to this amount.
3. Have an assistant help you get into the up position (bench press begins with arms extended overhead, elbows locked; leg press begins with legs extended and knees locked).
4. Bend the joint slightly (only two to three inches) on the first repetition.
5. Continue taking the weight downward further each time until, on the 7th repetition, you are unable to return the weight to the up position without assistance.
6. Complete three sets of seven repetitions every other day.

At the end of each week, redetermine your 1 RM and repeat these steps using the new weight.

Circuit Weight Training (CWT)

This system involves a series of weight training exercises of approximately 12 to 15 repetitions each using a moderate amount of weight (about 40 to 60 percent of 1 RM). The exerciser moves quickly from one station to another with minimal rest (15 to 30 seconds) between stations. Generally, the 2 or 3 circuits of 10 exercises is designed so that the total workout time is between 25 and 30 minutes. CWT increases aerobic capacity by approximately 5 percent, compared with 15 to 25 percent for other aerobic exercise programs. Lean-body mass also increases from 1 to 3.2 kg, and fat decreases 0.8 to 2.9 percent. Strength improves 7 to 32 percent. The energy costs of CWT are similar to jogging at 5 mph. Improvement in strength and maximum oxygen uptake (VO_2 max) depends on work performed, not on the equipment used. CWT will not develop high levels of aerobic fitness, but it can help maintain fitness.

Competitive Weight Lifting

There are two distinct categories of weight lifting. The first is the Olympic Games competition consisting of three specific overhead lifts: the military press, the snatch, and the clean and jerk. The other category is referred to as power lifting, which involves the squat, deadlift, and bench press. In either category, the primary objective is to lift as much weight as possible in each of the competitive events. Male lifters are divided into 11 body-weight divisions ranging from flyweight (114½ pounds) to super-heavyweight (over 242½ pounds). Women have 9 weight divisions, from flyweight (96½ pounds) to heavyweight (over 181 pounds).

Bodybuilding

Body builders are generally more concerned with flex appeal (size, shape, definition, proportion) than muscle strength. They use dumbbells, barbells and resistance-designed machines to carve out and define individual muscles. Beauty of physique is much more important than feats of strength. Competitors perform posing routines and are judged on symmetry (body parts having been equally developed top and bottom, left and right), muscle definition, and poise. Females finish up their competition by engaging in a brief freestyle routine to music, a kind of cross between sport and cabaret.

FREQUENTLY ASKED QUESTIONS

Do conditioning levels continue to improve throughout an athletic season?

No. Although you should continue to gradually improve, this is not the case. In fact, by Super Bowl Sunday it is estimated that players are functioning at about 65 to 70 percent of their early season efficiency. Numerous factors account for this:

1. Injuries and loss of practice and playing time
2. A change to less rigorous practice routines that emphasize strategy and the expected action of opponents
3. Rigorous travel schedules
4. Lack of a systematic maintenance program for muscular strength and endurance and anaerobic and aerobic endurance

For team sports, maintenance programs are essential. One weight training session weekly using near maximum lifts will help to maintain the strength acquired in the preseason. Anaerobic and aerobic endurance will also decrease unless time is set aside two or three times weekly for the purpose of maintaining these areas.

Can I do anything to improve my sprinting speed for my sport?

Yes. Speed in short distances can be improved by:

1. Taking faster steps
2. Taking longer steps
3. Taking faster and longer steps
4. Accelerating to maximum speed faster

With proper training, runners can increase their stride length (longer steps) and their stride rate (more steps per second). The interested reader is referred to *Sportspeed: The #1 Speed Improvement Program for All Athletes* (Dintiman and Ward 1988)

What is maximum effort training?

Maximum effort training involves the use of high-intensity exercises that tax each individual to complete exhaustion. They serve the purpose of producing psychological toughness, increasing the pain threshold, and improving physiological development beyond that occurring from regular training. Only the best mentally and physically conditioned athletes will be capable of incorporating this type of training into their schedules.

This type of training also is one of the few good methods of equalizing exercise effort among athletes of varying abilities and conditioning levels. It offers training geared to the individual, with everyone working against his or her own previous distance or time record and each coping with his or her own stress and psychological barriers until, finally, only complete physical exhaustion causes cessation of exercise.

A maximum effort session should be a part of every practice, occurring at the close of the workout. It should tax every individual to maximum capacity. It is also helpful to keep records and to test periodically to determine individual progress.

Once you condition your mind to quit only when physically no longer able to continue, you have made great strides toward becoming a good athlete in any sport. Here is a simple basic program for daily use:

1. *All-out sprint.* Perform an all-out sprint at maximum speed until no longer able to continue. Record the distance.
2. *Distance hop.* Perform a one-legged hop at maximum speed until no longer able to continue. Record the distance and time. Repeat using the opposite leg.

The above basic exercises can be supplemented by a number of other exercises to add variety and intensity to the program:

1. *Running in place.* Lifting the knees to waist level, sprint in place until no longer able to continue. Record the time. Avoid pacing or barely lifting feet from the ground.
2. *300-yard run.* Record the time in a 300-yard sprint.
3. *Two-legged hop.* Record the distance covered in 45 seconds. Slowly increase the time limit.

What is the condition known as male anorexia?

Anorexia nervosa (self-imposed starvation) does occur in some males; however, this condition is a self-destructive pathological behavior exhibited mostly by men who constantly strive for faster times in road races and better performance in sports through long, intense training. This overemphasis on physical prowess in some men is being labeled an *ascetic disorder* comparable to anorexia nervosa in women. Extreme dieting is now recognized as an emotional disorder. Extreme training is still acceptable in all sports, although some experts feel the psychology underlying both behaviors is the same. Individuals who feel obligated to exercise under even dangerous conditions (illness, injury, adverse heat or cold) experience depression when unable to train. The number of these individuals seems to be increasing.

Is DMSO a quick cure or quack treatment?

Dimethyl sulfoxide (**DMSO**) surfaced publicly during two segments of CBS TV's "60 Minutes" in late 1979, during which wonder-drug claims were made by some of its users. Cures and relief were hinted at for practically any disorder including sprains, joint inflammation, arthritis, black eyes, muscle bruises, burns, athlete's foot, gum conditions, infections, painful breast conditions, and muscle pulls. Numerous athletes in track and field and football claimed regular use for more than ten years and swore by its miracle effect in relieving joint pain and speeding recovery.

DMSO, in liquid or gel form, comes in strengths of 50 to 100 percent. It is actually a derivative of lignin, a by-product of wood pulp, and has been around for a long time. Paper manufacturing companies use it as an industrial solvent (100 percent strength). Veterinary doctors apply it topically (90 percent strength) to the affected areas of horses and dogs to reduce swelling. In two states, the 50 percent strength DMSO is legally used to treat a type of human bladder condition. In Canada, Great Britain and European countries, DMSO has been used to treat a wide variety of human conditions. Illegal use (most states) for human conditions involves 70 percent DMSO.

Regardless of the strength, when applied topically to the skin, DMSO is rapidly absorbed (along with anything else on the skin) and circulated throughout the body. Within 15 to 20 minutes, it can be found in practically any organ in the human body. It also produces a garlic-like taste in the mouth and gives off a similar odor from the skin. DMSO can be mixed with hydrocortisone cream, crushed aspirin, or local anesthetic to aid as an analgesic and act as a chemical carrier to transmit these properties into the blood stream within minutes.

Proponents of DMSO argue that it is safer than aspirin and produces no serious side effects other than the garlic taste and skin redness in some users. Testimony from thousands of users over more than ten years is proof of its effectiveness on traumatized joints and muscles. Some physicians point out that DMSO has been both effectively and safely used on their patients. Since it has so many uses, the argument goes, it is grossly misunderstood. In addition, it is so inexpensive to produce that it would result in little profit for drug companies, thus explaining the lack of interest on the part of the FDA and pharmaceutical companies. Complicating the issue is the charge by some physicians that the FDA does have scientific evidence of its safety and effectiveness.

Opponents point out that the rapid absorption of anything through the skin is dangerous since any impurities in the drug (industrial DMSO is not purified and may contain pesticides and other impurities) or on the skin are carried into the blood stream. There is also some evidence of side effects such as nausea, headaches, skin rash, and possible eye damage. DMSO tests performed on rabbits, dogs, and pigs made the lenses of their eyes dense and left them nearsighted. Concern is also expressed for the rare hypersensitive person who could suffer serious consequences. At present, DMSO use is illegal in most states and there is a need for adequate testing on human subjects to determine its true value and side effects. Arthritis sufferers, for example, are easy prey to exploitation by testimonial data and tend to use untested drugs before dangers are revealed, often neglecting proven forms of treatment and thereby increasing pain and crippling.

One area of agreement by both sides is that care should be taken when applying DMSO directly to the skin. The injured area should be thoroughly cleaned (not with alcohol since it would be absorbed) before applying DMSO with a Q-tip or rubber gloves. The injured limb should be propped up for 15 to 20 minutes to allow the DMSO to soak into the system before it is completely wiped off to prevent absorption of the dye from clothing. The majority of enthusiasm for DMSO use in humans comes from testimonials. Although there is undoubtedly some evidence to support its value and safety, there is no guarantee from health hazards with long term use. The FDA has received numerous applications from drug companies and physicians to evaluate its effectiveness and safety. These studies will eventually reveal the value and the hazards. Until these findings are uncovered, it may be wise to play it safe.

Which is better, long-slow distance or speed training for road races?

A number of different training methods are used to improve speed in road races (5K and 10K). **Long-slow distance** (LSD), fartlek (alternating fast and slow running over varied terrain), and intervals are a few techniques purported to improve speed. Some apply only to running while others such as LSD and intervals can apply to walking, swimming, cycling, and running.

As a beginning exerciser, you will experience greater speed with nearly every workout as long as you do not overdo any one session. This increased speed is due primarily to increased muscle strength. There is a direct relationship between speed and strength in early training. Later, cardiovascular efficiency comes into play and improvement is slower.

Most individuals are satisfied with the fitness and speed developed through the LSD approach. For fitness purposes, long-slow distance is the only exercise routine required. It is both safe and effective in improving cardiovascular conditioning. Continued LSD training, however, may fail to develop speed, and prepare you only for running long, slow distances.

For racing purposes, experts argue that you must train at a speed faster than you actually desire to race. For middle- and long-distance cyclers, swimmers, and runners, this means short, fast distances at or below the eventual race pace. Milers in track, for example, will run fast quarter miles and half miles in training (overspeed training). For running, speed work that uses intervals is included in this chapter. Other techniques such as towing, downhill running, and fartlek are also valuable for developing speed.

Selecting the best speed training techniques for any activity is done by determining how closely the training simulates the actual event. Although calisthenic activities such as rope jumping, push-ups, and jumping jacks are good fitness activities, they will do little for developing speed in sports.

When I am near the end of a distance race and feel tired, should I increase my stride length or shorten it to maintain my speed?

Physiologically it is better to shorten the stride length and increase your number of steps per second (stride rate).

Is too much of a good thing harmful?

Although the affected person may ignore them, the physiological signs of overindulgence are usually easy to recognize. Resting pulse rates usually rise, joints become stiff and sore, fatigue is common, and sleeping, eating, and elimination habits are disturbed. Although the telltale signs of physiological overindulgence appear common, it is unlikely that any one person will experience all of them. Factors such as age, conditioning level, rest habits, diet, and health factors such as anemia, illness, and mental stress determine when and if symptoms appear.

Competition seems to be a common denominator for most exercise addicts. With the inclusion of age group categories in nearly all sports, special olympics for the aged, and continued emphasis on exercise beyond the college years, there is more motivation to seek higher levels of fitness than are necessary for health alone. There are, therefore, many who are seeking to capture past glories or seeking glories never received.

You can usually tell when you're addicted by your behavior. You are compulsive about exercise—not a day can be missed; daily schedules are made around exercise, and workouts often receive priority over everything. Whether such behavior is a result of the exercise or your own personality is unknown. It is generally agreed, however, that negative addiction is unhealthy and, as the name implies, should be avoided. The long-term results would seem to be harmful, both physiologically and psychologically.

MYTHS AND FALLACIES

Marathoners are immune to heart disease.

As was pointed out under the discussion of heart disease in Chapter 1, no one is immune to heart disease. The "immunity of marathoners" myth began during the early years of distance running when only the very fit ran marathons. As the sport grew in popularity, however, so did the chances of successful marathoners having heart disease.

Champion athletes are born, not made.

Champions are products of hard work, not heredity. You do not have to be seven feet tall and weigh 250 pounds to become a champion athlete, nor do you need to be born with superior skill. Keep in mind that heredity deals the cards, but environment plays the hand. Some athletes born with superior coordination and physical qualities never reach stardom, while others with only average qualities become champions. The difference is strong dedication to two broad areas: skill development for *every* aspect of the particular sport, and physical development through numerous training programs to allow the body to perform these perfected skills with maximum power, strength, agility, endurance and speed. Modern-day champions are hardworking, dedicated individuals. They do not develop superior skill or physical qualities in one year. For many, it means one to two workouts daily, and countless additional hours of practice time on skills over a period of 5–12 years. Those that eventually make it are the most persistent, dedicated, and hardworking, not necessarily the most genetically blessed (Dintiman and Ward, 1988).

Sprinting speed cannot be improved.

The preponderance of slow or fast twitch fiber in the muscle groups involved in sprinting determines your genetic potential for speed. Muscle biopsy has revealed the existence of as much as 94 percent slow twitch fiber in some marathoners, and over 90 percent fast twitch fiber in some champion sprinters. Unfortunately, few individuals, regardless of their genetic makeup, ever reach their speed potential unless they follow a holistic speed improvement program. Coaches at all levels of competition are now well aware that speed can be improved in every athlete. Improvements in the 40-yard dash times of as much as 6 tenths of a second have occurred in individuals who followed the Seven Step Model for Speed Improvement (Dintiman and Ward 1988). Even at the professional level, athletes such as Bill Bates of the Dallas Cowboys, Carl Bland of the Detroit Lions, and others have improved their speed in short distances. Dramatic improvements have also occurred in high school athletes in various sports. Although it may be impossible to transform a 14.0 second 100-meter sprinter into an Olympic Champion, the proper training program can significantly reduce this slow time.

It is impossible to develop equal skill in both my right and left hands and feet?

There is only one reason why very few athletes in any sport are equally adept on both sides of the body—neglect. Observation of most athletes during a practice session reveals the tendency to repeat movements and actions with the dominant hand or limb. Few basketball players devote equal practice time, even in the off-season, to recessive hand shooting, dribbling, and passing. Soccer players do not devote near enough time to recessive limb goal kicking, trapping, and passing. Few baseball and football players can catch, let alone throw, with either hand. Years ago, a young basketball player at Southern Connecticut State University broke his dominant arm near the end of the season. During the next three months, he participated in pick-up games daily, unable to use his casted dominant arm. When this player returned the following season, his skill in his recessive hand was so good that it was impossible to tell whether he was right or left handed. This same skill development could occur in any dedicated athlete.

BIBLIOGRAPHY

Combs, Laura. *Winning Women's Bodybuilding.* Chicago: Contemporary Books, 1983.

Dintiman, George, and Robert Ward. *Train America: Achieving Peak Performance and Fitness for Sports Competition.* Dubuque, Iowa: Kendal-Hunt, 1988.

Dintiman, George, and Robert Ward. *Sportspeed: The #1 Speed Improvement Program for All Athletes.* Champaign, Illinois: Leisure Press, 1988.

Kirkley, George W. *Weight Lifting and Weight Training.* New York: Arco, 1981.

Lyon, Lisa, and Douglas Kenthal. *Lisa Lyon's Body Magic.* New York: Bantam, 1981.

Marshall, John L., and Heather Barbash. *The Sports Doctor's Fitness Book for Women.* New York: Delecorte, 1981.

Mentzer, Mike, and Ardy Friedberg. *Complete Book of Weight Training.* New York: William Morrow, 1982.

Schwarzenegger, Arnold. *Arnold's Bodybuilding for Men.* New York: Simon and Schuster, 1981.

Unitas, John, and George B. Dintiman. *The Champion's Edge.* West Point, N.Y.: Leisure Press, 1984.

Weider, Joe. *Muscle and Fitness Bodybuilding, Nutrition and Training Programs.* Chicago: Contemporary Books, 1981.

Willoughby, David P. *The Super Athletes.* New York: A. S. Barnes, 1970.

LABORATORY 11.1

A Personalized Fitness Program

PURPOSE: To design a total personalized fitness program.

SIZE OF GROUP: Alone

PROCEDURE

1. Establish a goal for each of the fitness areas you wish to develop. For example:
   a. Be able to run a 10K in under 40 minutes.
   b. Be able to finish in the top 10 percent of my age group in a triathlon.
   c. Improve my strength by 15 percent.
   d. Reduce my percent of body fat to 15 percent.
   e. A combination of all of the above.

2. Establish some specifically stated objectives. For example:
   a. Over a 10-week period, I will do a track workout once a week using the interval schedule from this chapter.
   b. Using the Set System and Groves' Super Overload, I will lift three times a week until I reach my goal.
   c. Using my personal fitness program and information from the nutrition chapter, I will modify my diet to lose ___ pounds in six months.

3. Establish some rewards for accomplishing your goals and objectives.

4. Using the goals, objectives, and information from this entire book, establish a total fitness program.

5. Write down your daily workouts including an objective for each day.
   a. Be sure to follow the concepts established in Chapter 3.
   b. The workouts should be for at least a three-month period.

LABORATORY 11.2

Personal Log

PURPOSE: To design a personal daily log.

SIZE OF GROUP: Alone

PROCEDURE

1. This lab is to be completed after Laboratory 11.1.

2. Using the example log in Chapter 3 and the information from Laboratory 11.1, design a personal log to record your progress (a 5-by-7 inch spiral notebook is a good size for recording information).

3. Information that will be helpful to record includes:
   a. Date and time
   b. Weather conditions, if appropriate
   c. Time and/or distance covered
   d. If doing intervals, the length of each repetition, the total number of repetitions, the time, and the rest interval
   e. General impressions and special considerations such as any unusual pains
   f. Nutritional information including everything eaten each day

Fitness Testing Prerequisites

Physical fitness testing requiring maximum effort is an important first in designing your personal exercise program. It is, however, a potential source of difficulty if carried out haphazardly. It is important to minimize any potential physical harm during the test, and to be fully aware of expected discomfort and pain several hours or days after the test. Although you may have had a medical examination, it is still necessary to use a preconditioning program for two to three weeks involving large muscle activity (walking, jogging, swimming, cycling), and progressively more use of other muscles to be tested (abdominal, shoulder, and arm). Such an approach reduces the incidence and severity of muscle soreness following various tests, as well as the risk of physical harm from overexertion.

The 1.5-mile run-walk test is potentially dangerous if you are over 30 years of age or overweight, have high blood pressure or high blood lipids, or have been inactive for several months or more. Avoid this test if you fall into any of these categories and assume that your aerobic fitness level is very poor. You can first choose an exercise program and slowly progress from low to high fitness levels.

Even with preconditioning, you may experience some discomfort during and after the test.

DURING THE TEST

Nausea may occur in the unconditioned person during or immediately following strenuous activity. It is a harmless functional disorder and does not suggest any health hazard. In many cases, nausea can be prevented by preconditioning for several weeks prior to the test, and through the use of explicit instructions on how to perform a particular test item such as the 1.5-mile run-walk.

A general muscular soreness may also occur that is present immediately, but then disappears three to four hours after exercise stops. The exact cause of this soreness is unknown, but it happens more often to unconditioned people. It appears that muscle pain occurs from muscles working without adequate blood supply, resulting in failure to remove waste products. The pain then supposedly results from the accumulation of lactic acid metabolites that irritate the receptor organs of pain located in the muscle. Proper warm-up and preconditioning can reduce the number of cases of general muscle soreness.

Headache, dizziness, fainting, digestive upset, undue pounding, or uneven heart beat are additional symptoms that could occur in some poorly conditioned people. You should take long, warm-to-hot showers, and allow sufficient time to cool down. Where symptoms persist, you should seek appropriate first aid or medical treatment.

Excessive breathlessness that persists long after exercise may also be a reason to see a medical professional. Additional signs during exercise that may indicate a need for medical treatment include bluing of the lips (except in cold weather), pale or clammy skin in the presence of normal temperatures, unusual shakiness or weakness persisting for more than 10 minutes following vigorous exercise, and muscle twitching (tetany), either localized, or generalized. Unusual reactions are not necessarily abnormal reactions, and you should not be alarmed; however, testing offers an opportunity for special diagnosis, and the potential to identify difficulties early.

An injury due to muscle strain or collisions can be avoided with proper warm-up and meticulous test planning designed for optimum safety.

Broken sleep may occur the night after the test. Muscles may ache somewhat from such unaccustomed exercise. This is an indication that the exercise was too severe for your conditioning level, and that the sore muscles were not accustomed to such activity. Again, it is a normal occurrence, and will certainly not continue for successive evenings.

Muscle soreness is the most common complaint the day following exercise. The older you are, the longer the period between exercise and muscle soreness. At age 17, it may appear within a few hours, at age 25, the following day, and, at age 50, not for two to three days. This localized soreness is sometimes explained as being caused by injury of fibers or of the sarcolemma, which transmits the contraction to the tendon. Damaged tissues are then repaired, resulting in a stronger muscle that is less vulnerable. However, it is unrealistic to believe that fibers are so sensitive and weak as to be ruptured by mild or moderate ex-

ercise. A more accepted theory is that fluid builds up, causing swelling and stiffness. The fluid compresses and irritates the nerve endings and causes pain. Soreness can generally be relieved by:

1. Determining which muscles are sore
2. Consulting a book on anatomy to locate the origin and insertion attachments of the sore muscles
3. Holding the attachments as far apart as possible for 1½ to 3 minutes (repeat twice, waiting 1 to 2 minutes between the two repetitions; for pain in the calf, for example, sit with your leg extended fully, and push your toes toward your knee)
4. Performing the above every four hours until pain is relieved

The risk of soreness can be reduced by warming up properly, avoiding bouncing-type stretching exercises, and slowly increasing your exercise effort rather than overextending yourself early in a workout or training program. The location of muscle soreness indicates either the area of least trained muscles, or the greatest exercise concentration. Again, muscle soreness is a common occurrence that almost always occurs when maximum effort testing involves previously unexercised muscles or unaccustomed intensity.

APPENDIX B

Your Fitness Profile

Name _____ Age _____ Ht. _____ Wt. _____ Date _____

Resting heart rate _____ Maximum heart rate (220 − age) _____ Target heart rate _____
THR = 60% of the distance between your resting and maximum HR (see Chapter 1)

Major Fitness Area	Test Item	Your Score	Interpretation	Page Reference
Aerobic fitness	1.5 mile run-walk test	_____	_____	Chapter 3, page 70
Muscular strength	Bench press (1 RM)	_____	_____	Chapter 4, page 78
	Shoulder press (1 RM)	_____	_____	Chapter 4, page 78
	Biceps curl (1 RM)	_____	_____	Chapter 4, page 78
	Leg press (1 RM)	_____	_____	Chapter 4, page 78
	Grip strength	_____	_____	Chapter 4, page 79
	Pull-ups	_____	_____	Chapter 4, page 79
	Modified pull-ups	_____	_____	Chapter 4, page 79
	Bar dips	_____	_____	Chapter 4, page 79
	Sit-ups	_____	_____	Chapter 4, page 80
Flexibility	Sit-and-Reach test	_____	_____	Chapter 5, page 124
Body composition	Body weight	_____	_____	Chapter 7, page 165
	Triceps skinfold	_____	_____	Chapter 7, page 168
	Biceps skinfold	_____	_____	Chapter 7, page 168
	Subscapula skinfold	_____	_____	Chapter 7, page 168
	Suprailiac skinfold	_____	_____	Chapter 7, page 168
Blood lipids[1]	Serum Cholesterol	_____	_____	Chapter 1, page 17
	LDL cholesterol	_____	_____	Chapter 1, page 17
	HDL cholesterol	_____	_____	Chapter 1, page 17
	HDL/LDL ratio	_____	_____	Chapter 1, page 17

[1]Blood samples to be drawn and analyzed by your physician.

APPENDIX C

Potassium and Sodium Content of Various Foods

TABLE C.1   WHOLE UNPROCESSED FOOD VERSUS PROCESSED FOODS— POTASSIUM AND SODIUM CONTENTS

Food	Amount	Potassium (mg)	Sodium (mg)	Potassium Sodium Ratio
Milk Foods				
Milk	1 c	370	122	3:1
Chocolate pudding (cooked from mix)	1 c	354	343	1:1
Chocolate pudding (instant)	1 c	335	820	1:2
Meats				
Beef roast (cooked)	3 oz	279	42	7:1
Corned beef (canned)	3 oz	51	803	1:16
Chipped beef	3 oz	170	3660	1:22
Vegetables				
Corn (cooked)	1 c	304	71	4:1
Creamed corn (canned)	1 c	248	671	1:3
Sugar-coated cornflakes	1 c	27	262	1:10
Fruits				
Peaches (fresh)	1 peach	202	1	202:1
Peaches (canned)	1	333	5	67:1
Peach pie	1 piece	201	201	1:1
Grains				
Whole-wheat flour	1 c	444	4	100:1
Whole-wheat bread	1 slice	68	132	1:2
Doughnut, snack cake	1	23	125	1:5

TABLE C.2 POTASSIUM IN FOODS

Foods Ranked by Potassium Per Serving	Potassium Per Serving (mg)	Energy Per Serving (kCal)	Foods Ranked by Potassium Per 100 kCalories	Potassium Per Serving (mg)	Potassium Per 100 kCal (mg)
Peach halves, dried (10)	1,295	311	Bok choy cabbage, cooked (1 c)	630	3,150
Lima beans, cooked (1 c)	1,163	260	Spinach, cooked (1 c)	838	2.044
Winter squash, baked (1 c)	1,071	96	Celery, outer stalk (1)	114	1,900
Pear halves, dried (10)	932	459	Romaine lettuce, chopped (1 c)	162	1,800
Sirloin steak, lean (8 oz)	928	480	Parsley, chopped fresh (1 c)	322	1,610
Potato, microwaved w/skin (1)	903	212	Zucchini squash, cooked (1 c)	455	1,569
Pinto beans, cooked (1 c)	882	265	Red radishes (10)	104	1,486
Baked potato, whole (1)	844	220	Looseleaf lettuce (1 c)	148	1,480
Spinach, cooked (1 c)	838	41	Mushrooms, raw sliced (1 c)	260	1,444
Cantaloupe melon (½)	825	94	Cauliflower, cooked (1 c)	400	1,333
Kidney beans, canned (1 c)	673	230	Asparagus, cooked (1 c)	558	1,268
Bok choy cabbage, cooked (1 c)	630	20	Tomatoes, whole canned (1 c)	529	1,126
Prunes, dried (10)	626	201	Winter squash, baked (1 c)	1,071	1,116
Peas, dry split, cooked (1 c)	592	230	Cabbage, raw shredded (1 c)	172	1,075
Butternut squash, baked (1 c)	583	83	Tomato, whole raw (1)	255	1,063
Blackeyed peas, cooked (1 c)	573	190	Beets, cooked (1 c)	532	1,023
Watermelon (1 sl)	560	152	Summer squash, cooked (1 c)	346	961
Asparagus, cooked (1 c)	558	44	Cantaloupe melon (½)	825	878
Beets, cooked (1 c)	532	52	Green beans, cooked (1 c)	373	848
Tomatoes, whole canned (1 c)	529	47	Green peppers, whole (1)	144	800
Orange juice, fresh (1 c)	496	111	Carrot, whole fresh (1)	233	752
Apricot halves, dried (10)	482	83	Butternut squash, baked (1 c)	583	702
Zucchini squash, cooked (1 c)	455	29	Apricots, fresh pitted (3)	313	614
Banana, peeled (1)	451	105	Brewers yeast (1 tbsp)	152	608
Nonfat milk or yogurt (1 c)	406	86	Apricot halves, dried (10)	482	581
Cauliflower, cooked (1 c)	400	30	Broccoli, cooked (1 c)	254	552
Green beans, cooked (1 c)	373	44	Wheat bran (¼ c)	103	542
Whole milk (1 c)	370	150	Nonfat milk or yogurt (1 c)	406	472
Summer squash, cooked (1 c)	346	36	Peach, fresh medium (1)	171	462
Parsley, chopped fresh (1 c)	322	20	Orange juice, fresh (1 c)	496	447
Apricots, fresh pitted (3)	313	51	Lima beans, cooked (1 c)	1,163	447
Sole/flounder, baked (3 oz)	272	120	Banana, peeled (1)	451	430
Mushrooms, raw sliced (1 c)	260	18	Potato, microwaved w/skin (1)	903	426
Tomato, whole raw (1)	255	24	Peach halves, dried (10)	1,295	416
Broccoli, cooked (1 c)	254	46	Orange, fresh medium (1)	237	395
Orange, fresh medium (1)	237	60	Baked potato, whole (1)	844	384
Carrot, whole fresh (1)	233	31	Watermelon (1 sl)	560	368
Chicken breast, roasted (½)	220	142	Pinto beans, cooked (1 c)	882	333
Peanuts, dried unsalted (1 oz)	204	161	Prunes, dried (10)	626	311
Cabbage, raw shredded (1 c)	172	16	Blackeyed peas, cooked (1 c)	573	302
Peach, fresh medium (1)	171	37	Kidney beans, canned (1 c)	673	293
Romaine lettuce, chopped (1 c)	162	9	Peas, dry split, cooked (1 c)	592	257
Apple, fresh medium (1)	159	80	Whole milk (1 c)	370	247
Brewers yeast (1 tbsp)	152	25	Sole/flounder, baked (3 oz)	272	227
Looseleaf lettuce (1 c)	148	10	Pear halves, dried (10)	932	203
Green peppers, whole (1)	144	18	Apple, fresh medium (1)	159	199
Celery, outer stalk (1)	114	6	Sirloin steak, lean (8 oz)	928	193
Red radishes (10)	104	7	Chicken breast, roasted (½)	220	155
Wheat bran (¼ c)	103	19	Peanuts, dried unsalted (1 oz)	204	127
Whole wheat bread (1 sl)	50	70	Whole wheat bread (1 sl)	50	71
Cheddar cheese (1 oz)	28	114	Cheddar cheese (1 oz)	17	25

Reprinted by permission from *Understanding Nutrition, 4th ed.* page 401. Copyright © 1988 by West Publishing Company. All rights reserved.

A Guide to Nutritive Value*

This guide was designed to relate the nutritive value of food to individual nutritional needs, and to compare the nutritive value of commonly eaten foods (see Table D.1). The standard used for these comparisons is the U.S. Recommended Daily Allowance (U.S. RDA).

UNDERSTANDING THE U.S. RECOMMENDED DAILY ALLOWANCE (U.S. RDA)

The U.S. RDA is the standard used in nutrition labeling. It is based on the Recommended Dietary Allowances (RDAs) set by the National Research Council. The RDAs are judged by the Council to be adequate for nearly all healthy persons, and generous for most.

	U.S. RDA
Protein	65 grams[1]
Vitamin A	5,000 International Units
Vitamin C	60 milligrams
Thiamin	1.5 milligrams
Riboflavin	1.7 milligrams
Calcium	1 gram
Iron	18 milligrams

The U.S. RDA for all these nutrients, exce; calcium, is the *highest* RDA for all sex-age cate gories. For many individuals, therefore, the U. RDAs are higher than the amount of nutrients re ommended by the National Research Council for their sex and age. (Table D.2 adjusts the U.S. RDA to fit individual nutrient needs. To illustrate: a five-year-old needs only 50 percent of the U.S. RDA for protein. Thus, an intake of 2 cups of milk, furnishing 40 percent of the U.S. RDA, almost meets the child's protein needs.)

USING THE GUIDE

Percentages of the U.S. RDA are shown for seven major nutrients: protein, vitamin A, vitamin C, thiamin, riboflavin, calcium, and iron. Food energy is expressed as calories.

Percentages are given to the nearest 2 percent up to 10 percent, to the nearest 5 percent up to 50 percent, and to the nearest 10 percent above 50 percent. A dash indicates only a trace or none of the nutrient.

Numbers given are averages compiled from tables of food composition. When several foods are listed on the same line, the figures may not fit all the foods included equally well. Important differences are explained in footnotes.

*Reprinted from "A Guide to Nutritive Value." A Cornell Cooperative Extension publication of the Division of Nutritional Sciences. Cornell University; Ithaca, New York. 1981. Used with permission.

[1]65 grams is the U.S. RDA for a mixed diet of animal and plant proteins; 45 grams is the U.S. RDA for a diet of mainly animal proteins: meat, fish, poultry, eggs, and milk.

TABLE D.1 PERCENTAGE U.S. RDA OF SOME COMMON FOODS[1] (BOLDFACE NUMBERS INDICATE SIGNIFICANT SOURCES OF NUTRIENTS)

Food	Amount or Description	Metric Weight (grams)	Calories	Percentage U.S. RDA						
				Protein	Vitamin A	Vitamin C	Thiamin	Riboflavin	Calcium	Iron[2]
Milk and Milk Products										
Milk, whole; yogurt	1 cup	(240)	160	**20**	**6**	2	**6**	**25**	**30**	—
skim, unfortified; buttermilk	1 cup	(240)	90	**20**	—	2	**6**	**25**	**30**	—
modified skim (99% fat free), fortified	1 cup	(240)	120	**25**	**10**	2	**6**	**25**	**30**	—
evaporated, undiluted	½ cup	(120)	160	**20**	**8**	2	**4**	**25**	**30**	—
nonfat dry solids, fortified	3 tbsp.; 1 cup reconstituted	(23; 240)	90	**20**	**10**	2	**6**	**25**	**30**	—
Milkshake, chocolate	10 ounces (1 cup whole milk)	(345)	400	**25**	**15**	2	**6**	**35**	**40**	4
Cheeses: cheddar; American; Swiss; processed	1 ounce (1¼" cube)	(30)	115	**15**	**6**	—	2	**8**	**20**	—
Cheese, cottage creamed	½ cup	(115)	120	**30**	4	—	2	**15**	**10**	—
Ice cream (10% fat)	½ cup	(115)	130	6	6	—	2	**8**	**10**	—
Milk pudding, vanilla	½ cup	(130)	140	**10**	4	—	2	**12**	**15**	—
Cream, half-half	¼ cup	(60)	80	4	6	—	—	6	6	—
Vegetables										
Important Sources of Vitamins A and/or C[3]										
Broccoli	½ cup cooked	(75)	20	4	**40**	**120**	6	**10**	**8**	4
Brussels sprouts; green pepper	½ cup cooked; 1 medium pepper	(75; 90)	25	4	**10**	**110**	4	4	2	6
Cabbage; cauliflower	⅔ cup raw; ½ cup cooked	(90)	15	2	2	**50**	2	2	4	2
Carrots	½ cup cooked or raw	(80)	30	2	**150**	**10**	4	2	2	2
Greens: beet; chard; collards; kale; mustard; spinach; turnip	½ cup cooked	(100)	20	2	**100**	**50**	6	**10**	**10**[4]	8
Plantain, green or ripe	½ cup cooked	(100)	140	2	**25**	**10**	4	1	—	2
Squash, winter; pumpkin; calabaza	½ cup cooked	(100)	60	2	**90**	**20**	4	6	2	4
Sweet potato; yam, yellow	½ cup cooked	(100)	120	2	**120**	**20**	4	2	2	4
Tomatoes; raw; canned; juice	1 small; ½ cup	(100)	20	2	**15**	**35**	4	2	—	4

Food	Amount or Description	Metric Weight (grams)	Calories	Percentage U.S. RDA						
				Protein	Vitamin A	Vitamin C	Thiamin	Riboflavin	Calcium	Iron[2]
Other Vegetables										
Asparagus	½ cup cooked	(80)	15	2	**15**	**30**	8	8	2	4
Beans, lima	½ cup cooked	(80)	95	**10**	4	**20**	**10**	4	4	10
Beans, snap	½ cup cooked	(60)	15	2	8	**15**	4	4	4	4
Beets; onions	½ cup cooked	(80)	30	2	—	8	2	2	—	2
Celery; cucumber; radishes	½ cup sliced	(50)	10	—	—	8	—	—	—	—
Corn	½ cup cooked; 1-5 inch ear	(80; 140)	85	4	6	8	2	4	—	4
Lettuce, crisp head; loose leaf	1 cup shredded	(55)	8	—	8	8	2	4	—	4
Peas, green	½ cup cooked	(80)	65	8	**10**	**25**	**15**	6	2	8
Turnips; rutabaga	½ cup cooked	(80)	20	2	6	**25**	2	2	2	2
Mushrooms	½ cup cooked	(120)	20	4	—	2	—	**15**	—	2
Potatoes, white	One: 4 per lb.	(100)	85	2	—	**25**	6	2	2	4
Potatoes, white, mashed	½ cup, milk and butter added	(100)	90	4	—	**20**	6	4	2	2
Squash, summer: zucchini; crookneck	½ cup cooked	(100)	15	2	8	**15**	4	4	2	2
Viandas[5]	½ cup cooked	(100)	90–130	2	4	4	4	2	—	4
Fruits										
Important Sources of Vitamins A and/or C[3]										
Apricots, canned in syrup	½ cup	(130)	110	—	**35**	6	—	2	—	2
Cantaloupe	¼ (5 inch diameter)	(230)	40	—	**90**	**70**	2	2	—	2
Grapefruit, white (edible portion); juice	½ (4 inch diameter); ½ cup	(120)	50	—	—	**70**	4	2	2	2
Mangos, raw	½ cup sliced	(80)	55	—	**80**	**45**	2	2	—	2
Orange (edible portion); juice	1 (2½ inch diameter); ½ cup	(120)	65	—	4	**100**	6	2	4	2
Peaches, raw	One: 4 per lb.	(100)	40	—	**25**	**15**	2	4	—	2
Strawberries, raw; frozen, sweetened	1 cup	(150; 250)	60; 250	—	2	**150**	2	6	4	8
Watermelon	1 cup diced	(160)	40	2	**20**	20	4	2	2	4
Other Fruits										
Apples; applesauce, sweetened	One: 3 per lb.; 1 cup	(150; 240)	85; 200	—	2	**10**	2	2	—	2
Bananas	1 medium; 1 cup sliced	(175)		2	4	**20**	**4**	**4**	2	4

Food	Portion	(g)	Cal.								
Blueberries; raspberries	½ cup unsweetened	(65)	40	—	—	25	—	—	2	—	4
Canned fruit in syrup: cocktail; pears	½ cup	(120)	80	—	2	2	—	—	—	2	4
Grapes	½ cup	(75)	60	—	—	6	—	2	—	2	2
Pears	One: 2½ per lb.	(180)	100	—	—	10	2	—	4	2	2
Pineapple, raw	½ cup diced	(75)	40	—	—	20	4	2	—	—	2
Prunes, dried; juice	5 medium; ½ cup	(30; 120)	80; 120	—	10	2	2	2	2	2	10
Raisins, seedless	⅓ cup; 1½ oz. package	(45)	120	2	2	—	2	2	2	2	8
Meat, Fish, Poultry, Eggs, Legumes											
Beef; veal; lamb	3 ounces cooked, lean only	(90)	180–225	**50**	—	—	6	6	**10**	—	15
Chicken, fried	1 drumstick and thigh	(125)	250	**50**	—	—	4	4	**10**	—	8
Chicken; turkey	3 ounces, no skin	(90)	180	**50**	—	—	4	4	**10**	—	8
Fish: clams; shrimp	3 ounces meat, no fat/breading	(90)	100	**50**	—	—	4	4	6	8	15[6]
haddock; perch; cod	3 ounces, no fat added	(90)	100	**50**	—	—	4	4	6	2	6
tuna, canned	3 ounces, in water; in oil	(90)	110; 170	**50**	—	—	4	4	6	2	15
Hamburger	3 ounces cooked	(90)	250	**45**	—	—	6	6	6	—	6
Hot dogs; bologna; cold cuts	1 hot dog; 2 ounces	(60)	160	**15**	—	—	10	10	**10**	—	**25**
Liver	2 ounces, no fat added	(60)	135	**35**	**500**	**15**	15	40	**120**	—	15
Pork, ham	3 ounces cooked, lean only	(90)	300	**45**	—	—	**40**	4	**10**	—	2
Pork sausage, cooked	1 link: 16 per lb.	(20)	95	6	—	—	10	4	2	—	6
Eggs	1 large	(50)	80	**15**	**10**	—	2	10	**8**	2	15
Legumes: dried beans; peas	1 ounce dried; ½ cup cooked	(30; 90)	125	**15**	—	—	10	4	4	4	4
Peanut butter; nuts	2 tbsp. peanut butter; ¼ cup	(30)	190	**15**	—	—	4	4	4	—	—
Cereal Products, Whole Grain/Enriched[7]											
Bread; toast; bagel	1 slice; ½ bagel	(25)	70	4	—	—	6	4	**6**	2	8
Cereals: oatmeal; wheat	1 cup cooked	(240)	110	4	—	—	10	4	**10**	—	6
ready-to-eat	1 ounce	(30)	100	refer to label on package							
Corn grits; corn meal	1 cup cooked	(240)	125	4	2	—	8	—	**8**	—	6
Hamburg roll	1 medium	(40)	120	6	—	—	10	6	**10**	2	10
Spaghetti; macaroni; noodles, rice	1 cup cooked	(150–200)	200	8	—	—	15	—	**15**	2	8

[1]References: *Composition of Foods.* Agriculture Handbook No. 8, USDA, 1963; *Nutritive Value of American Foods in Common Units,* Agriculture Handbook No. 456, USDA, 1975; *Food Values of Portions Commonly Used,* Bowes and Church, Lippincott, 1974; California Prune Advisory Board, 1973; *Tabla de Composicion de alimentos de use corriente en Puerto Rico,* Reguero y Santiago, University of Puerto Rico, 1973.

[2]See "Using The Guide" for explanation about lack of boldface in iron column.

[3]Highest vitamin A content is found in darker yellow-orange and green vegetables and fruits.

[4]Some calcium in spinach, swiss chard or beet greens may combine with a plant acid and may not be absorbed.

[5]Yautia (white tanier), ñame (white yam), malanga (taro, dasheen), yuca (cassava). Yuca has somewhat more vitamin C than listed.

[6]Clams provide 30% iron.

[7]Values for thiamin, riboflavin and iron are based on enrichment levels specified by FDA, October 1973.

Note: Some figures represent judgments made to help the user identify the most dependable sources of individual nutrients.

TABLE D.2 PERCENT OF U.S. RDA YOU NEED

Ages	Children					Women		Men
	4–6	7–10	11–18	19–50	51+	Pregnant	Nursing	19+
Protein	50	50	85	70	70	$+45^2$	$+30^2$	85
Vitamin A	50	65	100	80	80	$+20^2$	$+40^2$	100
Vitamin C	75	75	100	100	100	$+35^2$	$+65^2$	100
Thiamin	60	80	95	75	65	$+25^2$	$+35^2$	100
Riboflavin	60	80	100	75	70	$+20^2$	$+30^2$	100
Calcium	80	80	120	80	80	$+40^2$	$+40^2$	80
Iron	55	55	100	100	55	100+	100	55

[1]This table adjusts the U.S. RDA to fit individual needs based on age and sex.

[2]To be added to the percentage for females of appropriate age.

ADAPTED FROM *Nutrition Labeling: Tools for Its Use*, USDA, Agriculture Information Bulletin No. 382, 1975, and are based on the 1980 Recommended Dietary Allowances (RDA), National Academy of Sciences, National Research Council.

Highly significant sources of a nutrient are indicated by boldface type. In general, this designation is merited if a serving of food contains 10 percent or more of the U.S. RDA. Less than 10 percent is considered significant when more than one serving daily is common (for example, vitamin A in milk). Obviously, if the amount eaten is large enough, foods may be significant for some nutrients even though they are not indicated in bold.

No boldface is used in the iron column because judging which foods are especially significant is more complex for iron than for other nutrients. The amount of iron absorbed from foods varies with the types of food eaten and the individual's need for iron. The U.S. RDA assumes an average availability of 10 percent of food iron. Present knowledge indicates that iron in meat, fish, poultry, and soybeans is *more* than 10 percent available; iron in eggs, whole grains, nuts, and dried beans is *less*.

The percentage of protein contributed by foods depends on whether the food comes from plants or animals. Animal protein is more efficiently used than plant protein. Thus, 45 grams is the U.S. RDA basis for estimating percent protein in meat, fish, poultry, milk, and eggs. Sixty-five grams is the basis for cereals, legumes, and other vegetables.

Table D.3 lists total recommended calorie allowances. Calorie needs depend on age, sex, size, and activity. Body weight is the best measure of adequacy; weight gains indicate excess calories.

Calorie values of several foods not included in Table D.1 are listed in Table D.4. In general, these foods have relatively few nutrients in relation to calories. For food mixtures, the exact calorie value depends on ingredients used, especially amounts of fat or sugar.

TABLE D.3 RECOMMENDED CALORIE ALLOWANCES

	Ages	Calorie Range
Children	4–6	1300–2300
	7–10	1650–3300
Women[1]	11–14	1500–3000
	15–18	1200–3000
	19–22	1700–2500
	23–50	1600–2400
	51+	1200–2200
Men	11–14	2000–3700
	15–18	2100–3900
	19–22	2500–3300
	23–50	2300–3100
	51+	1650–2800

[1]Add 300 calories if you are pregnant, 500 if you are lactating.

ADAPTED FROM *Nutrition Labeling: Tools for Its Use*, USDA, Agriculture Information Bulletin No. 382, 1975, and are based on the 1980 Recommended Dietary Allowances (RDA), National Academy of Sciences, National Research Council.

TABLE D.4 CALORIE VALUES

Description	Amount	Calories
Bacon, crisp	2 slices	100
Beverages		
Beer	12 oz.	150
Carbonated, sweetened	12 oz.	130–150
Liquor 70–100 proof	1½ oz.	100–120
Dry wine	3 oz.	75
Sweet wine: sherry, port	3 oz.	120
Butter, margarine	1 tablespoon	100
Cake, angel	2 × 3 × 1½"	120
Cake, shortened, frosted	3 × 3 × 2"	400
Candy bar, milk chocolate	1 oz.	145
Cookies, chocolate chip	2	100
Crackers, saltine	1	15–20
Cream;		
Heavy	1 tablespoon	55
Sour	1 tablespoon	25
Cream Cheese	1" cube	60
Donuts, Danish	1 medium	150–175
Gelatin dessert	½ cup	80
Gravy	2 tablespoons	80
Jam, jelly, syrup, molasses, honey	1 tablespoon	50–60
Oils	1 tablespoon	125
Pie	1/6 of 9" pie	350–400
Popcorn with oil	1 cup	40
Potato chips	10–2" chips	110
Potatoes, French fried	10 fries	140
Pretzels	10–3" sticks	25
Salad dressings:		
French	1 tablespoon	70
Mayonnaise	1 tablespoon	100
Salad dressing	1 tablespoon	65
Sherbet	½ cup	130
Sugar	1 teaspoon	15

OTHER NUTRIENTS IN FOODS

Many nutrients other than those listed in Table D.1 are important. No single food, not even one that is highly enriched, provides all the nutrients needed for optimum health. Eating a wide variety of foods is therefore advisable.

Fast Food Nutrition

Food Description	Weight (g)	Energy (Kcal)	Protein (g)	Carbohydrates (g)	Fat (g)	Cholesterol (mg)
ARBY'S						
Roast Beef, reg	147	350	22	32	15.0	39.0
Roast Beef, jr.	86	218	12	22	8.0	20.0
Roast Beef, super	234	501	25	50	22.0	40.0
Roast Beef, deluxe	247	486	26	43	23.0	59.0
Beef 'n Cheddar*	190	490	24	51	21.0	51.0
Chicken Breast Sandwich	210	592	28	56	27.0	57.0
Potato Cakes (2)	85	201	2	22	14.0	1.3
French Fries	71	211	2	33	8.0	6.0
King Roast Beef	192	467	27	44	19.0	49.0
Bac'n Cheddar Deluxe	225	561	28	36	34.0	78.0
Hot Ham 'n Cheese	161	353	26	33	13.0	50.0
Turkey Deluxe	197	375	24	32	17.0	39.0
Baked Potato, Plain	312	290	8	66	0.5	0
Superstuffed Potato, Deluxe	312	648	18	59	38.0	72.0
Broccoli and Cheddar	340	541	13	72	22.0	24.0
Mushroom and Cheese	300	506	16	61	22.0	21.0
Taco	425	619	23	73	27.0	145.0
Vanilla Shake	250	295	8	44	10.0	30.0
Chocolate Shake	300	384	9	62	11.0	32.0
Jamocha Shake	305	424	8	76	10.0	31.0
Roasted Chicken Breast	150	254	43	2	7.0	200.0
Roasted Chicken Leg	161	319	41	1	16.0	214.0
Chicken Salad Sandwich	156	386	18	33	20.0	30.0
Chicken Salad & Croissant	150	472	22	16	36.0	12.0
Chicken Salad w/Tomato & Lettuce	270	515	25	24	36.0	12.0
Chicken Club Sandwich	210	621	26	57	32.0	108.0
Rice Pilaf	120	123	3	23	2.0	—
Scandinavian Vegetables, sauce	120	56	2	9	2.0	—
Tossed Salad, plain	210	44	3	7	tr	0
Tossed Salad w/20 Calorie Italian Drsg	240	57	3	9	1.0	0

SOURCE: Arby's Inc. Atlanta, Georgia. Nutritional analyses by Arby's Laboratory and other independent testing laboratories.

Food Description	Weight (g)	Energy (Kcal)	Protein (g)	Carbohydrates (g)	Fat (g)	Cholesterol (mg)
BURGER KING						
Whopper Sandwich*	285	640	27	42	41	94
Whopper* w/Cheese	289	723	31	43	48	117
Double Beef Whopper*	351	850	46	52	52	—
Double Beef Whopper* w/Cheese	374	950	51	54	60	—
Whopper Junior*	138	370	15	31	17	41
Whopper Junior* w/Cheese	158	420	17	32	20	52
Hamburger	109	275	15	29	12	37
Cheeseburger	120	317	17	30	15	48
Bacon Double Cheeseburger	159	510	33	27	31	104
French Fries, reg	74	227	3	24	13	14
Onion Rings, reg	79	274	4	28	16	0
Apple Pie	125	305	3	44	12	4
Chocolate Shake, med	273	320	8	46	12	—
Vanilla Shake, med	273	321	9	49	10	—
Vanilla Shake, added syrup	284	334	9	51	10	—
Chocolate Shake, added syrup	284	374	8	60	11	—
Whaler Fish Sandwich	189	488	19	45	27	84
Whaler w/Cheese	201	530	21	46	30	95
Ham and Cheese	230	471	24	44	23	70
Chicken Sandwich	230	688	26	56	40	82
Chicken Tenders*	95	204	20	10	10	47
B'kfast Croissanwich*						
Bacon, Egg, Cheese	119	355	15	20	24	249
Sausage, Egg, Cheese	163	538	19	20	41	293
Ham, Egg, Cheese	145	335	18	20	20	262
Scrambled Egg Platter	195	468	14	33	30	370
Scrambled Egg Platter						
w/Sausage	247	702	22	33	52	420
w/Bacon	206	536	18	33	36	378
French Toast Platter						
w/Bacon	117	469	11	41	30	73
w/Sausage	158	635	16	41	46	115
Salad, plain	148	28	2	5	0	0
w/House Dressing	176	159	3	8	13	11
w/Bleu Cheese	176	184	3	7	16	22
w/1000 Island	176	145	2	9	12	17
w/French	176	152	2	13	11	0
w/Golden Italian	176	162	2	7	14	0
w/Creamy Italian	176	—	—	—	—	—
w/Reduced-Calorie Italian	176	42	2	7	1	0
Cherry Pie	128	357	4	55	13	6
Pecan Pie	113	459	5	64	20	4

SOURCE: Burger King Corp. Inc. Nutritional analyses by Hazelton Laboratory of America (formerly Raltech Scientific Services Inc.), Madison, Wisconsin, and Campbell Laboratories, Camden, New Jersey.

Food Description	Weight (g)	Energy (Kcal)	Protein (g)	Carbohydrates (g)	Fat (g)	Cholesterol (mg)
DAIRY QUEEN						
Cone, sm	85	140	3	22	4	10
Cone, reg	142	240	6	38	7	15
Cone, lg	213	340	9	57	10	25
Dipped Cone, sm	92	190	3	25	9	10
Dipped Cone, reg	156	340	6	42	16	20
Dipped Cone, lg	234	510	9	64	24	30
Sundae, sm	106	190	3	33	4	10
Sundae, reg	177	310	5	56	8	20
Sundae, lg	248	440	8	78	10	30
Shake, sm	291	490	10	82	13	35
Shake, reg	418	710	14	120	19	50
Shake, lg	588	990	19	168	26	70
Malt, sm	291	520	10	91	13	35
Malt, reg	418	760	14	134	18	50
Malt, lg	588	1060	20	187	25	70
Float	397	410	5	82	7	20
Banana Split	383	540	9	103	11	30
Parfait	283	430	8	76	8	30
Peanut Buster Parfait	305	740	16	94	34	30
Double Delight	255	490	9	69	20	25
Hot Fudge Brownie Delight	266	600	9	85	25	20
Strawberry Shortcake	312	540	10	100	11	25
Freeze	397	500	9	89	12	30
Mr. Misty*, sm	248	190	0	48	0	0
Mr. Misty*, reg	330	250	0	63	0	0
Mr. Misty*, lg	439	340	0	84	0	0
Mr. Misty* Kiss	89	70	0	17	0	0
Mr. Misty* Freeze	411	500	9	91	12	30
Mr. Misty* Float	411	390	5	74	7	20
Buster Bar	149	460	10	41	29	10
Dilly Bar	85	210	3	21	13	10
DQ Sandwich	60	140	3	24	4	5
Single Hamburger	148	360	21	33	16	45
Double Hamburger	210	530	36	33	28	85
Triple Hamburger	272	710	51	33	45	135
Single w/Cheese	162	410	24	33	20	50
Double w/Cheese	239	650	43	34	37	95
Triple w/Cheese	301	820	58	34	50	145
Hot Dog	100	280	11	21	16	45
Hot Dog w/Chili	128	320	13	23	20	55
Hot Dog w/Cheese	114	330	15	21	21	55
Super Hot Dog	175	520	17	44	27	80
Super Hot Dog w/Chili	218	570	21	47	32	100
Super Hot Dog w/Cheese	196	580	22	45	34	100
Fish Filet Sandwich	170	400	20	41	17	50
Fish Filet Sandwich w/Cheese	177	440	24	39	21	60
Chicken Sandwich	220	670	29	48	41	75
French Fries, sm	71	200	2	25	10	10
French Fries, lg	113	320	3	40	16	15
Onion Rings	85	280	4	31	16	15

SOURCE: International Dairy Queen Inc., Minneapolis, Minnesota. Nutrient analyses by Hazelton Laboratory of America (formerly Raltech Scientific Services Inc.), Madison, Wisconsin.

Food Description	Weight (g)	Energy (Kcal)	Protein (g)	Carbohydrates (g)	Fat (g)	Cholesterol (mg)
HARDEE'S						
Hamburger	110	305	17	29	13	—
Cheeseburger	116	335	17	29	17	—
Big Deluxe*	248	546	29	48	26	77
¼-Pound Cheeseburger*	190	508	28	41	26	61
Roast Beef Sandwich	143	377	21	36	17	57
Big Roast Beef*	167	418	28	34	19	60
Hog Dog	120	346	11	26	22	42
Hog Ham & Cheese	148	376	23	37	15	59
Fisherman's Fillet Sandwich*	196	514	20	50	26	41
Chicken Fillet	192	510	27	42	26	57
Bacon Cheeseburger	224	686	35	42	42	295
Sausage Biscuit	1123	413	10	34	26	29
Sausage & Egg Biscuit	162	521	16	34	35	293
Steak Biscuit	134	419	14	41	23	34
Steak & Egg Biscuit	162	527	20	41	31	298
Ham Biscuit	108	349	12	37	17	29
Ham & Egg Biscuit	184	458	19	37	26	293
Bacon & Egg Biscuit	114	405	13	30	26	305
French Fries, sm	71	239	3	28	13	4
French Fries, lg	113	381	5	44	21	6
Apple Turnover	87	282	3	37	14	5
Milkshake	326	391	11	63	10	42

SOURCE: Hardee's Food Systems Inc., Rocky Mount, North Carolina. Nutrient analyses by Webb Food Laboratory, Raleigh, North Carolina.

Food Description	Weight (g)	Energy (Kcal)	Protein (g)	Carbohydrates (g)	Fat (g)	Cholesterol (mg)
JACK IN THE BOX						
Hamburger	98.0	276	13.0	30.0	12	29.0
Cheeseburger	113.0	323	16.0	32.0	15	42.0
Jumbo Jack*	205.0	485	26.0	38.0	26	64.0
Jumbo Jack* w/Cheese	—	630	32.0	45.0	35	110.0
Bacon Cheeseburger Supreme	231.0	724	34.0	44.0	46	70.0
Swiss & Bacon Burger	—	643	33.0	31.0	43	99.0
Ham & Swiss Burger	—	638	36.0	37.0	39	117.0
Mushroom Burger	178.7	477	28.0	30.0	27	87.0
Moby Jack*	137.0	444	16.0	39.0	25	47.0
Regular Taco	81.0	191	8.0	16.0	11	21.0
Super Taco	135.0	288	12.0	21.0	17	37.0
Club Pita	177.0	284	22.0	30.0	8	43.0
Chicken Supreme	228.0	601	31.0	39.0	36	60.0
Supreme Crescent	146.0	547	20.0	27.0	40	178.0
Sausage Crescent	156.0	584	22.0	28.0	43	187.0
Pancakes Breakfast	630.0	626	16.0	79.0	27	85.0
Scrambled Eggs Breakfast	720.0	719	26.0	55.0	44	260.0
Breakfast Jack*	126.0	307	18.0	30.0	13	203.0
Cooked Bacon, 2 slices	—	70	3.0	0	6	10.0

Food Description	Weight (g)	Energy (Kcal)	Protein (g)	Carbohydrates (g)	Fat (g)	Cholesterol (mg)
JACK IN THE BOX, *Continued*						
Chicken Strips Dinner	180.0	689	40.0	65.0	30	100.0
Shrimp Dinner	165.0	731	22.0	77.0	37	157.0
Sirloin Steak Dinner	—	699	38.0	75.0	27	75.0
Cheese Nachos	—	571	15.0	49.0	35	37.0
Supreme Nachos	—	718	23.0	66.0	40	65.0
Canadian Crescent	134.0	472	18.6	24.6	31	226.0
Pasta Seafood Salad	15.0	394	15.0	32.0	22	47.5
Taco Salad	358.0	377	31.0	10.0	24	102.0
French Fries, reg	68.0	221	2.0	27.0	12	8.0
Onion Rings	108.0	382	5.0	39.0	23	27.0
Hash Brown Potatoes	90.0	68	2.0	15.0	0	0
Vanilla Shake	317.0	320	10.0	57.0	6	25.0
Strawberry Shake	328.0	320	10.0	55.0	7	25.0
Chocolate Shake	322.0	330	11.0	55.0	7	25.0
Apple Turnover	119.0	410	4.0	45.0	24	15.0

SOURCE: Jack in the Box Restaurants, Foodmaker, Inc., San Diego, California. Nutrient analyses by Hazelton Laboratory of America (formerly Raltech Scientific Services Inc.), Madison, Wisconsin.

Food Description	Weight (g)	Energy (Kcal)	Protein (g)	Carbohydrates (g)	Fat (g)	Cholesterol (mg)
KENTUCKY FRIED CHICKEN						
Original Recipe						
Wing[1]	56.0	181	11.8	5.77	12.3	67.0
Side Breast	95.0	276	20.0	10.1	17.3	96.0
Center Breast[1]	107.0	257	25.5	8.0	13.7	93.0
Drumstick[1]	58.0	147	13.6	3.4	8.82	81.0
Thigh[1]	96.0	278	18.0	8.4	19.2	122.0
Extra Crispy						
Wing[1]	57.0	218	11.5	7.81	15.6	63.0
Side Breast*	98.0	354	17.7	17.3	23.7	66.0
Center Breast*	120.0	353	26.9	14.4	20.9	93.0
Drumstick[1]	60.0	173	12.7	5.9	10.9	65.0
Thigh[1]	112.0	371	19.6	13.8	26.3	121.0
Kentucky Nuggets (one)	16.0	46	2.82	2.2	2.88	11.9
Kentucky Nugget Sauce (oz)						
Barbeque	1.0[2]	35	0.3	7.1	0.57	1.0
Sweet and Sour	1.0[2]	58	0.1	13.0	0.56	1.0
Honey	0.5[2]	49	0	12.1	0.01	1.0
Mustard	1.0[2]	36	0.88	6.04	0.91	1.0
Kentucky Fries	119.0	268	4.8	33.3	12.8	1.8
Mashed Potatoes w/Gravy	86.0	62	2.1	10.3	1.4	1.0
Mashed Potatoes	80.0	59	1.9	11.6	0.6	1.0
Chicken Gravy	78.0	59	2.0	4.4	3.7	2.0
Buttermilk Biscuit	75.0	269	5.1	31.6	13.6	1.0
Potato Salad	90.0	141	1.8	12.6	9.27	11.0
Baked Beans	89.0	105	5.1	18.4	1.2	1.0
Corn on the Cob	143.0	176	5.1	31.9	3.1	1.0
Cole Slaw	79.0	103	1.3	11.5	5.7	4.0

[1] edible portion
[2] measured in ounces

SOURCE: Kentucky Fried Chicken Corp. Nutrient analyses by Hazelton laboratory of America (formerly Raltech Scientific Services Inc.), Madison, Wisconsin.

Food Description	Weight (g)	Energy (Kcal)	Protein (g)	Carbohydrates (g)	Fat (g)	Cholesterol (mg)
LONG JOHN SILVER'S						
3 Pc Fish & Fryes	—	853	43	64	48	106
2 Pc Fish & Fryes	—	651	30	53	36	75
Fish & More	—	978	34	82	58	88
3 Pc Fish Dinner	—	1180	47	93	70	119
3 Pc Chicken Planks Dinner	—	885	32	72	51	25
4 Pc Chicken Planks Dinner	—	1037	41	82	59	25
6 Pc Chicken Nuggets Dinner	—	699	23	54	45	25
Fish & Chicken	—	935	36	73	55	56
Seafood Platter	—	976	29	85	58	95
Clam Dinner	—	955	22	100	58	27
Batter Fried Shrimp Dinner	—	711	17	60	45	127
Scallop Dinner	—	747	17	66	45	37
Oyster Dinner	—	789	17	78	45	55
3 Pc Kitchen-Breaded Fish Dinner	—	940	35	84	52	101
2 Pc Kitchen-Breaded Fish Dinner	—	818	26	76	46	76
Fish Sandwich Platter	—	835	30	84	42	75
Seafood Salad	—	426	19	22	30	113
Ocean Chef Salad	—	229	27	13	8	64
A La Carte Items						
Batter-Fried Fish	86	202	13	11	12	31
Kitchen-Breaded Fish	58	122	9	8	6	25
Chicken Plank	62	152	9	10	8	X
Batter-Fried Shrimp	17	47	2	3	3	17
Clam Chowder	185	128	7	15	5	17
Cole Slaw	98	182	1	11	15	12
Fryes	85	247	4	31	12	13
Hush Puppies	47	145	3	18	7	1

SOURCE: Long John Silver's Inc., Lexington, Kentucky. Nutrient analyses by Department of Nutrition and Food Science, University of Kentucky.

Food Description	Weight (g)	Energy (Kcal)	Protein (g)	Carbohydrates (g)	Fat (g)	Cholesterol (mg)
McDONALD'S						
Chicken McNuggets*	109	323	19.1	13.7	21.3	72.8
Hamburger	100	263	12.4	28.3	11.3	29.1
Cheeseburger	114	328	15.0	28.5	16.0	40.6
Quarter Pounder*	160	427	24.6	29.3	23.5	81.0
Quarter Pounder* w/Cheese	186	525	29.6	30.5	31.6	107.0
Big Mac*	200	570	24.6	39.2	35.0	83.0
Filet-O-Fish*	143	435	14.7	35.9	25.7	45.2
Mc D.L.T.*	254	680	30.0	40.0	44.0	101.0
French Fries, reg	68	220	3.0	26.1	11.5	8.6
Biscuit w/Sausage, Egg	175	585	19.8	36.4	39.9	285.0
Biscuit w/Bacon, Egg, Cheese	145	483	16.5	33.2	31.6	263.0
Sausage McMuffin*	115	427	17.6	30.0	26.3	59.0
Sausage McMuffin* w/Egg	165	517	22.9	32.2	32.9	287.0
Egg McMuffin*	138	340	18.5	31.0	15.8	259.0
Hot Cakes w/Butter, Syrup	214	500	7.9	93.9	10.3	47.1
Scrambled Eggs	98	180	13.2	2.5	13.0	514.0

Food Description	Weight (g)	Energy (Kcal)	Protein (g)	Carbohydrates (g)	Fat (g)	Cholesterol (mg)
McDONALD'S *Continued*						
Sausage	53	210	9.8	0.6	18.6	38.8
English Muffin w/Butter	63	186	5.0	29.5	5.3	15.3
Hash Brown Potatoes	55	125	1.5	14.0	7.0	7.2
Vanilla Shake	291	352	9.3	59.6	8.4	30.6
Chocolate Shake	291	383	9.9	65.5	9.0	29.7
Strawberry Shake	290	362	9.0	62.1	8.7	32.2
Strawberry Sundae	164	320	6.0	54.0	8.7	24.6
Hot Fudge Sundae	164	357	7.0	58.0	10.8	26.6
Caramel Sundae	165	361	7.0	60.8	10.0	31.4
Apple Pie	85	253	1.9	29.3	14.3	12.4
Cherry Pie	88	260	2.0	32.1	13.6	13.4
McDonaldland* Cookies	67	308	4.0	49.0	10.8	10.2
Chocolate Chip Cookies	69	342	4.0	45.0	16.3	17.7

SOURCE: McDonald's Corp., Oak Brook, Illinois. Nutrient analyses by Hazelton laboratory of America (formerly Raltech Scientific Services Inc.), Madison, Wisconsin.

Food Description	Weight (g)	Energy (Kcal)	Protein (g)	Carbohydrates (g)	Fat (g)	Cholesterol (mg)
WENDY'S						
Single Hamburger, multigrain bun	119	340	25	20	17	67
Single Hamburger, white bun	117	350	21	27	18	65
Double Hamburger, white bun	197	560	41	24	34	125
Bacon Cheeseburger, white bun	147	460	29	23	28	65
Chicken Sandwich, multigrain bun	128	320	25	31	10	59
Kid's Meal Hamburger, 2 oz	75	220	13	11	8	20
Chili, 8 oz	256	260	21	26	8	30
French Fries, reg	98	280	4	35	14	15
Taco Salad	357	390	23	36	18	40
Frosty Dairy Dessert	243	400	8	59	14	50
Hot Stuffed Baked Potatoes						
Plain	250	250	6	52	2	tr
Sour Cream & Chives	310	460	6	53	24	15
Cheese	350	590	17	55	34	22
Chili & Cheese	400	510	22	63	20	22
Bacon & Cheese	350	570	19	57	30	22
Broccoli & Cheese	365	500	13	54	25	22
Ham & Cheese Omelet	114	250	18	6	17	450
Ham, Cheese, & Mushroom Omelet	118	290	18	7	21	355
Ham, Cheese, Onion, & Green Pepper Omelet	128	280	19	7	19	525
Mushroom, Onion, & Green Pepper Omelet	114	210	14	7	15	460
Breakfast Sandwich	129	370	17	33	19	200
French Toast, 2 slices	135	400	11	45	19	115
Home Fries	103	360	4	37	22	20

SOURCE: Wendy's International Inc., Dublin, Ohio. Nutrient analyses entrée items, Hazelton laboratory of America (formerly Raltech Scientific Services Inc.), Madison, Wisconsin: other items, US Department of Agriculture Handbook #8.

*Registered Trademark.

APPENDIX F

Energy Costs of Common Activities

TABLE F.1 ENERGY COST OF COMMON ACTIVITIES

Activity	Approximate Calories (per hour)	Activity	Approximate Calories (per hour)
Rest (basal metabolism)	70	Tennis (singles)	450
Sitting at rest	100	Sawing wood	480
Hand sewing	105	Swimming	500
Bricklaying (6 per min.)	105	Fencing	539
Dressing and undressing	118	Field Hockey	546
Singing	122	Basketball	564
Typewriting rapidly	140	Skiing	791
Ironing (5-lb. iron)	144	Handball/squash	864
Dishwashing	144	Wrestling	791
Sweeping	169	Football	900
Driving car	170	Ice Hockey	930
Shoemaking	180	Walking (up stairs)	1100
Walking slowly (2.6 mph)	200	Jogging/Running:	
Volleyball	210	5.8 mph	570
Carpentry, metal working	240	8.0 mph	760
Dancing (fox trot)	266	10.0 mph	900
Archery	268	11.4 mph	1300
Gymnastics	270	13.2 mph	2330
Golf	290	14.8 mph	2880
Walking (3.75 mph)	300	15.8 mph	3910
Badminton	396	17.2 mph	4740
Cycling (9.4 mph)	408	18.6 mph	7790
Horseback riding (gallop)	441		

The chart does not include the 200 to 350 additional calories that will be burned immediately following exercise for five to eight hours due to increased metabolic rate.

APPENDIX G

Prevention and Emergency Treatment of Common Exercise Injuries

TABLE G.1   INJURY AND TREATMENT INFORMATION

Injury	General Comments	Prevention and Treatment	Need for a Physician
EXTREMITIES			
Ankle	Most injuries involve inversion sprains (outer edge of foot turns inward). Ankles are not strong enough for most sports, and are poorly supported by muscles and ligaments that often stretch and tear from high-speed direction changes, cutting, and contact.	Improved support muscle strength offers some protection, along with preventive taping (inversion sprains only). R-I-C-E therapy is the preferred treatment. Use crutches for two or three days if pain is severe.	If swelling or pain remains for three days If ligament or tendon damage is present If pain prevents walking If symptoms of fracture exist
Bruise (charley horse)	A charley horse is nothing more than a thigh contusion from a direct blow to a relaxed thigh muscle (the tissue is compressed against the bone). Bruises to other areas occur in similar fashion.	Prevention involves use of proper equipment in contact sports. R-I-C-E therapy is the preferred emergency and home treatment. Replace ice with heat on the third or fourth day.	If pain and discoloration do not disappear with rest, treatment, and mild exercise
Elbow (tennis and pitcher's)	The movement causing the condition is a forceful extension of the forearm and a twisting motion (serve in tennis, curve in baseball). The more you play and the older you are, the more likely you are to be afflicted. Pain is present over the outer (lateral epicondyle) or inner (medial epicondyle) elbow and radiates down the arm. Pain is produced by tears, inflammation and scar tissue at the attachment of the extensor muscles to the bony prominence of the elbow.	Prevention centers around use of warm-up, correction of poor stroke mechanics, avoiding use of wet tennis balls and heavy, inflexible rackets, and reducing the frequency of curve ball pitches (should be greatly restricted in little league baseball with growing youngsters).	If condition remains more than two or three weeks If pain makes exercise impossible If severe swelling is present

TABLE G.1 INJURY AND TREATMENT INFORMATION—Continued

Injury	General Comments	Prevention and Treatment	Need for a Physician
Fractures	A fracture should be suspected in most injuries where pain and swelling exist over a bone.	Apply ice packs, protect and rest the injured part for 72 hours. In severe cases, splint the bone where the victim lies and transport to emergency room.	If limb is cold, blue, or numb If pelvis or thigh are involved If limb is crooked or deformed If shock symptoms are present If rapid, severe swelling occurs
Hamstring strains	The large muscle group in the back of the upper leg is commonly strained during vigorous exercise. Pain is severe and prohibits further activity. In a few days, discoloration may appear.	Prevention includes proper stretching before exercise, proper diet, improved flexibility, and care in running around wet areas. For treatment, use R-I-C-E therapy followed by heat application in three to four days.	If severe discoloration occurs If pain and discomfort remain after 10 to 15 days of treatment
Knee	The knee is a vulnerable joint that depends on ligaments, cartilage, and muscles for support. *Chondromalacia* of the patella, or roughing of the undersurface of the kneecap, is the most common injury; kneecap pain and grating symptoms are evident. A tear of the *cartilage* is the second most common injury. Pain is evident along the inner or outer part of the knee joint, along with swelling. *Ligament* tears are less common but occur from a blow to the leg. Swelling and knee instability result.	Prevention involves flexibility and strength. Exercises should stretch and strengthen the hamstrings, quadriceps, and Achilles tendon. Chondromalacia is treated through use of arch supports, or by building up the inner part of the heel of the shoe. Aspirin and quadriceps exercises also help. Serious knee injury (cartilage and ligament damage) requires an examination by an orthopedic surgeon. Use of the arthroscope to examine and insert small tools through puncture wounds offers effective treatment and rapid recovery.	If swelling and pain persist more than three to five days If ligament or cartilage damage is suspected If chondromalacia is suspected
Shin splints	A shin splint is merely an inflammation of the anterior and posterior tendons of the large bone in the lower leg. It is an overuse syndrome developing in poorly conditioned individuals in the beginning of their training program. Hard surfaces add to the problem.	Avoid hard surfaces, too much mileage, doing too much too soon, using improperly fitted shoes, and running on banked tracks or road shoulders. R-I-C-E therapy is recommended for two to four days, followed by taping and heat therapy, and stretching exercises.	If condition remains more than two to three weeks If condition reoccurs after reconvening your exercise routine
Tendonitis	The location of the pain and swelling of the tendon varies in different sports. With considerable running, the Achilles tendon is affected. In those involving repeated movement of the upper arms (swimming, baseball), it is the shoulder tendon. When a snapping or rotation of the elbow is involved (tennis/handball), it is the elbow tendon.	For both prevention and treatment, stretch the involved tendon daily and exercise lightly until pain disappears. R-I-C-E therapy is helpful in the early stages for three to four days. See *Elbow* in this appendix. Pain may disappear during a workout, only to return and grow worse later.	If pain and inflammation continue after two to three weeks of treatment

TABLE G.1   INJURY AND TREATMENT INFORMATION—Continued

Injury	General Comments	Prevention and Treatment	Need for a Physician
Varicose veins	Varicose veins are nothing more than abnormally lengthened, dilated veins. Surrounding muscles support deep veins, whereas superficial veins get little support. In some individuals, vein valves that prevent blood from backing up become defective, enlarged, and lose their elasticity. The condition is uncommon in young people.	Prevention and treatment for those with symptoms or a family history include bed rest and leg elevation, avoiding long periods of standing, use of elastic bandages and support stockings, surgery for severe cases, and removal of intra-abdominal pressure (obesity, tumor, or tight girdles).	If pain is severe enough to make walking difficult If cosmetic problem is bothersome
FEET AND HANDS			
Athlete's foot	Athlete's foot is caused by a fungus, and is accompanied by a bacterial infection. Itching, redness, and a rash on the soles, toes, or between the toes is common.	Prevention and treatment are similar; wash between the toes with soap and water, dry thoroughly, use medication containing Tinanctin twice daily, and place fungistatic foot powder in shoes and sneakers.	If treatment does not relieve symptoms in two to three weeks
Blisters	Blisters are produced by friction causing the top skin layer to separate from the second layer. Blisters can become severely inflamed or infected unless properly treated. A porous inner sole can be purchased that almost completely eliminates getting blisters on the feet.	Use clean socks, comfortably fitting shoes, and vaseline to reduce friction. Avoid breaking open blisters (skin acts as a sterile bandage). If the blister breaks, trim off all loose skin and apply antibiotic salve. Avoid use of tincture of benzoin, and of powder which increases friction, since that is more likely to cause blisters than prevent them.	If inflammation and soreness develop If redness occurs in the involved limb If pain or sensitivity occur under the arms or in the groin area
Bunions	Bunions are merely growths on the head of the first or fifth toe that produce inflammation (swelling, redness, and pain).	Bunions can be prevented by using properly fitted shoes.	If symptoms of infection occur
Corns	Hard corns may result from poorly fitted shoes. Inflammation and thickening of soft tissue (top of toes) occur. Soft corns are often caused by excessive foot perspiration and narrow shoes. The corn forms between the fourth and fifth toe in most cases.	Prevention and treatment involves use of properly fitted shoes, soaking feet daily in warm water to soften the area, and protecting the area with a small felt or sponge rubber doughnut. Trim and file corns to reduce pressure.	If a change of shoes and treatment does not improve the condition

TABLE G.1   INJURY AND TREATMENT INFORMATION—Continued

Injury	General Comments	Prevention and Treatment	Need for a Physician
Heel bruise	The most common cause of heel pain is plantar fascitis—inflammation of the broad band of fibrous tissue that runs from the base of the toes back to the heel and inserts on the inner aspect of the heel. Mild tears and severe bruises are also common.	Prevention involves proper stretching and use of a plastic heel cup. Aspirin should be used to reduce inflammation (two tablets, four times daily); rest is indicated for five to seven days.	If pain persists for more than five to seven days after rest and treatment
Ingrown toenails	The edge of the toenail grows into the soft tissue, producing inflammation and infection.	Prevention and treatment involves proper nail trimming, soaking the toe in hot water two to three times daily, and inserting a small piece of cotton under the nail edge to lift it from the soft tissue.	If infection occurs
Stress fracture	A stress fracture is a small crack in a bone's surface, generally a foot, leg, or hand. Unexplained pain may exist over one of the small bones in the hand or foot. X-ray will not reveal small cracks until the bone heals and a callus (scar tissue) forms.	Prevention involves not running too many miles, not increasing mileage too fast, running on soft surfaces, and taking care to progress slowly in your fitness program. Treatment requires rest and proper equipment (especially footwear).	If unexplained pain exists in the lower back, hip, ankle, wrist, hands, or feet
HEAD AND NECK			
Cauliflower ear	A deformed painful outer ear is common in wrestling, rugby, and football from friction, hard blows, and wrenching in a headlock position. With poor circulation to the ear, fluid is absorbed slowly, and the ear remains swollen, sensitive, and discolored.	Use protective ear guards, apply vaseline to reduce friction, and apply ice as soon as a sore spot develops. Once a deformed ear develops, only a plastic surgeon can return the ear to normal appearance.	If symptoms of infection develop If cosmetic surgery is desired
Concussion	Any injury to the head producing dizziness or temporary unconsciousness should be considered serious.	Apply ice to the area. Observe the patient for 72 hours for alertness, unequal pupil size (although about one person in four has unequal pupil size all the time), and vomiting. Pressure inside skull may develop in 72 hours.	If unconsciousness occurred If bleeding occurs from ears, eyes, or mouth If there is unequal pupil size, lethargy, fever, vomiting, convulsions, speech difficulty, stiff neck, or limb weakness

TABLE G.1   INJURY AND TREATMENT INFORMATION—Continued

Injury	General Comments	Prevention and Treatment	Need for a Physician
Dental injuries	Common in basketball and contact sports from elbow contact.	Chipped tooth—avoid hot and cold drinks. Swelling due to abscess—apply ice pack. Excessive bleeding of socket— place gauze over socket and bite down. Toothache—aspirin and ice packs.	If tooth is chipped, abscess is present, or bleeding of socket or toothache present
Eye (object in eye, contusion from a ball or elbow)	Eye injuries are more common in racket sports and handball from ball contact, and in contact sports from elbow contact. In racket sports, the ball may ricochet off the top of the racket into the eye, or the victim may turn to see where his or her partner is hitting the ball in doubles play.	Protective eye guards should be used in racketball and handball. Never turn your head in doubles play. Avoid rubbing—you could scratch the cornea. Close both eyes to allow tears to wash away a foreign body. Grasp the lashes of the upper lid and draw out and down over the lower lid. If it feels like an object is in eye but none can be, cornea scrape probably occurred, and will heal in 24 to 48 hours. To remove object, moisten corner of handkerchief and touch object lightly.	If object is on the eye itself If object remains after washing If object could have penetrated the globe of the eye If blood is visible in eye If vision is impaired If pain is present after 48 hours
Nasal fracture	Some noses are better targets than others. The blow may come from the side or front. The side hit causes more deformity. Hemorrhage is profuse (mucous lining is cut), and swelling is immediate.	Prevention involves use of a face guard in football. In other sports, it is a matter of luck. Bleeding should be controlled immediately (see Nosebleed).	If bleeding continues If deformity and considerable swelling are present
EXTREMITIES **Neck**	Neck injuries are more common in contact sports, and require immediate and careful attention. Assume a vertebrae is involved, and avoid movement of any kind until a physician or rescue squad arrives.	Neck flexibility exercises should be a part of your warm-up routine. Neck strengthening exercises are a necessity for contact sport participants.	If any injury to the neck occurs
Nosebleed	Nosebleed may occur even from mild contact to the nose.	Do not lie down when bleeding starts. Squeeze the nose between the thumb and forefinger just below the hard portion for 5 to 10 minutes while seated with the head tilted back. Avoid blowing the nose or placing cold compresses on the bridge of the nose.	If bleeding occurs frequently and is associated with a cold If victim has a history of high blood pressure If emergency treatment fails to stop the bleeding

TABLE G.1   INJURY AND TREATMENT INFORMATION—Continued

Injury	General Comments	Prevention and Treatment	Need for a Physician
TORSO			
Back	The first 7 vertebrae control the head, neck, and upper back. The next 12 provide attachments for the ribs. The 5 lumbar vertebrae of the lower back support the weight of the upper half of the body. It is this area that plagues millions of Americans.	Avoid exercise motions that arch the back. Back pain may be caused by muscular and ligamentous sprains, mechanical instability, arthritis, and ruptured discs. Most problems will improve with rest, heat, pain medication, and an exercise program.	If pain, weakness, or numbness in legs is present. If pain remains after rest and heat therapy. If aching sensation occurs in buttocks, or further down the leg
Chest pain	Chest pain provides a heart attack scare to everyone over age 30. Actually, pain could be in the chest wall (muscle, rib, ligament, or rib cartilage), the lungs or outside covering, or the gullet, diaphragm, skin, or other organs in the upper part of the diaphragm. Sharp pain that lasts a few seconds, pain at the end of a deep breath, or one that worsens with a deep breath, pain upon pressing a finger on the spot of discomfort, and painful burning when the stomach is empty are all symptoms that are probably not associated with a heart attack.	Any of the symptoms to the right require immediate hospitalization and physician care.	If any of the following symptoms are present: mild to intense pain with a feeling of pressure, or squeezing on the chest; pain beneath the breastbone; accompanying pain in the jaw, or down the inner side of either arm; accompanying nausea, sweating, dizziness, or shortness of breath; or pulse irregularity
Groin strain	The groin muscles (area between the thigh and abdominal region) are easily torn from running, jumping, and twisting. It is a difficult injury to prevent and cure. Pain, weakness, and internal bleeding may occur.	Prevention involves proper stretching prior to exercise. R-I-C-E therapy is suggested for treatment.	If symptoms remain after several weeks of rest and mild exercise
Hernia	The protrusion of viscera (body organs) through a portion of the abdominal wall is referred to as a hernia. Hernias associated with exercise and sports generally occur in the groin area.	Prevention involves attention to proper form in weight lifting and weight training, and care in lifting heavy objects.	If a protrusion is located that protrudes further with coughing
Hip pointer	A hard blow to the iliac crest or hip produces what is commonly called a hip pointer. The injury is severely handicapping, and produces both pain and spasm.	Prevention involves the use of protective hip pads in contact sports. R-I-C-E therapy is suggested for treatment.	If symptoms of a fracture are present

TABLE G.1 INJURY AND TREATMENT INFORMATION—Continued

Injury	General Comments	Prevention and Treatment	Need for a Physician
Jock itch	Jock itch is acquired by contact and is associated with bacteria, fungi, molds, and ringworm.	Prevention and treatment involve practicing proper hygiene (showering in warm water, use of antiseptic soap, powder, and proper drying); drinking enough water; regularly changing underwear, supporter, and shorts; disinfecting locker benches, mats and other equipment; and avoiding long periods of sitting in warm, moist areas.	If condition persists for more than 10 days
Wind knocked out	With a hard blow to the right place, such as a relaxed midsection, breathing is temporarily hampered. Although you will have trouble convincing the victim, breathing will return. The blow has only increased abdominal pressure, produced pain, and interferred with the diaphragmatic cycle reflex due to nerve paralysis or muscle spasm.	The victim should be told to try to breath slowly through the nose (no easy task for someone who is gasping, dizzy, and 100 percent convinced death is only seconds away). Clothing is loosened at the neck and waist, and ice is applied to the abdomen.	If breathing is still not normal in one or two minutes If breathing stops (start CPR) If pain persists in the midsection
SHOULDER **Tendonitis**	Tendonitis is common in tennis and baseball. Soreness results on the front of the shoulder when elevating the arm from the side.	Ice and aspirin are used. Prevention and treatment involves flexibility and weight training exercises (see Chapters 4 and 5). Flexibility movements concentrate on back stretching while weight training choices are lateral lifts, military, and bench presses.	If soreness remains for 7 to 10 days
THORAX **Rib fracture and bruises**	Fractures may occur from direct contact or, uncommonly, from muscular contraction. A direct blow may displace the bone and produce jagged edges that cut the tissue of the lungs, producing bleeding or lung collapse.	The type of contact helps reveal rib fracture. Pain when breathing and palpatation are also signs. R-I-C-E therapy should be initiated immediately.	If pain is present when breathing after a direct blow to the thorax If fracture is suspected
MISCELLANEOUS INJURIES AND ILLNESSES **Abrasions**	Superficial skin layers are scraped off. Injury imposes no serious problem if cleaned properly.	Clean with soap and warm water. Use a bandage if the wound oozes blood. Remove loose skin flaps with sterile scissors if dirty; allow to remain if clean.	If all dirt and foreign matter cannot be removed If infection develops

TABLE G.1   INJURY AND TREATMENT INFORMATION—Continued

Injury	General Comments	Prevention and Treatment	Need for a Physician
Common cold	Handshaking with an infected person or breathing in particles after a sneeze are two ways of transmitting a cold virus. Contributing factors may be low resistance, improper nutrition, tension, bacteria entering the respiratory track, and remaining indoors in winter months, which increases the likelihood of close contact with a contagious person.	A cold will typically last about seven days. There is no known protection or cure. Antihistamines, decongestants, and cold tablets are of little value. Aspirin (for those over 16 years of age) or acetaminophen (for those under 16), combined with rest, and plenty of fluids are sound advice. Exercise only lightly and include one or two days of rest.	If fever or sore throat lasts more than a week If pain is present in one or both ears
Fainting and dizziness	Lack of blood flow to the brain commonly occurs with increasing age, and may result in temporary loss of vision or lightheadedness	Place the victim in a lying position with the feet elevated. If it is not possible to lie down, an alternative position is a sitting posture with the head lowered between the legs.	If loss of consciousness occurs If dizziness occurs frequently
Frostbite	Frostbite, a destruction of tissue by freezing, is more likely to occur on small parts of the nose, cheeks, ears, fingers, and toes.	See the section "Dressing Properly for the Weather" in Chapter Nine for prevention. Thaw rapidly in a warm water bath. Avoid rubbing areas with snow. Water should be comfortable to a normal, unfrozen hand (not over 104°F). When a flush reaches the fingers, remove the frostbitten part from the water immediately. For an ear or nose, use cloths soaked in warm water.	Always see a doctor
Heat exhaustion/ heat stroke	The body loses heat to the environment and maintains normal temperature by: *Evaporation*—Sweat evaporates into the atmosphere. *Radiation*—With body temperature higher than air temperature, heat loss occurs. *Convection*—As body heat loss occurs, air is warmed. This warmed air rises and cooler air moves in to take its place, cooling the body. *Conduction*—Heat moves from deeper body organs to skin through blood vessels. The skin acts as a radiation surface for heat loss to the air.	Symptoms of heat exhaustion include nausea, chills, cramps, and rapid pulse. Prevention involves following the steps outlined in the section "Dressing Properly for the Weather" in Chapter 9. Treatment requires immediate cooling with ice packs to the head, torso, and joints, and maintaining proper water and electrolyte balance.	If rapid improvement is not evident If multiple cramps occur If core temperature does not immediately return to normal

TABLE G.1   INJURY AND TREATMENT INFORMATION—Continued

Injury	General Comments	Prevention and Treatment	Need for a Physician
Hypothermia	With extremely cold temperatures and high wind chill, core body temperature may drop below normal levels.	Prevention involves following the steps outlined in the section "Dressing Properly for the Weather" in Chapter Nine. Treatment calls for warming with blankets, heating pads, replacing wet clothing, and administering warm drinks.	If core temperature drops below 94°
Infected wounds	Bacterial infection in the bloodstream (septicemia).	Keep area clean, changing the bandage and soaking and cleaning in warm water twice daily. Up to 10 to 12 days may be needed for normal healing.	If fever is above 100° If thick pus and swelling occur the second day
Minor cuts	Minor cuts can develop into serious problems if mistreated or neglected. Avoid use of antiseptics that may destroy tissue and actually retard healing.	Clean the wound with soap and water or hydrogen peroxide, removing all dirt and foreign matter. Use a butterfly bandage or steri-strip to bring the edges of the wound tightly together without trapping the fat or rolling the skin beneath.	If cut occurs to face or trunk If deep cut involves tendons, nerves, vessels, or ligaments If blood is pumping from a wound If tingling or limb weakness occurs If cut cannot be pulled together without trapping the fat If direct pressure fails to stop the bleeding
Muscle cramps	Muscular cramps commonly occur in three areas: back of lower leg (calf), back of upper leg (hamstring group), and front of upper leg (quadriceps group). Cramps may be related to fatigue, tightness of the muscles, or fluid, salt, and potassium imbalance.	Stretch before you exercise and drink water freely. If cramp occurs, stretch area carefully.	If multiple cramps occur If symptoms of heat exhaustion are present
Muscle soreness	You may experience two different types of soreness: general soreness that appears immediately after your exercise session and disappears in 3 to 4 hours, or localized soreness appearing 8 to 24 hours after exercise. The older you are, the longer the period between exercise and soreness.	You can help prevent soreness by warming up properly, avoiding bouncing-type stretching or flexibility, exercises and progressing slowly in your program. Doing too much too soon is a common cause. You can expect to have some soreness after your first few workouts, especially if you have been inactive. Don't stop exercising, it will only reoccur later.	If muscle soreness persists after the second week

Correct Posture

It is important to recognize that individual differences do exist in the area of body mechanics because of the heterogeneity of anatomical structure (size, weight, and body build included). Researchers have already clearly identified these differences from individual to individual in the realm of normal posture with respect to the shape of the vertebral column and lumbar spine, pelvic structure, height of arches, foot/leg alignment, shoulder/neck area, abdominal contour, thoracic cavity, and upper back. Normal posture has been defined as the mechanical correlation of the various body systems (skeletal, muscular, visceral) and their neurological association. Ideal posture, then, may be described as a position permitting maximum efficiency of the body organs and systems. It is obvious that slight deviations from the ideal described below are perfectly normal, in spite of the fact that investigators are in general agreement on a description of what constitutes good and poor posture.

Correct standing posture demands that the body is perfectly erect, resisting the downward pull of gravity at all points. The point of balance is located approximately midway between the heel and the ball of the foot. An imaginary straight line connects the major body segments at the center of the area, beginning at the lobe of the ear and extending downward through the tip of the shoulder, the waistline, the hip joint, and the side of the kneecap and ending at the outside ankle bone. Such alignment places all points in one vertical line for optimum erectness, balance, ease of maintenance, and appearance. This position is maintained with ease by the tone of the muscles rather than by voluntary muscle contraction. More specifically, the feet remain slightly separated, with the toes pointing forward (slightly outward also constitutes normal position). The knees are extended in a relaxed manner without rigid locking. The slight forward pelvic tilt and the natural curve in the lumbar area are not exaggerated. The chest is held high and the abdomen flat and below the chest. Shoulders are comfortably drawn backward with the blades nearly flat. The head remains erect with the chin level horizontal to the floor and the neck drawn backward.

Sitting posture must encourage both relaxation and optimum function of the musculature without undue strain and fatigue. The two most common faults in sitting posture are failure to push the hips back in the chair and rounding the back. The head, neck, and trunk remain in the position described previously, with the hips contacting the back of the chair. The head is held erect by the neck and shoulder muscles. It is also essential that reading materials be held correctly to prevent a forward tilt of the head and neck and rounding of the shoulders. The entire length of thigh and buttocks must be supported by the seat, with the heels and toes resting firmly on the floor.

Walking posture parallels that described for ideal standing. Sideward motion of any type should be avoided as the legs and arms coordinate their movements swinging straight forward from the hips and shoulder joints. The heel of the lead leg contacts the surface first before weight is shifted to the outer borders of the other foot by pushing off with the toes. Both the leg and arm swing should be free and easy to minimize jarring, avoid unnecessary movement, and maintain proper body alignment without twisting. Again, correct walking posture varies from individual to individual.

Foot care may seem elementary in nature; however, shoe selection as a preventive measure against foot defects is extremely important and represents an area of concern to all. Follow these 10 suggestions for judging a proper fit:

1. There should be no excessive pressure on any part of the foot.

2. There should be no looseness to create friction.

3. The soles should be only sufficiently sturdy to protect from injury and moisture, not so thick and rigid as to immobilize the toes in walking. The soles should be flat, not of the rocker type that hinders plantar flexion of the toes.

4. The inner border of the shoe should be straight from the ball forward so as to allow the big toe to lie straight.

5. The heel should be broad, low, and of rubber surfacing to absorb jar.

6. The shank should be narrow enough to fit under the inner side of the arch in passive standing. Many oxfords are proportioned to fit the higher arch. This is a problem for women particularly.

7. The toe cap should be full enough to allow free action of the toes.

8. There should be a space of ½ inch (¾ inch for growing children) from the end of the longest toe to the end of the toe cap. This is necessary to provide toe room after the foot has become warm. Without this allowance a shoe that was thought to be long enough when first fitted will later prove to be too short.

9. The shoe should lace up the front so as to be readily adjustable.

10. The shoe should be good, porous leather, but not too heavy. Patent leather and suede are not porous enough to permit adequate ventilation of the feet. Excessive accumulation of perspiration makes the feet damp and clammy. This factor is further exaggerated by already weak feet, which perspire more than normal.

COMMON POSTURE AND BODY MECHANICS DEFECTS

The defects discussed in Table H.1 represent the majority of conditions that can be aided by the joint efforts of the medical and physical education offices. A multitude of exercises may be used to improve each condition, and no attempt is made to provide complete listings. Rather, the approach or focal point of attack is provided for each impediment.

TABLE H.1   DESCRIPTION OF COMMON POSTURAL DEFECTS

Condition	Description	Posture and Body Mechanics Emphasis
Spinal Deviations		
Cervical lordosis (poke neck)	The chin is held both high and forward, and accompanied by a round upper back. Flexibility is limited in the area of cervical extension in most cases.	The anterior cervical and posterior cervical-dorsal muscles should be strengthened.

TABLE H.1 DESCRIPTION OF COMMON POSTURAL DEFECTS—Continued

Condition	Description	Posture and Body Mechanics Emphasis
Dorsal kyphosis (Round upper back)	The upper back is rounded, with the normal curve changed in a backward or reverse direction and with flexion of the spine in the thoracic region. Shoulder blades tend to bulge. Severe cases result in a depressed sternum, lowered rib cage, and deviation of normal positions of heart, lungs, and abdominal viscera.	The strength of the thoracic spinal extensors should be elevated to assist in support of the thoracic cavity. There should be upper arm and shoulder strength improvement.
Kyphosis (forward head)	The head, face, chin, and neck tilt downward, mainly from the junction of the seventh cervical and first thoracic vertebrae. The individual may be forced to roll up the eyeballs to focus straight ahead. Long hours of sitting, reading, typing, and writing over a desk tend to encourage such a position.	Exercises should improve the flexibility in the cervical area and the strength of the muscles of the upper back and neck.
Kypholordosis (round hollow back)	Both round upper back and lordosis exist, with upper and lower curves nearly equal.	Correction is difficult since treatment of one tends to aggravate the other.
Lordosis (hollow back)	The lumbar spine remains in a forward position while the pelvic tilt is exaggerated, providing a marked hollowness beginning at approximately the shoulder blade area and continuing to the buttocks. This condition may be of two types: (1) flexible hollow back—correct mechanical position can be attained with forced effort, or (2) stiff, or fixed, hollow back—correct position cannot be assumed.	For both types, increased abdominal strength and tone are prescribed. Stiff hollow back is assisted also by stretching the lumbar spine extensors and hip flexors and by improving strength in the hip extensors.
Lumbar kyphosis (flat back)	The normal curve of the lumbar spine area is decreased, providing a flat area or backward bulge, which reduces the shock absorption ability of the lumbar curve and induces more rapid fatigue. This is often accompanied by other fatigue-inducing defects, such as prominent abdomen, flat chest, and forward head.	Abdominal and spine extensor muscles should be strengthened.

TABLE H.1   DESCRIPTION OF COMMON POSTURAL DEFECTS—Continued

Condition	Description	Posture and Body Mechanics Emphasis
Round shoulders	The upper back is both rounded and forward (scapulae abducted) from the normal perpendicular line. The shoulder adductors, rhomboids, and trapezius muscles are lengthened and the pectoral muscles shortened, resulting in an imbalance in muscle pull and alignment.	Back extensor and shoulder retractor muscle strength should be improved. Increased flexibility of the pectoral and anterior seratus muscles will help.
Scoliosis (lateral curvature)	Asymmetry of the level of the shoulders and hips, with a vertical spinal column and equal waistline contours are noticeable when viewing an afflicted individual from the front or back. In early stages a line drawn from the first cervical vertebra to the lumbar sacral area may simulate a "C," with an "S" deviation forming later in life through upper body compensation. Shortened leg, poor trunk muscle strength, injury, poor posture, occupation, disease, visual or auditory difficulties, or congenital factors may be the underlying cause of scoliosis. There are seven characteristics of lateral asymmetry of which two or more may be present: a displacement or an imbalance of whole segments over the feet, "C" or "S" curve, spinal column rotation, shoulder asymmetry, hip and waistline contour asymmetry, vertical and lateral flexibility of the spine, and pain.	The strength of the abdominal muscles and back musculature should be increased. Asymmetrical strength is also important, along with development of means to decrease the pelvic tilt. Careful consultation with a physician is imperative because of the seriousness of this type of impediment.

Foot Deviations

Condition	Description	Posture and Body Mechanics Emphasis
Achilles tendon	Difficulty in this area may take the form of bursa irritation (inflammation and swelling at the insertion of the tendon), tenosynovitis (inflammation and swelling of the tendon), and rupture (tearing of the tendon).	In general, improvement of the foot conditions listed may take the form of partial or complete rest, corrective footwear, improved foot strength, and establishing proper habits of standing, walking, and running. Exercises should attempt to improve muscle strength, gait, circulation, and flexibility. All activity is performed without shoes or socks for proper execution and rapid inspection during performance. Hallux valgus (bunion) cure is extremely difficult, with surgery the only really effective measure. Preventive efforts are most effective.
Angulation of gait	Toeing in (pigeon-toed) or out places a burden on the longitudinal arches.	

TABLE H.1   DESCRIPTION OF COMMON POSTURAL DEFECTS—Continued

Condition	Description	Posture and Body Mechanics Emphasis
Anterior arch	A weakness in the anterior arch is characterized by fatigue, discomfort, and callus under the heads of the second, third, and fourth metatarsal bones. Both longitudinal and anterior arch weakness may be caused by injury, obesity, inadequate muscle tone and strength, or footwear that is too tight, large, or short.	
Hallux valgus (bunion)	This condition is characterized by a deviation of the direction of the large toe which is turned toward the remaining toes. Calcium forms at the site of the irritation as a healing effort, increasing the size of the joint and compounding the problem.	
Corns	This condition may be caused by excessive pressure caused by faulty mechanics of the feet or by improper footwear.	
Inadequate foot flexibility	This is caused by a rigidity of the gastronemius (calf) and Achilles tendon, which may cause pronation.	
Longitudinal arch	Weakness in the longitudinal arch may be accompanied by pronation, abduction, eversion, or inward hip rotation.	
Pronation	This condition is inward rotation of the ankles, whereby increased body weight is forced upon the inner border of the longitudinal arches. The condition can also be caused by inadequate foot muscle tone and ligament strength.	
Supination	This is outward rotation of the ankles whereby increased body weight is forced upon the outer borders of the longitudinal arches. This condition is generally not associated with insufficient muscle strength in the areas involved.	

APPENDIX I

Lower Back Exercises

The exercises described below are designed to help prevent lower back problems. They are mainly flexion exercises to improve lumbar (lower back) and gluteal (buttocks) musculature. Don't overdo it. Starting position for all exercises: knees and hips bent with back flat and neck comfortably supported; arms to the side; feet flat on the floor.

1. Take in a deep breath, exhale slowly. Tighten the stomach and buttock muscles and hold the back flat against floor for a count of five. Relax. Repeat very slowly 5 times.

2. With both hands on **one** knee, bring the knee up as near to the chest as possible. Return it slowly to the starting position. Relax. Repeat, alternating with each leg, 10 times.

3. Tighten the abdominal muscles and hold the back flat, then bring **both** knees up to the chest, grasp the knees with the hands, and hold the knees against the chest about 30 seconds. Return slowly to the starting position. Relax. Repeat 5 times.

4. Bring one knee to the chest; straighten that knee, extending the leg as far as possible; bend knee and return to original position. Relax. Alternate with the opposite leg. Repeat 5 times. Note: This exercise is *not* recommended for patients with sciatic (nerve) pain.

5. Lie on back with knees bent; feet flat on floor. Pull up to a sitting position. Hold for a count of five. Return to starting position. Relax. Repeat 5 times.

APPENDIX J:

Girth Control Exercises

Every college student seems to want a flat "tummy." In fact, a flat stomach has become strongly associated with fitness and wellness. A large belly can make young men or women appear much older than they really are. It also can be a sign of poor health; evidence of accumulating fat that may lead to hypertension, stroke, heart disease, diabetes, and other ailments. Some fat around the midsection is not necessarily unhealthy. Practically everyone acquires at least a small "spare tire" (fat on both sides of the hips) and some abdominal fat after the college years. Becoming obsessed with this somewhat natural change is a mistake. In fact, as you reach the third and fourth decades of life, obtaining the flat stomach you had in high school or college may be impossible.

Many people attempt to solve the girth control problem by using unnatural and worthless devices such as girdles, corsets, weighted belts, rubberized workout suits, and special exercise equipment that promises a flat stomach with just minutes of use each day. Unfortunately, re-acquiring lost youth in the abdominal area is not quite so easy. The only way to firm a sagging stomach area is to combine a negative caloric balance with a sound calisthenic program. You will need several months of both diet control and exercise to shrink the fat cells, and notice a difference in the way your stomach muscles look and feel.

Before beginning an exercise program, measure your waist with a tape measure, and take skinfold measures on the point of both hips, and next to the navel. Remember, you must also follow the suggestions in Chapter 7 to reduce your caloric intake if fat cells are to decrease in size. This reduction, combined with exercise, can be effective at any age. A negative caloric balance shrinks fat cells, and calisthenics improve the tone of the underlying muscle tissue.

Consider the use of high repetitions of the exercises listed below, working toward 100 repetitions of each exercise daily. Begin with the maximum number you can perform in one set. Add 2 to 5 repetitions each day until you reach 100.

1. *Sit-ups*—Lie flat on your back, with knees slightly bent, and both hands resting on your chest. Pull chin to chest, and sit up slowly to approximately 60 degrees.

2. *Crunches*—Lie flat on your back, with the knees bent and pulled toward the chest. Raise your head and shoulders off the floor as you thrust your upper body towards the knees and return to the starting position.

3. *Twisting crunches*—Lying flat on your back, hands behind your head, touch opposite elbow to opposite knee while the other leg straightens; keep feet flexed.

4. *Alternate knee kicks*—Lie flat on your back, with hands under buttocks. Bend

one knee with other leg straight and raised 6″ off the floor. Straighten bent knee, and bend other leg as in walking or marching.

5. *Side Raise*—Lie on your side, with arm extended and head on bicep. Hold both legs 6″ off the floor, feet together. Raise top leg up and return to leg-together position.

6. *Back Scissors*—Lie on your stomach, with hands at sides, palms down for support.

Start with legs apart and feet off floor; and bring feet together, then apart.

Do these exercises every day, and expect to work for three or four months, at which time you will be able to measure and see results. Remember that abdominal exercise only strengthens muscles that lie beneath fat. Unless you reduce calories to eliminate fat, you will merely have firm abdominal muscles beneath the fat.

GLOSSARY

Additives Substances added to foods to improve their taste or to alter or preserve them

Adipose tissue Body fat

Aerobic Conditioning Developing the circulatory system

Aerobics Activities which will help develop the circulatory system

Afterburn The calories expended due to an increase in metabolic rate following exercise

Aging The deterioration of the body due to years of wear and tear

Amino acids Protein building blocks needed for the body to function well

Amphetamines A stimulant that increases metabolic rate and decreases appetite

Anaerobics An activity performed at such a high intensity (for example, sprinting) that there is insufficient time for the utilization of atmospheric oxygen at the tissue level, and thus an oxygen debt is created

Androgenic hormones Male sex hormones, primarily testosterone; found in varying amounts in both men and women

Angina pectoris Insufficient blood supply and oxygen to a portion of the heart muscle, resulting in chest pain and tissue damage

Anorexa Nervosa An extreme underweight condition brought about by compulsive starvation dieting; occurring mainly in young women due to nervous or psychogenic loss of appetite

Antagonist muscles Muscles that are in direct opposition, such as the biceps and the triceps; the biceps muscle contracts (agonist) while the triceps (antagonist) muscle relaxes as the arm is flexed at the elbow

Anti-gravity muscles The larger extensor muscles of the body that give support to the skeletal framework and combat the pull of gravity

Antipyretic The diminishing of fever

Arrhythmia Irregular heart rate; varying intervals between heart beats

Arteriosclerosis A condition in which the arteries have hardened, become thick, and lost elasticity

Artery A blood vessel that carries blood away from the heart

Ascetic A person who renounces comfort to lead a life of self-denial

Atherosclerosis A condition in which arterial walls contain deposits of soft, spongy, or hard calcified substances that produce narrowing or blocking

Athlete's foot A foot fungus often accompanied by a bacterial infection that causes itching, redness, and a rash on the soles, toes, or between the toes

Atrophy A weakened condition of muscle tissue generally characterized by decrease in size and strength

Ballistic exercises Flexibility exercises employing bouncing and jerking movements at the extreme range of motion

Barbiturates A depressant that slows down body functions

Basal metabolism The number of calories expended to maintain vital functions while at complete rest

Basic food groups Four major food categories (milk, meat, vegetables and fruits, and breads and cereals) necessary for a balanced diet

Behavioral contract A written agreement between two parties (or with oneself) to behave in a prescribed manner

Blood Fat Fat which is circulating in the circulatory system—some good (HDL), and some bad (LDL)

Blood Pressure Pressure on the vessel walls; normal blood pressure is 120/80—the upper number is when the heart contracts, and the lower is the pressure when the heart is at rest

Body Building   Designed to build and accentuate the muscles for looks rather than strength

Body composition   The major structural components of the human body: muscle, fat, and bone

Bone Jolt   The stress or G force created with each step in walking or running

Bulimia   Believed to be a form of anorexia nervosa, bulimic individuals repeatedly gorge themselves with food, and then deliberately induce vomiting or bowel movement

Bulk   Muscle mass accumulated through strength training

Bunion   An inflammatory growth on the head of the first or fifth toe

Caffeine   A stimulant drug present in coffee, tea, cola drinks, and some other sodas

Calcium   A mineral that is the main component of the bones and teeth

Calf Muscle   The muscle at the back of the lower leg which when contracted lifts the body up on the toes

Caloric balance   A condition achieved when the calories acquired from food exactly equal the calories expended

Calorie   A unit used to measure the amount of heat released from food; one calorie supplies the quantity of heat required to raise the temperature of one gram of water one degree centigrade

Carbohydrate loading   An attempt to reduce carbohydrate intake to near zero for three days (depletion stage) before resorting to a high carbohydrate diet for three days in order to raise glycogen stores in skeletal muscle and the liver and to increase energy levels the day of the contest

Carbohydrates   Organic compounds composed of carbon, hydrogen, and oxygen, including starches, sugars and cellulose

Cardiac output   The volume of blood ejected into the aorta, usually expressed as liters per minute

Cardiovascular efficiency   The ability of the heart, lungs and blood vessels to supply oxygen and nutrients to working muscles while removing waste products created by muscular contractions

Carotid pulse   Located on either side of the neck just under the jawbone; key location for determining heart rate

Carryover activity   Physical activity that can be continued in later life with little risk and high fitness value

Cartilage   Fibrous connective tissue between the surfaces of movable and immovable joints

Cauliflower ear   A deformed, painful outer ear caused by repeated friction and trauma

Cellulite   A label given to lumpy deposits of fat commonly appearing on the back and front of the legs and buttocks in overweight individuals; it is actually just fat

Cerebrovascular accident (CVA)   A stroke (see stroke)

Charley horse   An injury caused by a blow to a contracted or relaxed muscle

Cholesterol   A chemical substance found in animal fats that is believed to play a part in clogging the arteries

Chondromalacia   Roughing of the undersurface of the kneecap, producing pain and grating

Circulatory System   The heart, lungs, and blood vessels

Collateral blood vessels   Blood vessels that develop around a blocked artery; they compensate in part for the loss of blood supply to the heart

Complete Protein   Food source containing all essential amino acids in the correct proportions

Concentric contraction   A muscle contraction in which the muscle shortens while overcoming resistance

Connective Tissue   Tissue which connects muscles to bones (tendons), and bone to bones (ligaments)

Cool-down   The use of 5 to 10 minutes of very light exercise movements at the end of a vigorous workout to slowly cool the body to near normal core temperature

Core Temperature   The body's internal temperature surrounding the vital organs, which is measured most accurately using a rectal thermometer

Coronary arteries   The blood vessels that supply the heart muscle with blood

Coronary thrombosis   Blockage of a coronary blood vessel due to a clot

Creatine   An energy-rich compound that plays a key role in providing energy for instant muscle contraction

Crude Fiber   The portion of food that remains undisolved after being subjected to acids and bases in the laboratory; always less than the dietary fiber in the same food

DMSO   The controversial drug, dimethyl sulfoxide, originally used by veterinarians to reduce joint inflammation in animals, and presently used by some athletes for joint and soft tissue injuries

Daily Log   An accounting of daily activity

Degenerative diseases   Common diseases of adults

such as coronary heart disease, high blood pressure, diabetes, and rheumatism

Diastolic blood pressure The pressure of the blood against the walls of the arteries while the heart is in the relaxation phase (between beats)

Dietary Fiber The undigestible portion of food after it is exposed to the body's enzymes; always higher than the crude fiber in the same food

Diuretic A chemical substance that increases the secretion and discharge of urine and other body fluids

Diverticulosis Outward ballooning of the intestinal wall in the descending colon

Dorsal kyphosis Round upper back

Dysmenorrhea Painful menstruation

Eccentric contraction A muscle contraction in which the muscle gradually lengthens while combating the pull of gravity

Electrolytes Chemical compounds in solution in the human body capable of producing electric current; important in the prevention of heat cramps, heat exhaustion, and heat stroke

Embolus A clot that breaks free from a vessel wall and travels in the bloodstream until it reaches an area it is unable to pass

Emphysema Swelling and inflammation of tissue resulting in tearing of the alveoli and decreased lung efficiency

Endorphins A group of hormones that are very similar in composition to morphine; normally produced and released by the pituitary gland to help reduce great pain, anxiety, and stress

Enkephalins Hormones similar to endorphins with similar tranquilizing properties; the level of both drugs in the blood rises during strenuous exercise

Enriched Returning the mineral Iron, and the B vitamins Thiamin, Riboflavin, and Niacin to refined products

Essential Amino Acids Amino acids that cannot be manufactured by the body, and therefore must be acquired through food sources

Fartlek A form of training also known as speed play which alternates fast and slow running over varied terrain for three to four miles

Fats Food components that store energy and vitamins in the body

Fat-soluble vitamins Vitamins not necessarily eliminated from the body but rather stored in the fatty tissues

Fiber A nonnutritive substance in food which combines with water to form stools and to aid digestion

Fibrin A sticky substance that combines with blood cells to form a clot in the healing of a cut

Flexibility The range of motion at a joint

Fluorides Mineral salts often added to drinking water for the prevention of tooth decay

Fortified Nutrients added to food that may or may not have been in the original product

Frequency How often one engages in exercise, preferably a minimum of three times per week on alternate days

Frostbite Destruction of tissue by freezing

Full-range movement Movement that starts from a fully extended, pre-stretched position and continues to a fully contracted position

Glucose (glycogen) Sugar which can be used by the body for energy

Good Samaritan law A law existing in some states that protects a person giving first aid from being sued unduly; it recognizes a moral obligation of common decency to assist other human beings in need

Gram (g) Approximately one-fifth a level teaspoon

Hallux valgus A bunion

Hamstring Muscles The muscles at the back of the upper leg which when contracted will flex the knee joint

Health-related Fitness Fitness which is necessary to sustain life, consisting of five components: cardiovascular efficiency, muscular strength, muscular endurance, flexibility, and body composition

Heart attack Death of heart muscle due to an occlusion or to an insufficient blood supply that fails to meet the oxygen needs of the heart muscle

Heart Rate The number of heart (beats) contractions in one minute

Heat exhaustion Collapse due to water loss and electrolyte imbalance

Heat stroke Failure of the body to regulate heat after exposure to high temperatures

Hernia The protrusion of part of an organ through a portion of the abdominal wall

High Biological Value A protein source such as meat that contains all eight essential amino acids in the correct proportions

High-density lipoproteins (HDL) The part of serum cholesterol responsible for transporting fats out of the bloodstream; increases with exercise and considered beneficial to one's health

Hip pointer An injury to the iliac crest (hip)

Hunger A physiological response of the body indicating a need for food

Hyperplasia   New fat cell formation

Hypertension   Often termed high blood pressure; exists when the systolic pressure exceeds 140 mm Hg and/or the diastolic blood pressure exceeds 90 mm Hg

Hypertrophy   An enlargement of a tissue or organ due to exercise

Hypokinetic disease   A disease that relates to or is caused by the lack of regular physical activity

Hypothermia   An abnormal drop in core body temperature

Incomplete Protein   Food sources that do not contain all essential amino acids, or contain several in incorrect proportions

Indicator Nutrients   The eight nutrients that must be listed on all food labels: Protein, Vitamin A, Thiamin (B1), Riboflavin (B2), Niacin, Vitamin C, Calcium, and Iron

Infarct   Tissue death in a body part due to lack of oxygen

Intensity   The minimum heart rate necessary to bring about cardiovascular conditioning

Interval training   A training routine consisting of four elements: intensity, duration, repetitions, and rest intervals

Iron   One of the body's essential minerals

Ischemia   Inadequate blood supply (oxygen) to a body part

Isokinetic contraction   A muscular contraction performed against a controlled maximum resistance throughout the full range of motion

Isometric contraction   A muscular contraction in which muscle length remains unchanged while force is exerted on an immovable object

Isotonic contraction   A muscular contraction in which muscle length shortens while resistance is overcome

Ketosis   A condition brought about by restricted carbohydrate intake resulting in excessive acetones or other ketones being secreted by the liver—stored fat becomes more available for energy, aiding in the loss of body fat

Kilocalorie   A unit used to measure the amount of heat released from food; 1,000 small calories; *also* Calorie

Kypholordosis   Round hollow back

Kyphosis   Forward head

Lactic acid   A chemical causing fatigue produced by the metabolism when oxygen supply is insufficient to meet oxygen needs during exercise

Long, Slow Distance (LSD)   A training theory under which runners cover long distances at a slow pace in order to build strength and endurance

Ligament   A band of tissue connecting bones or supporting internal organs

Lipid   Refers to all fats and fatty substances

Lipoproteins   Circulating proteins that become attached to blood lipids

Lordosis   Hollow back

Low-density lipoproteins (LDL)   The part of serum cholesterol responsible for the fatty buildup on arterial walls, which may lead to a heart attack

Low Biological Value   A protein source such as corn and wheat that does not contain all eight essential amino acids, or contains some in low proportions

Low In Kcalories   No more than 40 Calories per serving, or 09 Kcal per gram

Lumbar kyphosis   Flat back

Lumbar region   The lower back area

Maintenance load   The amount of exercise that enables an individual to maintain his present level of conditioning

Marathon   A race covering 26 miles, 385 yards

Maximal oxygen uptake   The best measure of cardiovascular or aerobic fitness; the amount of oxygen one is capable of utilizing at the tissue level during vigorous exercise

Maximum repetition (RM)   The amount of weight with which an individual can perform a specified number of repetitions; for example, 8 RM is the amount of weight with which one can perform only 8 repetitions

Medical Exam   A series of tests designed to determine one's readiness to participate in a vigorous fitness program

Megavitamins   Vitamins containing extremely large doses

Metabolic rate   (*See basal metabolism*)

Metabolism   The chemical transformations of the body; for example, conversion of food into body tissue, muscle contraction, and maintenance of chemical machinery

Microgram   1 thousandth of a milligram (1 millionth of a gram)

Mile and One-half Test   A running test used to estimate one's aerobic capacity

Milligram (mg)   1 thousandth of a gram

Minerals   Components of various hormones, enzymes, and other substances that help regulate chemical reactions in cells

Morton's Foot   The second toe is longer than the

great toe, creating impact stress with each step, particularly in the stopping action

Motor Fitness Designates fitness components such as coordination, speed, agility, reaction time, and balance which are necessary for competitive athletic success

Muscular endurance A muscle's ability to continue submaximal contractions against a resistance

Muscular strength The amount of force a muscle can exert for one repetition

Muscular tone The firmness of a muscle group in a relaxed state

Negative Addition A compulsive, unhealthy approach to exercise characterized by a need to constantly push oneself beyond healthy limits

Negative consequences Events and situations that follow a behavior and are unpleasant; punishments

Negative resistance The lowering phase of weight lifting

Nonessential Amino Acids Amino acids that can be manufactured by the body (not necessarily needed in food sources)

Nutrition Density Foods that are high in nutrients and low in calories

Obesity A condition characterized by a higher than normal percentage of body fat

Overload A training principle through which the system to be trained is made to work at a level beyond normal demands

Overtraining Excessive, hard training day after day; failure to alternate light and heavy workouts

Oxygen debt The difference between the ideal amount of oxygen for performing an exercise task and the actual amount of oxygen taken in

Oxygen uptake The volume of oxygen (VO_2) extracted from the inspired air, usually expressed as liters per minute

Passive Stretch *See Reciprocal Stretch*

Physiological fitness Fitness levels in each of the following areas: cardiovascular efficiency, muscular strength and endurance, flexibility, and body composition

Plaque Strands of fibrous tissue that attach to the inside of arteries to form soft and mushy (if mostly fat particles) or hard (if scar tissue) atheromatous buildup; also refers to bacteria that form on the teeth

Polyunsaturated fats Fats derived from vegetables, lean poultry, fish and cereal

Positive consequences Events and situations that follow a behavior and are pleasant; rewards

Pre-stretched When a relaxed muscle is pulled into a position of increased tension prior to the start of contraction

Progressive Overload A theory of gradually increasing the work load during each workout in order to build muscular strength

Protein A basic food component critical to all living things

P:S ratio A comparison of the amount of saturated and polyunsaturated fats consumed on a daily basis; it is desirable to consume two to three times more polyunsaturated than saturated fats

RDA Recommended Daily Allowances; guidelines for certain nutrients established by the National Research Council of the National Academy of Sciences and judged to be adequate for all healthy persons and generous for most

Radial pulse The pulse taken at the wrist

Range of Motion Associated with flexibility, it is the movement possible around a joint

Reciprocal stretch A flexibility technique whereby a muscle group is isometrically contracted immediately before passive stretching of their antagonists takes place

Reduced-calorie Food At least a third lower in calories than the food it most closely resembles

Reduced Sodium Processed to reduce the regular amount of sodium by 75% or more

Residual Soreness Soreness which arises as a result of an exercise bout (can be present from one to several days afterwards) which is associated with new activity or unusual intensity

Risk Factor Any factor which is associated with an increased incidence cardiovascular disease

Road Racing Competitive running using roads as a course

Round shoulders Postural defect in which the tips of shoulders are drawn forward in front of the gravity line

Satiety The feeling of fullness or satisfaction after a meal, which prompts an individual to stop eating

Saturated fats Fats found in animal products and linked to plaque buildup in the arteries

Sciatica Pain in the buttocks, hip, thigh, leg, or foot at the site of the great sciatic nerve

Scoliosis Lateral curvature of the spine

Second wind A sudden relief from signs of fatigue such as breathlessness, rapid pulse, and muscular discomfort

Sedentary The lifestyle of individuals who spend most of their time in passive work and recreation

Sets   Groups of muscular repetitions performed for a particular movement or exercise

Set Point Theory   The body's tendency to defend an individual's body weight, and resist dieting efforts to change

Sit-and-reach   A test used to measure back and hamstring flexibility

Skinfold measures   A procedure to estimate total body fat by measuring the thickness of a fold of two layers of skin and the fatty tissue attached

Sodium Free   Less than 5 mg sodium/serving

Somatotype   A classification of body types from ectomorph (skinny), to mesomorph (muscular), to endomorph (fat)

Specificity   The characteristic that the physiological effects of training are unique to the exercise or sport one is involved in and do not fully condition the body for different sports or exercises

Sprinting   Running as fast as possible for short distances

Static flexibility exercises   Exercises in which a position is held steady for a designated period of time at the extreme range of motion

Steady state   A condition in which the oxygen demands of activity are exactly equal to oxygen intake; no oxygen debt occurs

Stress fracture   A small crack in a bone's surface; generally occurs in the feet, legs, or hands

Stroke   A lack of blood supply to the brain resulting from blockage or the rupture of a blood vessel

Stroke volume   The amount of blood pumped by the heart per beat

Systolic blood pressure   The pressure of the blood against artery walls as it is forced out of the heart

Target heart rate   A heart rate 60 to 70 percent of the distance between the resting and maximum rates; must be maintained during exercise to produce a training effect

Tendon   A fibrous cord which attaches a muscle to a bone or other structure

Tendonitis   Inflammation of tendons such as those in the heel, shoulder, and elbow

Time   The amount of time necessary to maintain a conditioning heart rate (intensity) which is high enough to have a training effect

Transitory ischemic attack (TIA)   A mild stroke that occurs when the brain is deprived of adequate blood supply for a short period of time

Triathlon   A race which has three parts: a swim; a bicycle ride; and a run

Triglyceride   A chemical compound consisting of glycerol and fatty acids; linked to atherosclerosis

Type A behavior pattern   A complex of personality traits which has been related to the development of coronary heart disease; these traits include aggressiveness, competitiveness, impatience, a harrying sense of time urgency, and free-floating hostility

Type B behavior pattern   A complex of personality traits believed to be possessed by those not likely to develop coronary heart disease; these personality traits are the opposite of those possessed by type A behavior pattern people

United States Recommended Dietary Allowances (U.S. RDA)   A simplified RDA appearing on food labels showing the percent of the RDA by serving

Unsalted   Processed with the normally used amount of salt

Variable resistance   Resistance that varies in direct proportion to the force exerted

Varicose veins   Abnormally lengthened, dilated veins in the legs

Vein   A blood vessel that carries blood toward the heart

Very Low Sodium   35 mg or less sodium per serving

Warm-up   The preparation of the body for vigorous activity through stretching, calisthenic, and running movements designed to raise core temperature

Water-soluble vitamins   Vitamins which combine with water and are easily eliminated from the body

Weighted vest   A specially designed garment that contains compartments to hold varying amounts of weight

Work hypertrophy   The principle upon which our body responds to training and gradually becomes capable of more sustained exercise

Workload   The amount of weight designated for performing a particular exercise

INDEX